ADVANCES IN VETERINARY SCIENCE AND COMPARATIVE MEDICINE

VOLUME 30

ADVISORY BOARD

W. I. B. Beveridge C. E. Hopla
J. H. Gillespie Norman D. Levine
W. R. Hinshaw C. A. Mitchell
W. R. Pritchard

CONTRIBUTORS TO THIS VOLUME

Howard L. Bachrach A. Heldstab
K. Benirschke R. Ippen
T. A. Bertram Bill L. Lasley
Catherine G. Fabricant Kenneth M. Meyers
Bruce Glick C. Miller

ADVANCES IN VETERINARY SCIENCE AND COMPARATIVE MEDICINE

Edited by

CHARLES E. CORNELIUS
California Primate Research Center
University of California
Davis, California

CHARLES F. SIMPSON
Department of Preventive Medicine
College of Veterinary Medicine
University of Florida
Gainesville, Florida

Volume 30

1985

ACADEMIC PRESS, INC.
Harcourt Brace Jovanovich, Publishers

Orlando   San Diego   New York
Austin   London   Montreal   Sydney   Tokyo   Toronto

COPYRIGHT © 1985 BY ACADEMIC PRESS, INC.
ALL RIGHTS RESERVED.
NO PART OF THIS PUBLICATION MAY BE REPRODUCED OR
TRANSMITTED IN ANY FORM OR BY ANY MEANS, ELECTRONIC
OR MECHANICAL, INCLUDING PHOTOCOPY, RECORDING, OR
ANY INFORMATION STORAGE AND RETRIEVAL SYSTEM, WITHOUT
PERMISSION IN WRITING FROM THE PUBLISHER.

ACADEMIC PRESS, INC.
Orlando, Florida 32887

United Kingdom Edition published by
ACADEMIC PRESS INC. (LONDON) LTD.
24–28 Oval Road, London NW1 7DX

LIBRARY OF CONGRESS CATALOG CARD NUMBER: 53-7098

ISBN 0–12–039230–5

PRINTED IN THE UNITED STATES OF AMERICA

85 86 87 88   9 8 7 6 5 4 3 2 1

CONTENTS

CONTRIBUTORS ix
PREFACE xi

New Approaches to Vaccines
HOWARD L. BACHRACH

I. Introduction 1
II. Impetus for the New Vaccines 2
III. Prospects for the New Vaccines 3
IV. Recombinant DNA Subunit Vaccines 4
V. Other Approaches to Vaccines 23
VI. Conclusions 32
References 33

Atherosclerosis: The Consequence of Infection with a Herpesvirus
CATHERINE G. FABRICANT

I. Introduction 39
II. Initial Experiments 42
III. Pathogenetic Mechanisms of MDV-Induced Atherosclerosis 52
IV. Evidence of MDV Infection in Cells Comprising Arterial Lesions 59
V. Immunization Protects against MDV-Induced Atherosclerosis 60
VI. Preliminary Evidence for a Herpesvirus Role in Human Atherosclerosis ... 62
VII. Summary and Conclusions 63
References 65

The Ontogeny and Microenvironment of the Avian Thymus and Bursa of Fabricius: Contribution of Specialized Cells to the Avian Immune Response
BRUCE GLICK

I. Introduction 67
II. Bursal Ontogeny and Microenvironment 68
III. Nonbursal Site for Immunoglobulin Synthesis 73
IV. Identifying the Nonbursal Site and Associated Cells 76
V. The Role of the Avian Thymus 82

VI. The Multipotential Stem Cell	82
VII. Thymic Ontogeny	83
VIII. The Thymic Microenvironment	84
References	87

Neutrophilic Leukocyte Structure and Function in Domestic Animals

T. A. BERTRAM

I. Introduction	91
II. Neutrophil Morphology	92
III. Neutrophil Metabolism and Antimicrobial Systems	103
IV. Neutrophil Migration and Activation	110
V. Phagocytosis and Degranulation	114
VI. Granulocytopoiesis	116
VII. Neutrophils of the Circulating Blood (Neutrophil Heterogeneity)	117
VIII. Neutrophil Function in Inflammatory and Immunologic Processes	118
IX. Summary	121
References	122

Pathobiology of Animal Platelets

KENNETH M. MEYERS

I. Introduction	131
II. Acquisition	132
III. Ultrastructure	134
IV. Basic Platelet Response	138
V. Modulators	151
VI. Agglutinating Agents	155
VII. Platelet Membrane Glycoproteins	156
VIII. Tumor Cells	157
IX. Thrombocytopenia	159
References	159

The Pathology of Prosimians, Especially Lemurs

K. BENIRSCHKE, C. MILLER, R. IPPEN, AND A. HELDSTAB

I. Introduction	167
II. Review of the Literature	168
III. General Considerations	172
IV. Perinatal Mortality	173

V.	Congenital Anomalies	180
VI.	Infections	184
VII.	Hemosiderosis; Hepatoma	187
VIII.	Hyperplasia of the Islets of Langerhans	195
IX.	Pectus Excavatum	196
X.	Miscellaneous Conditions	200
XI.	Conclusions	205
	References	206

Methods for Evaluating Reproductive Function in Exotic Species
BILL L. LASLEY

I.	Introduction	209
II.	The Estrogen/Testosterone Ratio	212
III.	Evaluation of Estrogenic Components	214
IV.	Bioactive Luteinizing Hormone Measurements	220
V.	Direct Assays for Steroid Conjugates	222
VI.	Pregnanediol-3-Glucuronide	223
VII.	Estrone Conjugates	226
	References	228

INDEX 229

CONTRIBUTORS

Numbers in parentheses indicate the pages on which the authors' contributions begin.

HOWARD L. BACHRACH, U.S. Department of Agriculture, Agricultural Research Service, Plum Island Animal Disease Center, Greenport, New York 11944 (1)

K. BENIRSCHKE, Zoological Society of San Diego, San Diego, California 92112, and Departments of Pathology and Reproductive Medicine, University of California San Diego, La Jolla, California 92093 (167)

T. A. BERTRAM,[1] National Animal Disease Center, Ames, Iowa 50010 (91)

CATHERINE G. FABRICANT, Department of Microbiology, New York State College of Veterinary Medicine, Cornell University, Ithaca, New York 14853 (39)

BRUCE GLICK, Poultry Science Department, Mississippi State University, Mississippi State, Mississippi 39762 (67)

A. HELDSTAB, Institute of Animal Pathology, University of Bern, 3001 Bern, Switzerland (167)

R. IPPEN, Akademie der Wissenschaften der DDR, Forschungsstelle für Wirbeltierforschung, 1136 Berlin, German Democratic Republic (167)

BILL L. LASLEY, Research Department, San Diego Zoo, San Diego, California 92112 (209)

KENNETH M. MEYERS, Department of Veterinary and Comparative Anatomy, Pharmacology, and Physiology, Washington State University, Pullman, Washington 99164 (131)

C. MILLER, School of Veterinary Medicine, University of California at Davis, Davis, California 95616 (167)

---

[1]Present address: Department of Veterinary Pathobiology, College of Veterinary Medicine, University of Illinois, Urbana, Illinois 61801.

PREFACE

The seven articles in this volume include the latest knowledge about animal vaccines, herpesvirus and atherosclerosis, the avian immune system, the importance and function of the neutrophil in animals, and the biology of animal platelets. Specific topics discussed are the pathology of prosimians and reproduction in certain exotic species.

In the first article by Bachrach there is a description of five general procedures that could lead to the production of practical vaccines for use in animals and man. Such vaccines could result in the control of certain untreatable diseases of today, such as cancer.

The second article by Fabricant contains substantial evidence that Marek's disease herpesvirus causes atherosclerosis in normocholesterolemic chickens, and that the lesion is similar to that seen in humans with chronic atherosclerosis.

Glick demonstrates that the chicken has contributed greatly to an understanding of the immune response in other species. The review deals in great detail with the ontogeny, microenvironment, and function of the bursa of Fabricius and thymus in avian immunity.

The article by Bertram, pertaining to neutrophils of domestic animals, delineates neutrophil morphology between species, the response of neutrophils to infectious agents, the process of enzyme release from granules, and the functions of the cell.

A detailed discussion of normal and abnormal animal platelets is contained in Meyers' article.

The sixth article by Benirschke, Miller, Ippen, and Heldstab is a very interesting review of the anatomic pathology of prosimians. Apparently, this work is the first report of the incidence of congenital disorders among prosimians. In addition, metabolic diseases and infections are identified.

The last article by Lasley is a summary of the role of endocrinology in reproduction among exotic species. Special emphasis is devoted to methods.

C. E. CORNELIUS
C. F. SIMPSON

New Approaches to Vaccines

HOWARD L. BACHRACH

U.S. Department of Agriculture, Agricultural Research Service, Plum Island Animal Disease Center, Greenport, New York

I.	Introduction	1
II.	Impetus for the New Vaccines	2
III.	Prospects for the New Vaccines	3
IV.	Recombinant DNA Subunit Vaccines	4
	A. Preparation of Immunogenic Genes for Cloning	5
	B. Recombinant DNA Protein Vaccine for Foot-and-Mouth Disease	6
	C. Recombinant DNA Protein Vaccines for Other Viral Diseases	10
	D. Recombinant DNA Protein Vaccines for Bacterial and Parasitic Diseases	21
V.	Other Approaches to Vaccines	23
	A. Chemically Synthesized Vaccines	24
	B. Recombinant Virus Vaccines	27
	C. Genetically Engineered Reassortants and Deletion Mutants	29
	D. Antiidiotype Antibody Vaccines	31
VI.	Conclusions	32
	References	33

I. Introduction

Recombinant DNA and other molecular biological and chemical methods are being applied to the development of new types of safe and effective vaccines for animals and humans. While most of these vaccines are still in developmental stages, some of them are expected to supplement or replace conventional whole-agent vaccines. The principal motivation for the new approaches stems from findings, made mostly in the 1970s, that the isolated surface proteins of infectious agents generally possess immunogenic activity. Five strategies are currently being applied to the generation of new types of vaccines: (1) recombinant DNA cloning of immunogenic surface proteins, (2) chemical synthesis of polypeptide vaccines, (3) construction of recombinant viruses having guest genes for foreign surface proteins, (4) genetic engineering of nonpathogenic mutant agents, and (5) production of monoclonal antiidiotype antibodies that mimic the major immunogenic epitopes of the surface proteins of infectious agents.

II. Impetus for the New Vaccines

Several factors are contributing to the recent interest in exploring new approaches to vaccine development. One factor is that the time-honored conventional methods of attenuation or inactivation of infectious agents have not produced effective vaccines for many diseases, including hepatitis A and B, most diseases caused by retro- and herpesviruses, malaria, trypanosomiasis, and other parasitic diseases. Also, the use of certain conventional whole-agent vaccines can give rise to serious complications. For example, attenuated virus vaccines can perpetuate their genomes in animal and human populations, producing acute infections or slowly progressive disease in immunodeficient individuals or in alternate animal species. Also, certain apparently avirulent virus strains can revert to virulence, either by host-induced proteolysis of surface proteins of the phenotype, as in the activation of the HN and F_0 proteins of Newcastle disease virus (Nagai and Klenk, 1977) and of the HA protein of influenza virus (Klenk *et al.*, 1975), or by mutations in the genotype, as in the reversion of attenuated oral Sabin poliovirus vaccines (Kew *et al.*, 1981). While the Sabin vaccine has been highly effective in the United States and several other countries, it produces a few cases each year in the United States of paralytic polio in vaccinees and their contacts (Kew *et al.*, 1981). Also, the attenuated virus can become established in the human population, and the antibody responses to attenuated poliovirus vaccine have been found to be uncertain in tropical climates (Salk and Salk, 1984). Owing to these complications and to the fact that poliovirus is usually absent in Finland and Sweden (one outbreak in 1984 and one case in 1977, respectively) where only inactivated vaccine has been used, a leading vaccinologist has recommended that the Sabin vaccine be replaced in the United States with an improved high-potency, single-dose, inactivated poliovirus vaccine. This proposal, however, poses the problem that supposedly inactivated vaccines sometimes contain infectious virus, as occurred in early commercial batches of poliovirus vaccines used in the United States. Similarly, so-called inactivated foot-and-mouth disease (FMD) virus vaccines are found to be infectious far too frequently. For example, at least 44% of the outbreaks of FMD in Europe from 1968 to 1981 were caused by incompletely inactivated vaccines or escape of virus from vaccine manufacturing facilities (FAO, 1981). Similarly, outbreaks of FMD in three South American countries in 1979 and 1980 were caused by three different vaccines that contained infectious virus (Casas, 1981). In addition, conventional whole-agent vaccines, particularly crude preparations, have been implicated in postvaccinal pyrogenic and allergic reactions, abortions, Guillain-Barré neurological syndromes, and other adverse sequelae. Another postvaccinal danger, even with inactivated virus vaccines (e.g., those for dengue-2, influenza, rabies, and others), is that of the immune enhancement of disease and of mortality when antibody levels have decreased sharply prior to subsequent infection with homologous viruses (Halstead, 1982).

III. Prospects for the New Vaccines

When perfected, the new vaccines should be most useful in controlling infectious diseases for which whole-agent vaccines have been lacking. Others may supplement or supplant vaccines which are dangerous to use because of potential infectiousness or the various postvaccinal adverse reactions mentioned above. In contrast to whole-virus vaccines, the presence of only one or two essential proteins of a virus in many of the new vaccines should eliminate the formation of antibodies against many irrelevant epitopes of the virus and of proteins and other antigens that contaminate crude and partially purified viral preparations. Consequently, the incidence of unwanted side reactions should be reduced. Also, it will be possible to freeze-dry protein vaccines for use in regions where refrigeration is lacking, and because the protein vaccines do not contain nucleic acid, the danger of producing disease is eliminated.

Replacements of conventional vaccines can be expected, however, to proceed slowly and with caution because of the natural resistance of pharmaceutical manufacturers and groups responsible for animal and human health to replace effective, time-tested products with new ones that lack comparable histories of clinical testing and field use. However, a few subunit protein vaccines are already in commercial use, including (1) detergent- or ether-split influenza A and B virus vaccines, (2) a hepatitis B vaccine composed of 22-nm protein particles (Australian antigen) purified from the blood of individuals recovered from hepatitis B, and (3) a vaccine composed of pilus proteins and a part of the toxin of enterotoxigenic *E. coli* that have been cloned in nontoxigenic *E. coli*. The crude subunit influenza vaccines produce high-antibody titers and apparently fewer side effects than whole-virus vaccines; however, two doses are needed to protect unprimed recipients (Jennings *et al.*, 1984). There is presently no whole-virus vaccine alternative to the 22-nm protein subunit vaccine for hepatitis B, although cloned, synthetic, and recombinant virus vaccines are under development. Many viruses, bacteria, and parasites possess surface proteins that retain their immunogenicity after isolation, making them promising candidates for subunit vaccines. The five approaches to the new vaccines mentioned above—recombinant DNA cloning, chemical synthesis, construction of recombinant viral vectors, nonpathogenic mutant agents, and antiidiotype antibodies—are being researched in many laboratories. The remainder of this article deals with progress being made on vaccines by these approaches against viral, bacterial, and parasitic diseases.

IV. Recombinant DNA Subunit Vaccines

The biosynthesis of the surface proteins of infectious agents by cloning and the expression of the encoding genes in single-celled or animal hosts using recombinant DNA (rDNA) methods are at the forefront of the newer approaches to vaccine development. Recombinant DNA technology, first described in 1973, deals with the splicing of the DNA gene encoding a known protein into a DNA vector, such as a double-stranded DNA virus or a bacterial plasmid, and subsequent transfer of the chimeric DNA into an alternate host cell for its replication and regulated expression of the guest gene. By means of recombinant DNA technology, genes (even those of RNA viruses after copying them into DNA using reverse transcriptase) can be transplanted between plants, animals, and microorganisms—events that occur rarely in nature, except for plasmid exchanges among microorganisms. Most of the modern advances in molecular biology and in nucleic acid and protein chemistry have contributed to the development of rDNA technology. These advances include the elucidation of the structure and function of bacterial plasmids and viruses; the discoveries of the DNA double helix, messenger RNAs, and the genetic code; the finding that retroviruses possess reverse transcriptase, which permits them to replicate by a recombinant DNA pathway; the discovery and isolation of restriction endonucleases that cleave DNA generally where thymine, cytosine, adenine, and guanine bases form palindromic sequences on opposite strands; the isolation of DNA ligases, S1 nuclease, and terminal deoxyribonucleotidyl transferases; the development of rapid protein- and DNA-sequencing procedures; and the finding that microorganisms such as *E. coli, Bacillus subtilis,* and yeasts can serve as alternate hosts for chimeric DNA vectors containing guest genes encoding foreign proteins. Harmless K12 strains of *E. coli* are the most common alternate hosts, but the protein products normally remain intracellular and are subject to cleavage by *E. coli* proteases and to contamination with bacterial toxins. Methods are now being developed for splicing secretory DNA sequences to the guest genes, which will permit some protein products to be secreted from *E. coli. Bacillus subtilis* secretes many proteins, but it has not gained wide use because of other factors. Yeasts are quite hospitable to eukaryotic genes and can carry out glycosylations that may be needed to simulate the structural authenticity of the glycoproteins of enveloped viruses.

A. Preparation of Immunogenic Genes for Cloning

While transplantation of eukaryotic genes into microorganisms has become routine in many laboratories, methods for isolating genes for transplantation are often variable and difficult. The methods used depend upon a number of factors: whether a gene is DNA or, as in many viruses, RNA; the size, segmentation, and strandedness of the genome; whether it has a plus or minus sense with respect to messenger RNA; the locus of the immunogenic gene(s) in the genome; the mix of introns (noncoding regions) and exons in the gene; and whether the messenger RNA transcribed is mono- or polycistronic. The genomes of message-sense RNA viruses (picorna, corona, calici, and toga), which are fully or partially polycistronic depending upon the viral family, translate to polyproteins that are precursors to viral proteins and enzymes. This replication strategy complicates the isolation of specific genes from messenger-sense RNA viruses. Moreover, once isolated, an RNA gene must be reversely transcribed into DNA before being cloned.

Three strategies for isolating specific genes from viruses are shown in Fig. 1. Strategies 1 and 2 begin with the dissociation of purified virions, followed by isolation and purification of the released immunogenic protein and viral DNA or RNA genomes. If the released genome is RNA, it must be transcribed to DNA. The DNA is amplified by cloning and then cleaved with appropriate restriction endonucleases to manageable fragments. At the same time, it is generally necessary to determine enough of the sequence of the immunogenic protein to be able to identify (using the genetic code in reverse) which of the DNA fragments code for it. In strategy 3, mRNA for the surface protein may

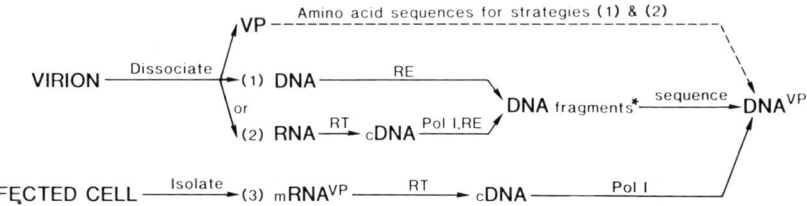

FIG. 1. Three strategies for isolating DNA fragments (DNA^{VP}) that encode a viral surface protein (VP), starting with purified virions or mRNA^{VP} isolated from infected cells. RT, reverse transcriptase; RE, restriction endonucleases; Pol I, DNA polymerase I; cDNA, complementary strand; ✶, amplify DNA fragments by cloning before sequencing them. From Bachrach (1982) with permission of the *J. Am. Vet. Med. Assoc.*

be isolated by several methods. In one method, an antibody specific for the immunogenic surface protein is used to precipitate nascent protein chains still attached to mRNA molecules. In a method called hybrid selection, authentic or synthetic DNA fragments specific for the immunogenic protein are used to "fish" homologous mRNA out of an infected cell lysate. If synthetic DNA fragements are used, it is generally necessary, because of code redundancies, to synthesize several DNA fragments for use in the mRNA "fishing" expedition. Alternatively, isolated mRNAs can be selected which have molecular weights close to those expected on the basis of the length of the proteins they encode. Unambiguous identification is then made either by sequencing the mRNAs or by programming a cell-free protein-synthesizing system with the mRNAs and comparing the synthetic products with authentic proteins by specific immunoprecipitation and/or tryptic-peptide mapping. As in strategy 2, the isolated mRNA is transcribed into complementary DNA and converted to double-stranded DNA with DNA polymerase I. In strategy 3 this DNA is the viral-specific DNA (Fig. 1). In strategies 1 and 2 the DNA fragments are amplified by cloning (not shown) before sequencing them, generally by the method of Maxam and Gilbert (1977). The cloned DNA fragments of interest are those that have coding sequences for the viral immunogenic surface protein. Comparisons of the physical and functional maps of viral genomes can be of help in this identification process.

B. Recombinant DNA Protein Vaccine for Foot-and-Mouth Disease

The production of cloned surface proteins of infectious agents for many important diseases of animals and humans is a very active area of research. A vaccine of this type for FMD (Kleid et al., 1981) was characterized by United States Secretary of Agriculture J. R. Block as the first effective vaccine produced by gene splicing for any disease of "animals or humans." Because the vaccine stimulates immunity in both cattle and swine that protects against infection with FMD virus, it holds considerable promise for reducing the incidence of FMD and thereby increasing the world's output of meat and other animal products. Although the initial cloned vaccine was for type A_{12} FMD, similar strategies with simplifying modifications have been used to clone and express the genes for the immunogenic surface proteins of 10 or more subtypes of FMD virus, including those for most of the 7 immunological types of this virus: A, O, C; SAT 1, 2, and 3; Asia 1. The cloned surface proteins for virus types A_{24}, A_{27}, A_{79}, and C_3 have been demonstrated to induce protection in cattle (P. D. McKercher, personal communication) equivalent to that reported for the cloned A_{12} protein (Kleid et al., 1981).

The strategy for cloning the type A_{12} protein vaccine is described here as an example of the process used for viruses. The genome of FMD virus (a picornavirus) is a single messenger-sense strand of infectious RNA approximately 8000 nucleotides long (Bachrach, 1977). It contains a genome-coded viral protein VP_g linked to its 5′ end followed successively by a short leader nucleotide tract, a 100–150 nucleotide poly(C) tract, a long open-frame coding region, and finally a 3′ poly(A) tract. The coding region translates to a polyprotein that is rapidly cleaved by both host-cell-coded and viral-coded proteases to capsid proteins VP_1, VP_2, VP_3, and VP_4 and noncapsid proteins VP_g, a protease (Pro), an RNA polymerase (Pol), and probably one or two additional unidentified proteins. The order of the genes in the FMD RNA genome is 5′ VP_4–VP_2–VP_3–VP_1–(?)–VP_g–Pro–Pol 3′. The major immunogenic protein of FMD virus is VP_1. (In previous publications by this author, this protein was termed VP_3 because it migrates as the third-slowest capsid protein in SDS/8 M urea polyacrylamide gel electrophoresis, but VP_1 is used herein in conformity with genome map assignments for FMD and polioviruses.) VP_1 has a molecular weight of approximately 24,000. By several measurements VP_1 appears to reside in an exposed position in the viral capsid: (1) when virions are treated with proteases for short periods, VP_1 is the only capsid protein cleaved; (2) when virions react with ^{125}I, VP_1 is the only capsid protein iodinated even though VP_2 and VP_3 together have twice as many tyrosine residues as VP_1 (Bachrach et al., 1978); and (3) VP_1 tends to be lost from virions that are repeatedly centrifuged in cesium chloride density gradients.

While VP_1 was rather large to be synthesized chemically, it was synthesized, along with other FMD viral proteins, by programming a cell-free ribosome system from Ehrlich ascites tumor cells with purified genomic FMD RNA (Chatterjee et al., 1976). However, as is well known, this procedure is not a production-scale method. For the preparation of vaccine quantities of VP_1, it was concluded (Bachrach et al., 1978) that it would be necessary to clone and express the gene for VP_1 by the then newly emerging recombinant DNA technology.

In preparation for cloning and expressing the VP_1 gene in *E. coli* K12, the immunogenicity of VP_1 isolated from virions was rigorously tested in swine and cattle (Bachrach et al., 1975, 1982), which are the most important domestic animal species naturally susceptible to FMD. Two inoculations of these animals with 100-μg doses of VP_1 in a modified incomplete Freund's oil adjuvant induced protective immunity against subsequent challenge with virus. In addition, it was determined that a 13-kDa fragment excised with CNBr from an internal region of VP_1 was also immunogenic in animals. (After cloning, it was found that the 13-kDa fragment occupied positions 55 through 179 in the 213 amino acid chain of VP_1.) Also, for the purpose of identifying VP_1-specific cloned DNA fragments, amino acid sequences were determined (Matheka and Bachrach, 1975; Bachrach et al., 1973, 1979, 1982) at the N- and C-termini of VP_1, at the N-terminus of the 13-kDa fragment, and the C-terminus of VP_3, which just precedes VP_1 in the genome of FMD virus (see above).

On the basis of the above information, the gene for VP_1 was cloned in *E. coli* K12 (Fig. 2) (Kleid et al., 1981). With oligodeoxyribothymidylic acid (oligo dT) as the primer, purified FMD viral genome RNA was transcribed into DNA using reverse transcriptase (step 1, Fig. 2) following strategy 2 of Fig. 1. One of the transcripts, amplified in a pBR322 vector in *E. coli* K12, was found by DNA sequencing to contain coding sequences for the C-terminus of VP_3 and all of VP_1, including its 13-kDa internal region. Moreover, the condons designated -2 and -1 in Fig. 2 for the C-terminus of VP_3 were contiguous with those for the N-terminus of VP_1 (codons 1, 2, 3, etc.). This demonstrated that cleavage at the -Gln-Thr- juncture of VP_3 and VP_1 is not followed by trimmings with exopeptidases, because the amino acid residues Gln and Thr had previously been determined to be C-terminal in VP_3 and N-terminal in VP_1, respectively (Bachrach et al., 1973, 1979, 1982). In addition, DNA sequencing revealed that the immunologically active 13-kDa fragment excised from VP_1 with CNBr commences at the amino acid following the methionine residue 54 and terminates at methionine residue 179 (not shown in Fig. 2). The actual residue molecular

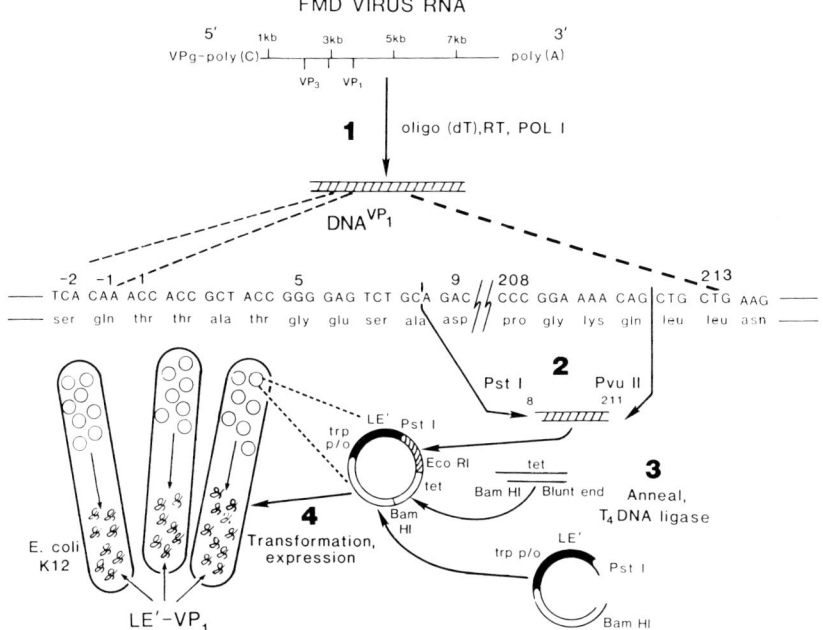

FIG. 2. Cloning and expression of foot-and-mouth disease virus protein VP$_1$ in *E. coli* K12. Step 1: strategy (2) of Fig. 1 was used to prepare DNA^{VP_1}. Its positive-sense strand contained coding sequences for the known C-terminus of VP$_3$ (codons −2, −1), N-terminus of VP$_1$ (condons 1, 2, 3, 4, 5, 6, . . .), C-terminus of VP$_1$ (213) and sequences for the 13-kDa CNBr fragment from VP$_1$ (codons for amino acids 55 through 179, not shown). Step 2: excision using *Pst*I and *Pvu*II of DNA segment coding for amino acids 8 through 211 of VP$_1$. Step 3: insertion together with a tetracycline-resistance marker (*tet*) into a pBR322 plasmid having a *trp* promoter–operator–LE′ leader. Step 4: transformation of *E. coli* K12 with the chimeric plasmid and expression of fusion protein LE′–VP$_1$. From Bachrach (1982) with permission of the *J. Am. Vet. Med. Assoc.*

weight of this region (13,480) was in very close agreement with the earlier 13,000 value estimated by polyacrylamide gel electrophoresis using molecular-weight markers (Bachrach *et al.*, 1979).

Step 2 (Fig. 2) involved the use of restriction endonucleases *Pst*I and *Pvu*II to excise a DNA fragment encoding amino acids 8 through 211 of VP$_1$. Step 3 consisted of the splicing of this fragment into a pBR322 plasmid having a tryptophan synthetase (*trp*) promoter–operator–LE′ leader and tetracycline-resistance gene (*tet*) marker, as shown (Fig. 2). After annealing the complementary sticky ends of the gene insert to the vector and bonding the blunt ends with T4 DNA ligase, the chimeric plasmid was used in step 4 to transform *E. coli* K12 in the presence of calcium ions. The transformed bacteria were grown to high concentration, during which the copy number of the chimeric plasmid also increased. Tryptophan was then depleted from the medium, causing expression of a fusion protein $LE'-VP_1$ with a molecular weight of approximatley 44,000. The $LE'-VP_1$ product, which was present at 1 to 2 million copies per bacterium, reacted with VP_1-specific antibody. More importantly, two 250-μg doses of the fusion protein in a modified Freund's incomplete oil adjuvant induced high levels of neutralizing antibody in swine (1.4 to 1.5 $\log_{10}PD_{50}$) and cattle (2.1 to 2.7 $\log_{10}PD_{50}$) and protected these livestock species against contact challenge with homologous virus (Table I) (Kleid et al., 1981). Two doses of the $LE'-VP_1$ fusion protein vaccine were as effective as two or three 100-μg doses of VP_1 or two 50-μg doses of the 13-kDa fragment of VP_1 isolated from virions. For obscure reasons, one steer vaccinated with virion-derived VP_1 responded with a low neutralizing antibody titer (1.6 $\log_{10}PD_{50}$) and was susceptible to the challenge virus, while two others vaccinated with the 13-kDa fragment had low postvaccination antibody titers but were nevertheless immune to challenge. In the whole-virus vaccine controls, as little as one 10-μg dose of acetylethylenimine-inactivated virus, containing approximatley 1.6 μg of VP_1 in situ, induced 3 $\log_{10}$ of neutralizing antibody in swine and protected the animals against challenge with infectious virus. All 30 unvaccinated swine and 7 unvaccinated cattle were susceptible to challenge exposure.

C. Recombinant DNA Protein Vaccines for Other Viral Diseases

Examples of immunogenic surface proteins of viruses that have potential or demonstrated usefulness as subunit vaccines are given in Table II. These isolated proteins have been reported to possess one or more of the following activities: (1) reaction with neutralizing antibody, (2) induction of neutralizing or viral-precipitating antibodies, and (3) induction of protective immunity in animals or humans against viral challenge. Table II also shows whether or not the genes for these proteins are being cloned in alternate hosts. In addition to the cloned protein vaccine for FMD already discussed (Section IV,B), other cloned vaccines in various stages of development include those for hepatitis A and B; feline, porcine, canine, and mink parvovirus diseases; bovine papillomas (warts); herpes simplex 1 and 2; Epstein–Barr-virus-associated diseases and cancers; bovine rhinotracheitis; pseudorabies; Rift valley fever; rabies; vesicular stomatitis; swine transmissible gastroenteritis; and bovine leukemia. These developments are discussed

TABLE I

NEUTRALIZING ANTIBODY AND IMMUNE RESPONSES OF SWINE AND CATTLE TO NATIVE AND CLONED ANTIGENS OF FMD VIRUS, TYPE A_{12}[a]

Animal	Number of vaccinations	Neutralizing antibody ($-\log PD_{50}$)	Fraction immune
VP_1			
Swine	1	ND	1/10
Swine	2	ND	8/10
Swine	3	2.2	2/2
Cattle	2	1.6	0/1
Cattle	2	2.6–2.7	5/5
Cattle	3	2.6	2/2
13-kDa fragment			
Swine	2	1.3	3/3
Cattle	2	0.4	2/2
$LE'-VP_1$			
Swine	2	1.4, 1.5	2/2
Cattle	2	2.1, 2.7	6/6[b]
Virus [AEI]			
Swine	1	3.0	9/9
Swine	2	4.0	6/6
None			
Swine	ND	ND	0/30
Cattle	ND	ND	0/7

[a] VP_1, virus capsid protein 1 (24 kDa), 100 g/dose; 13-kDa fragment, from VP_1, 50 μg/dose; $LE'-VP_1$, 44-kDa fusion VP_1 cloned in *E. Coli* K12, 250 μg/dose; virus[AEI], FMD virus inactivated with acetylethylenimine, 10 μg/dose. Swine were revaccinated, as required, with VP_1, 13-kDa fragment, or inactivated virus on days 28 and 60 and were challenge exposed on day 56 or day 80, respectively. Cattle were revaccinated, as required, on days 14 and 28 and were challenge exposed on day 72. Revaccinations with $LE'-VP_1$ were on day 24 for swine and 28 for cattle; challenge exposures were on days 32 and 42, respectively. Prechallenge neutralizing antibody titers of sera were determined as PD_{50}/ml in suckling mice. ND, not done. Adapted from Bachrach (1982) with permission of the *J. Am. Vet. Med. Assoc.*

[b] One steer developed a single small foot lesion, not generalized disease.

below in the order of the viral replication classes (Bachrach, 1978) listed in Table II.

1. DNA and DNP Viruses

a. Class I: Double-Stranded DNA Viruses. Class I DNA viruses (Papova-, Adeno-, and Herpetoviridae) possess immunogenic surface proteins. Two large, open reading frames, L1 and L2, in the nontransforming region of the bovine papilloma (wart) virus genome have

TABLE II

Candidates for Subunit Vaccines for Viral Diseases[a]

Class	Family	Virus	Immunogenic proteins	Cloned
I_{DNA}	Papova	Bovine papilloma	Surface proteins	Yes
		SV40	T	Yes
	Adeno	Adeno	Hexons, penton fibers	Yes[b]
	Herpes	Marek's, turkey	2–3 Glycoproteins	NR[c]
		IBR, pseudorabies	Glycoproteins	IP[c]
		Herpes simplex 1 and 2	gpC and gpD	Yes (gpD)
		Herpes zoster	gp118	NR
		Epstein–Barr	gp340	IP
I_{DNP}	Orthopox	Rabbitpox, vaccinia	Proteins and HA	NR
II	Parvo	Feline, mink, porcine	Capsid proteins	Yes
III	Reo	Reo	$\sigma 1, \sigma 3, \lambda 2$	Yes[b]
	Orbi	Bluetongue	P2	IP
	Rota	Simian, human, bovine	Proteins	Yes
IV	Picorna	FMD, polio, hepatitis A	Capsid proteins	Yes[b]
		Coxsackie B3	VP_2	NR
	Calici	Vesicular exanthema	p61	NR
	Corona	TGE	Glycoproteins	Yes
	Toga: Alpha	Semliki Forest	Split virus E_{1-3}	NR
	Flavi	Tick-borne enceph	Glycoprotein VP_3	NR
	Pesti	Hog cholera, BVD	Split virus E_{1-2}	NR
	Rubi	Rubella	Split virus E_{1-2}	NR
V_{seg}	Orthomyxo	Fowl plague, influenza	Split virus, HA_{1-2}	Yes
	Bunya	Rift Valley fever	G_{1-2}	Yes
	Arena	Pichinde	Glycoproteins	Yes[b]

been cloned and expressed in *E. coli* for use of the products as vaccines (Pilacinski *et al.*, 1984). Because simian virus 40 (SV40) is a much used cloning vector, its tumor antigens (T and t) are readily cloned in both prokaryotes and eukaryotes, but these antigens are of little importance in human and veterinary medicine. The hexons and penton fibers of adenoviruses elicit neutralizing antibodies (Ginsberg, 1975), but minor interest has been shown in cloning them for vaccine use. For

TABLE II (Continued)

Class	Family	Virus	Immunogenic proteins	Cloned
V	Paramyxo	Sendai, Newcastle, PI-3	F, HN	IP
		Measles	F, H	Yes (H)
	Rhabdo	Rabies, VSV	G	Yes
VI	Retro	Friend	gp71	NR
		Maloney, human	gp 62 (human)	Yes
		Feline leukemia	Sol tumor cell antigen	Yes[b]
		Bovine leukemia	gp51	Yes[b]
Unclassified	Hepatitis B	Human	HBsAg	Yes

[a]The split influenza virus and HBsAg (isolated from blood) subunit vaccines are in use.

[b]Cloned genes for adeno, hepatitis A, arena, and leukemia virus proteins (except gp62 human) are not reported to be expressed. Reovirus σ3 protein has been expressed in *E. coli* alone and as a fusion protein; σ1 only as a fusion protein (W. K. Joklik, personal communication). Updated from Bachrach (1982) with permission of the *Am. J. Vet. Med. Assoc.*

[c]NR, not reported to author's knowledge; IP, in progress.

herpesviruses, two vaccinations with two proteins isolated from plasma membranes of cells infected with turkey herpesvirus produced protective immunity in chickens against Marek's disease (Kaaden and Dietzschold, 1974). Consequently, work preparatory to cloning and expressing the corresponding genes from both turkey and Marek's herpesviruses is in progress (K. Nazerian, personal communication). Surface glycoproteins prepared from infectious bovine rhinotracheitis (IBR) and porcine pseudorabies (PR) virions have been shown to elicit neutralizing antibodies and protective immunity in cattle (Lupton and Reed, 1980) and swine (Platt, 1982), respectively, against the homologous viruses. The latter vaccine was a mixture of proteins and glycoproteins extracted with detergent from PR virus and mixed with Freund's incomplete adjuvant. Work is underway on cloning and expressing the genes for the surface glycoproteins of IBR (Mayfield et al., 1983) and PR viruses.

A PR virus glycoprotein–β-galactosidase fusion protein expressed in *E. coli* is reported to protect mice from lethal challenge with PR virus (Robbins et al., 1984a,b). Glycoprotein gp300/350 isolated from Epstein–Barr virus induces both viral neutralizing antibodies and antibody-mediated cellular toxicity in experimental animals (Qualtiere et al., 1982). This same protein, called gp340 by Epstein (Morse, 1984), appears to prevent tumor development in cottontop tamarin monkeys challenged with Epstein–Barr virus. The gene encoding gp340 has been isolated and is being cloned for expression in *E. coli* (Morse, 1984). However, the greatest progress on cloning subunit protein vaccines for herpesviruses has been carried out with herpes simplex viruses. Monoclonal antibodies to glycoproteins gC and gD of herpes simplex virus 1 (HSV-1) are reported to be type restrictive and type common, respectively, in their ability to protect against HSV challenge (Dix *et al.*, 1981). In accord with this report, HSV-1 DNA specific for gD cloned in *E. coli* produced a gD-related polypeptide that elicited neutralizing antibodies to both HSV-1 and HSV-2 (Watson *et al.*, 1982). Subsequent to this work, the cloning of the gene for gD of HSV-2 was reported (Lasky and Dowbenko, 1984). The successes with HSV are expected to lead to a protein vaccine for veneral herpes and are also serving as models for the possible development of cloned vaccines for several herpesvirus diseases of animals and humans. These expectations may well include a protein vaccine for chickenpox and dermatomal zoster, because gp118 of varicella zoster virus has been shown to elicit complement-independent neutralizing antibodies (Friedricks and Grose, 1984).

b. Class I: Double-Stranded DNP Virus. The pox- and iridoviruses comprise the double-stranded deoxyribonucleoprotein (DNP) viruses. Unlike the infectiousness of DNA isolated from Class I DNA viruses, nearly intact virions containing core and capsid enzymes are required for the initiation of infection by Class I DNP viruses. There is no evidence that any one or a combination of surface proteins isolated from DNP viruses can induce immunity to infection. The orthopoxviruses possess as many as five important surface antigens (Baxby, 1982). Antigens solubilized from intracellular rabbitpox or vaccinia viruses are reported to elicit neutralizing antibodies to homologous intracellular virus but not to extracellular virus (Appleyard and Andrews, 1974; Balachandran *et al.*, 1980); however, animals having these antibodies are not protected against infection. It appears that immunological responses induced by a late hemagglutinin present in the envelope of extracellular virus and in plasma membranes of infected cells are necessary to the protective process. Ironically, while effective subunit protein vaccines have not been described for orthopoxviruses, extraordinary progress is being made in the use of vaccinia virus as a vector for carrying the genes of the surface proteins of other viruses (e.g., herpes, hepatitis B, influenza, and porcine TGE viruses) into animals, where expression of the guest genes induces protection against challenge with the corresponding infectious agent (Mackett *et al.*, 1982). Consequently, the notable success in eradicating smallpox using vaccinia virus vaccine presages the real possibility of using recombinant vaccinia viruses as live vaccines for the prevention of many other important diseases of animals and humans, an idea that no doubt never occurred to Edward Jenner.

c. Class II: Single-Stranded DNA Viruses. Considerable progress is being made in the cloning and expression of the genes for the surface proteins of viruses in Class II, which is composed solely of the Parvoviridae. These viruses contain separately encapsidated positive or negative single-stranded DNA genomes, which upon extraction become double stranded and infectious. In theory, but not yet proven, either strand alone should be infectious because the 3' ends of the DNA single strands act to self-prime their replication by way of double-stranded intermediates. The isolated surface proteins from both H-1 rat and canine parvoviruses have been reported to induce neutralizing antibodies in guinea pigs (S. Rhode, III, personal communication). The genes for the surface proteins of porcine, feline panleucopenia (FP), and Aleutian mink (Mayer *et al.,* 1983) parvoviruses are being cloned in *E. coli.* Testing of the immunogenicity of the proteins expressed by the porcine and FP parvovirus genes is in progress (Fox *et al.,* 1984; Carlson *et al.,* 1984). The single-stranded DNA of porcine parvovirus codes for three major proteins, 90, 65, and 60 kDa. The two smaller proteins are subsets of the largest, indicating that a common segment of the three could be a useful immunogen. An association has been reported very recently between rheumatoid arthritis and a human parvovirus (Simpson *et al.,* 1984). If this report is confirmed, the progress being made on the cloning of animal parvovirus surface proteins could hasten the development of a vaccine against human arthritis.

2. *RNA and RNP Viruses*

a. Class III: Double-Stranded RNP Viruses. Advances are also being made in cloning protein vaccines for Class III viruses, which include the double-stranded RNP Reo-, Orbi-, and Rotaviridae. These families are so similar in replication strategies that they could easily be considered a single family, with subdivisions based on host range and slight structural differences. Regardless, they are RNP and not RNA viruses, because the RNA polymerases coded by and present in the mature virions are essential for replication (Bachrach, 1978). This replication requirement also applies to the negative-stranded RNP viruses (Classes V_{seg} and V) discussed below. For reoviruses, the surface protein σ1 appears to be a vaccine candidate because it elicits neutralizing antibodies in animals; for certain serotypes σ3 and λ2 proteins also display this activity (Joklik, 1981). While most of the λ2 protein chain resides in the core of the reovirus, a segment penetrates through to the surface of the virion.

For orbiviruses, protein P2 of bluetongue virus was presumed to be immunogenic because a high correlation existed between P2-precipitating and neutralizing antibody titers (Huismans and Erasmus, 1981), and monoclonal antibody to P2 passively immunized sheep (Letchworth and Appleton, 1983). The isolated P2 protein has now been reported to elicit neutralizing antibodies in sheep and to induce protective immunity in these animals against challenge with high doses of infectious bluetongue virus (Huismans *et al.*, 1983). For rotaviruses, an unreduced p26 and a gp34 glycoprotein of simian SA11 virus elicit type-specific neutralizing antibodies (Bastardo *et al.*, 1981). Using monospecific polyclonal antiserums, the major neutralization-specific epitopes of calf rotavirus have been shown to reside in a minor protein designated VP7.2 present in the outer shell of the virion (Killen and Dimmock, 1982). The genes of human, bovine, and simian rotaviruses have been cloned in *E. coli* (Flores *et al.*, 1984). The rapid progress being made on the cloning of the genomes of the double-stranded RNP viruses (reo, orbi, and rota) is expected to lead to the production of amounts of surface proteins sufficient for thorough testing as candidate vaccines (Compans and Bishop, 1983).

b. Class IV: Single-Stranded RNA Viruses. The development of subunit protein vaccines for viruses containing messenger-sense, infectious, single-stranded RNA genomes will be discussed separately for the four families comprising this virus class. The four families have distinctively different architectures and protein compositions and slightly different replication strategies. For the picornaviruses, the prototype subunit vaccine work with proteins isolated from virions and proteins cloned in *E. coli* has been carried out with FMD virus (Bachrach *et al.*, 1975; Kleid *et al.*, 1981). The immunizing capacities of the 213 amino acid 24-kDa surface protein VP_1 isolated from subtype A_{12} and its 13-kDa CNBr-derived internal fragment (amino acids 55–179) as well as those of a 44-kDa $LE'-VP_1$ fusion protein (amino acids 8–211) cloned in *E. coli* have been described above in Section IV,B. Similar results have been obtained with cloned fusion proteins for FMD virus subtypes A_{24}, A_{27}, A_{79}, and C_3 (P. D. McKercher, personal communication). For reasons most likely having to do with protein conformation or proteolytic sensitivity, it has been more difficult to protect livestock with subtype O_1 subunit vaccines. For example, only two of three goats inoculated repeatedly with recombinant type O_1 surface protein developed neutralizing antibodies with no detectable or very low viremias and milder fevers than two control goats when challenged with virus (Hofshneider *et al.*, 1981). Also, peptides cleaved from the surface protein of type O_1 virus induced neutralizing antibodies in guinea pigs but only partial protection against spread of infection from the primary lesions when challenged with virus (Kaaden *et al.*, 1977). Work on chemically synthesized peptide vaccines for FMD stemming from the recombinant DNA successes will be discussed below in Section V,A. Following the work with FMD virus (Bachrach *et al.*, 1975, 1978), it was reported that VP_2 of Coxsackie virus B3 induces neutralizing antibodies (Beatrice *et al.*, 1980) and that the proteins of poliovirus possess immunogenic activity. Protein VP_1 isolated from poliovirus is reported to be a weak immunogen (Blondel *et al.*, 1982; Chow and Baltimore, 1982), and VP_2 and VP_3 are reported to have additional immunogenic activity (Wimmer *et al.*, 1984).

For caliciviruses, the single major protein that constitutes the capsid of vesicular exanthema virus of swine (Bachrach and Hess, 1973) may be a subunit vaccine candidate because two vaccinations of swine with the purified protein induced neutralizing antibodies (A. H. Dardiri and H. L. Bachrach, unpublished data). Consequently, similar activities could be expected using the isolated proteins of feline calicivirus and San Miguel sea lion virus (Bachrach and Hess, 1973).

Togavirus surface proteins have potential as subunit vaccines. For the *Alpha* genus, protection against challenge is obtained when the glycoprotein of Semliki Forest virus is in the form of multimeric micelles (Simons *et al.*, 1980). For the *Flavi* genus, glycoprotein V_3 isolated with detergent as polymeric complexes from tick-borne encephalitis virus elicits hemagglutination-inhibiting and neutralizing antibodies and, in comparison with whole-virus vaccines, is 10 times more active in competition radioimmunoassays and equally as effective in stimulating a protective immune response (Heinz *et al.*, 1981). For the *Pesti* genus, swine vaccinated repeatedly with glycoproteins, presumed to be E_1 and E_2 from detergent-split hog cholera (HC) virus or from infected cells, produced neutralizing antibodies and were protected against infection with HC virus (Dalsgaard and Overby, 1976). Detergent-split bovine diarrhea virus, which is analogous to HC virus for bovines, was less potent as a subunit vaccine against HC than were the HC virus glycoproteins. For the *Rubi* genus, detergent-split rubella virus (Cappel and Decuyper, 1976) appears to hold more promise as a subunit vaccine than hemagglutinin rosette or virosome preparations (Trudel and Payment, 1982).

Coronaviruses, which contain the longest messenger-sense single-stranded RNA genomes ($\sim$ 20,000 nucleotides), also have surface proteins that are subunit vaccine candidates. Using antiserums specific for each of three proteins of a human coronavirus, the slowest migrating protein ($\sim$ 13 kDa) elicits neutralizing antibody against one viral strain and both neutralizing and hemagglutination-inhibiting antibodies against another strain (Schmidt and Kenney, 1982). Also, two or three 1-mg doses in aluminum hydroxide or Freund's adjuvants of a

25-kDa immunogen (probably a glycoprotein) isolated from transmissible gastroenteritis (TGE) virus given intramuscularly to weanling pigs induce the formation of neutralizing antibodies (apparently including secretory IgA antibodies) and protect the pigs against infection with virulent TGE virus (Gough et al., 1983). Owing to these results, work is underway to develop a cloned protein vaccine for TGE of swine. The gene for the surface glycoprotein gp195 of TGE virus has been cloned and expressed in *E. coli* (Hu et al., 1984), and that for surface glycoprotein gp31 also appears to be a candidate for cloning.

c. *Class V_{seg}: Segmented Single-Stranded RNP Viruses.* These RNP viruses—Orthomyxo- (eight segments), Bunya- (three segments), and Arenaviridae (two segments)—have surface glycoproteins that are vaccine candidates. Influenza virus subunit vaccines split with detergents or ether are already in wide use. They effect seroconversions and appear to produce fewer side reactions than whole-virus vaccines, but two doses are required for unprimed recipients (U.S. Dept. HEW, 1976). The gene for the principal surface immunogen of fowl plague virus, the hemagglutinin (HA) gene, has been cloned and expressed in *E. coli* (Emtage et al., 1980), and that for wild-type human influenza virus has been expressed in both *E. coli* (Heiland and Gething, 1981; Davis et al., 1981) and eukaryotic cells in culture (Gething and Sambrook, 1981). Each reprogrammed eukaryote was reported to express more than 10^8 cell-associated HA molecules that absorbed specifically to red blood cells and to viral antibodies. When the gene for an anchorless mutant was cloned, the HA expressed was efficiently secreted into the extracellular fluid (Gething and Sambrook, 1982). However, cloned HA molecules have not yet been demonstrated to be effective vaccines against influenza; this is also the case for chemically synthesized segments of the HA, which will be discussed in Section V,A. Thus, more research is needed to solve the problems involved. Perhaps the inclusion of the neuraminidase (NA) of the viral envelope would be beneficial. Already, one such vaccine containing both the HA and NA moieties of influenza virus shows promise in mouse tests (Morein et al., 1982).

Glycoproteins G_1 and G_2 encoded by the mid-sized viral RNA segment are the principal immunogens of the Bunyaviridae (Gentsch et al., 1980). The genes for these two proteins in Rift Valley fever virus map G_2G_1 and have been cloned and partially expressed, i.e., the N-terminal two-thirds of G_2 and C-terminal two-thirds to three-fourths of G_1, leaving the sequences intermediate within G_2G_1 unexpressed (USAMRDC contract, 1982; J. Dalrymple, personal communication). The expressed segments elicit a low level of neutralizing antibodies

($\sim 10^{-1}$) in mice, and the mice are poorly protected (15–20%) against challenge of immunity with 28 LD_{50} of homologous virus. Perhaps the unexpressed central region in the G_2G_1 gene encodes the immunodominant epitopes of Rift Valley fever virus. The bisegmented arenaviruses also contain one or two surface glycoproteins. Although these glycoproteins have not been characterized fully for their immunogenicity, glycoprotein pGP-C encoded by the small RNA segment of Pichinde virus appears to be worth cloning as a candidate for a subunit vaccine (Ramsingh and Leung, 1982).

d. Class V: Nonsegmented Single-Stranded RNP Viruses. The surface glycoproteins of the nonsegmented negative-stranded RNP viruses (Paramyxo- and Rhabdoviridae) have also been examined for their immunogenicity. The paramyxoviruses have two surface glycoproteins: one of them possesses hemagglutinin (H) activity or both hemagglutinin and neuraminidase (HN) activities and the other has cell fusion and hemolytic activities (i.e., the F glycoprotein). The H protein isolated from measles virus (Bellini *et al.*, 1981) or the HN protein from Sendai, Newcastle disease, simian-5, and parainfluenza-3 (PI-3) viruses all elicit neutralizing antibodies (Merz *et al.*, 1980; Hosaka, 1980). The F proteins induce antibodies that inhibit the cell-to-cell spread of virus (Merz *et al.*, 1980). An oil-adjuvanted mixture of HN and F proteins isolated from PI-3 virus and formed into 30 S micelles induces serum antibodies and protective immunity in lambs against PI-3 virus pneumonia (Morein *et al.*, 1983). While several groups have been attempting for some time to clone the H, HN, F, and matrix proteins of the paramyxoviruses (Rozenblatt *et al.*, 1982; P. Choppin, personal communication), their efforts have met with limited success thus far. However, the cloning and characterization of DNA complementary to measles virus mRNA encoding the H and matrix proteins have been reported (Rozenblatt *et al.*, 1982). In addition, segments of the P, NP, and matrix genes of Sendai virus have been cloned in *E. coli* using plasmid pBR322, but expression has not been demonstrated (Gupta *et al.*, 1983). This slow progress with the paramyxoviruses is in marked contrast to reports for the rhabdoviruses, which have a glycoprotein G with both immunogenic and hemagglutinating activities. Both rabies virus subunits and the isolated glycoprotein G induce neutralizing antibodies and immunity in animals (Cox *et al.*, 1980). Moreover, the glycoprotein G genes of both rabies (Yelverton *et al.*, 1983) and vesicular stomatitis (VS) (Rose and Shafferman, 1981) have been cloned in *E. coli*. The VS G gene product from *E. coli* is precipitated by antibody to the virus, suggesting that it contains epitopes of the authentic G protein. Improvement in yields of the G-like protein has been obtained by cloning the gene in eukaryotic cells using an SV40 vector (Rose and Bergmann, 1982). In addition, a cloned anchorless form of the G protein of VS virus is slowly secreted from the eukaryotic cells. Tests are in progress to assess the immunogenicity in cattle of G protein isolated from VS virions and emulsified in complete Freund's adjuvant (Yilma, et al., 1985). Cattle that received a single intramuscular 100-µg dose of isolated G protein were resistant in varying degrees to intradermolingual challenge with 10^4 infectious units of VS virus. The biosynthetic G protein (Rose and Bergmann, 1982) and synthetic peptides (ca. 6–18 amino acid residues long) are also being tested for activity in stimulating immunity to VS.

e. Class VI: RNP Retroviruses. The retroviruses, which replicate by a DNA pathway analogous to cloning, possess envelope glycoproteins that are immunogenic. For example, glycoprotein gp71 isolated from the Friend murine leukemia virus immunizes mice against challenge infection with homologous virus (Ihle et al., 1976). Also, a vaccine composed of feline leukemia virus subunits and soluble tumor antigens has been reported to be about 80% effective in providing protection against viral challenge (Lewis et al., 1981). Analogous results for retrovirus diseases such as avian and bovine leukemias, equine infectious anemia, and human T cell leukemia/lymphoma (HTL) would constitute a breakthrough in cancer prevention. Because AIDS (acquired immunodeficiency disease syndrome) appears to be caused by retroviruses (LAV and HTLV-3) (Barré-Sinoussi et al., 1983; Gallo et al., 1984), examination of the envelope glycoproteins of these viruses for immunogenicity is definitely warranted. In the case of bovine leukemia, preliminary experiments indicate that neutralizing antibodies are elicited by a crude viral subunit vaccine and also by glycoprotein gp51 isolated from virions (J. F. Ferrer, personal communication). In addition, genes from bovine leukemia virus have been cloned in a λ phage vector (Kashmiri et al., 1984). Using the cloned DNA as a probe, a protein (~150 kDa) in the plasma of cattle infected with bovine leukemia virus was found to block the expression of the viral genome in infected lymphocytes *in vivo* at the transcriptional level (Gupta et al., 1984). Efforts are now being directed toward obtaining expression of the gp51 moiety.

3. Unclassified Viruses

Hepatitis B viruses are an unclassified five-member group of double-stranded DNA viruses which unexpectedly possess some of the replication characteristics of retroviruses (Summers and Mason, 1982). For example, (1) a DNA minus strand of duck hepatitis B virus is transcribed from an RNA template before the viral DNA plus strand is made, (2) the organization of the hepatitis B genome is similar to that of the proviral DNA of retroviruses, (3) at least a part of the hepatitis DNA genome appears to integrate into the chromosome of the host, and (4) the virus can apparently transform hepatic cells *in vivo* into hepatomas (Marx, 1982). Hepatitis B surface antigen (HBsAg) isolated from the virus affecting humans has been shown to protect chimpanzees against viral challenge (Dreesman et al., 1981). This antigen was subsequently purified from human sera and approved for use as a vaccine for humans (Hilleman et al., 1981). However, vaccination is so costly ($\sim$ \$100) that it is used primarily for medical and dental personnel at high risk of infection. The subunit vaccine is reported to induce cross-type neutralizing antibodies to all hepatitis B viruses that possess the "a" surface antigen (Szmuness et al., 1982). Recently, a vaccine has been tested in chimpanzees and humans that contains HBsAg derived from cultures of human hepatoma cells (McAleer et al., 1984). The gene for the HBsAg has been cloned in *E. coli* by several groups, and the expressed protein reacts with antibody to authentic HBsAg (Edman et al., 1981). Cloning in transformed monkey kidney cells using an SV40 vector results in the expression of partially glycosylated HBsAg molecules that also assemble into 22-nm particles (Laub et al., 1983). Cloning of the *HBsAg* gene in yeast produces 22-nm multimeric particles that simulate their natural counterparts (Valenzuela et al., 1982). A vaccine containing HBsAg produced by a rDNA strain of yeast is reported to elicit anti-HBsAg titers in human volunteers that are predominantly "a" epitope-specific (Scolnick et al., 1984). This is reportedly the first human trial of a vaccine prepared by rDNA technology. Trials in animals using chemically synthesized peptides corresponding to immunodominant regions of the HBsAg molecule have been carried out and are discussed in Section V,A.

D. Recombinant DNA Protein Vaccines for Bacterial and Parasitic Diseases

Recombinant DNA technology is also being applied to the preparation of protein vaccines for bacterial and parasitic diseases. Most of the early work has been concentrated on the somatic pili of enterotoxigenic *E. coli* (ETEC) that cause diarrhea in neonatal livestock and humans. The ETEC have somatic pili composed of 14- to 22-kDa protein molecules called pilin that adhere to the mucosal surface of the small intestines, initiating colonization by the bacteria. Immunologically distinct types of pili have been isolated from ETEC: K88 and 987P from swine;

K99 from cattle, sheep, and swine; CFA/1 and CFA/2 from humans; and type I and other common pili. Pili isolated from ETEC have been used as vaccines to prevent diarrheal disease in both humans and animals. Certain pilin genes appear to be encoded by bacterial chromosomes (type I and probably 987P), while others are derived from plasmids (K88, K99, and CFA/1 and 2) (Issacson, 1981). The production by cloning of pili encoded by plasmids has been reported, for example, for the K99 pili (DeGraaf et al., 1984), and cloned vaccines for animals have been developed in Western Europe (Trevis and Bertelsen, 1982) and the United States. The latter vaccine produced by rDNA technology has been approved by the United States Department of Agriculture (USDA) for use in swine (*Genetic Engineering News*, 1983). It contains three antigens that induce antibodies that block adhesion and colonization by the ETEC and one antigen that stimulates the production of an antitoxin. The vaccine is administered to pregnant sows shortly before parturition so that the piglets acquire immunity through the sows' milk.

An alternate method of protecting domestic animals against ETEC has been achieved through genetic engineering. Monoclonal antibody to K99 pilus antigen produced in hybridomas and amplified in mice significantly reduces both the severity of scours and the mortality of calves so treated. (Sherman et al., 1983). The product was successfully tested in Canada and has since been approved by the USDA for use in the United States.

A cloned pilus vaccine is being developed for use in humans against penicillin-resistant strains of *Neisseria gonorrhoeae* (WRAIR Res. Rep., 1982a; Meyer, 1982). A plasmid vector containing a segment of gonococcal DNA that encodes pili has been used to transform *E. coli*. The transformants have been detected with pili-specific monoclonal antibody, indicating that epitopes of gonococcal pili have been expressed by the cloned DNA. Additional progress in this direction could lead to an effective protein vaccine against gonorrhea.

A vaccine against syphilis has long evaded researchers, primarily because of the inability to culture the etiological agent of this disease, *Treponema pallidum, in vitro*. However, at least three groups of investigators have now cloned and expressed in *E. coli* genes encoding envelope antigens of this spirochete (Stamm and Bassford, 1982). It is anticipated that this work may lead to vaccines for syphilis and other diseases caused by spirochetes.

Immunogenic porin proteins in the membrane of *Brucella abortus* have been identified (Winter et al., 1983), but their genes have not yet been cloned and expressed in alternate hosts. The development of an effective nonviable vaccine for *Brucella abortus* through rDNA technology would constitute a major advance toward eradicating bovine brucellosis in the United States.

Work toward the production of rDNA protein vaccines against parasitic diseases is in progress, including those for avian coccidiosis (USDA, 1983) and malaria (Ellis *et al.*, 1983). The cloning and expression in *E. coli* of the malarial sporozoite surface antigen gene from *Plasmodium knowlesi* has been accomplished. There is also the possibility that rDNA technology may eventually play a role in the control of African sleeping sickness and other diseases caused by trypanosomes. Persons infected with *Trypanosoma rhodesiense* develop antibodies that react with the organism's surface glycoprotein, thereby initiating the killing of most of the parasitic population. However, resistant trypanosomes appear which display one or another of the 20 or more variant surface glycoproteins that can be encoded and expressed by *T. rhodesiense* (WRAIR Res, Rep., 1982b). The alternation between immunity to one variant of the parasite and reinfection with another generally continues until the host succumbs. The project of cloning the vast numbers of variant surface glycoproteins presented by trypanosomes is a task that no doubt will await progress on agents with less surface protein complexity. However, the finding of two types of antibodies against phospholipid regions of the *T. rhodesiense* membrane that may not undergo variation presents a new avenue of investigation for the control of African sleeping sickness and possibly also for cattle diseases caused by *Trypanosoma vivax, Trypanosoma congolense,* and *Trypanosoma brucei* (ILRAD Reports, 1983).

The control of diseases caused by trypanosomes may well be achieved by an application of rDNA technology that would involve the injection of cloned genes for immunotolerance into the germ plasm of animals. For example, if the tolerance of certain strains of cattle and sheep to trypanosomiasis (ILRAD Reports, 1983) is found to reside in a few distinct genes, it may be possible to insert the cloned genes into the germ lines of livestock by inoculation of the pronuclei in fertilized ova. As with mice that have been so endowed with human growth hormone genes (Palmiter *et al.*, 1983), the acquired trypano-tolerant genes should be transmitted to succeeding generations of livestock during the normal course of reproductive breeding.

V. Other Approaches to Vaccines

Breakthroughs in rDNA and other genetic engineering technologies have stimulated research on additional approaches to the development of vaccines. Four of these approaches are discussed below.

A. Chemically Synthesized Vaccines

Contrary to the title of this review article, the chemical synthesis of experimental polypeptide vaccines is neither new in concept nor execution. Over 20 years ago a synthetic hexapeptide identical to the C-terminus of tobacco mosaic virus (TMV) protein, cross-linked to serum albumin molecules, was shown to induce antibodies in rabbits that specifically precipitated and neutralized TMV (Anderer, 1963). Later, a peptide synthesized to correspond to the P_2 region of bacteriophage MS-2 coat protein was shown to induce neutralizing antibodies in rabbits almost as efficiently as the intact MS-2 coat protein (Langbeheim *et al.*, 1976), and one corresponding to the *conformational* antigenic determinant of egg-white lysozyme provoked antibody reactive with native lysozyme (Arnon *et al.*, 1971).

The recent renewed interest in synthetic peptide vaccines is due primarily to remarkable advances in protein and nucleic acid chemistry and in immunochemistry. Included in these advances are (1) powerful chromatographic and electrophoretic separation techniques, (2) the rapid automated synthesis of peptides and DNA sequences 15 and more residues long, (3) the ease of deriving amino acid sequences from the sequencing of encoding DNAs that have been produced by rDNA technology, (4) the development of highly sensitive radioimmunoassays, (5) the mapping of epitopes on proteins with monoclonal antibodies, (6) the finding that dominant epitopes can be continuous sites six to seven amino acid residues long or discontinuous sites of similar length composed of distant residues brought into juxtaposition by three-dimensional foldings of the protein, generally stabilized by disulfide bonds (Atassi, 1980), and (7) advances in experimental and predictive methods for locating surface antigenic sites, such as X-ray crystallography, isolation of active sites by chemical and enzymatic excisions, locating heterologous regions of amino acid sequences by comparing antigenic variants of a protein, calculation of sequences having high hydrophilicities (Hopp and Woods, 1981), and computer calculation of three-dimensional structures having the lowest free energies (Anfinsen and Scheraga, 1975).

The early studies on synthetic peptides for TMV, lysozyme, and MS-2 proteins coupled with the aforementioned rapid advances in molecular biology have stimulated a number of recent investigations of synthetic peptides that mimic immunodominant regions of viral and bacterial antigens. These include synthetic peptides for SV40 and the viruses of Maloney leukemia, hepatitis B, influenza, herpes diseases, FMD, and poliomyelitis. Thus, synthetic hepta- and undecapeptides corresponding to the N- and C-termini, respectively, of the large T antigen of SV40 virus are reported to induce antibodies in rabbits against the authentic T antigen (Walter et al., 1980). A synthetic pentadecapeptide corresponding to the encoding nucleotide sequence at the 3' end of Maloney leukemia virus was found to evoke antibody reactive with the native protein and a precursor protein present in infected cells (Sutcliffe et al., 1980). Several synthetic peptides mimic immunogenic activities of hepatitis B virus (HBV): (1) a peptide corresponding to residues 138 to 149 of HBsAg having a high computed hydrophilicity competes in radioimmunoassays with antibody to authentic HBsAg (Hopp and Woods, 1981), (2) other linear peptides corresponding to this general region and three other regions also elicit antibodies reactive with native HBsAg (Lerner et al., 1981), (3) cyclic polypeptides (corresponding to HBsAg cyclized residues 124–137 with side chains composed of residues 117–123 or 122–123) that induce neutralizing antibodies in mice after a single inoculation without being linked to a protein carrier (Dreesman et al., 1982) are scheduled for testing in chimpanzees, and (4) immunization of rabbits with a free or carrier-linked 26-mer corresponding to amino acid residues 120–145 located in the pre-S region of HBV DNA are reported to elicit high levels of group-specific antibodies, particularly when the peptide is covalently linked to liposomes (Neurath et al., 1984). It needs to be remembered, however, that while all these synthetic peptides can evoke antibodies that react with HBV and/or HBsAg particles, their protective capacities in vivo have yet to be fully demonstrated.

Synthetic peptides corresponding to regions of the hemagglutinin (HA) of influenza viruses have been examined by several groups of investigators. A peptide corresponding to residues 91–108 of type A H_3N_2 influenza virus conjugated to tetanus toxoid in the presence of Freund's oil adjuvant stimulated the production of neutralizing and hemagglutination-inhibiting antibodies and partial protection of mice against challenge with infectious mouse-adapted type A virus (Muller et al., 1982). These findings are in accord with the observation that the 91–108 sequence occupies a folded corner of the three-dimensional structure of the influenza HA molecule (Wiley et al., 1981). Also, 18 of 20 synthetic peptides, corresponding to 75% of the HA1 part of the HA molecule, are reported to induce antibodies reactive with authentic HA1 over its entire three-dimensional structure. Antibody to HA1 failed to react with any of the 20 peptides, emphasizing the importance of native protein conformation in the presentation of epitopes (Green et al., 1982). Also, peptides mimicking the first 11 amino acids at the N-terminus of the cell fusion region of the HA2 of influenza A and B viruses were found to bind to both human antibodies and anti-HA monoclonal antibodies. However, antipeptide antibodies, while binding to both HA and virus, failed to neutralize viral infectivity (Atassi and Webster, 1983). Consequently, as with attempts to clone protein vaccine for influenza (see Section IV,C,2,c), additional work is required to perfect synthetic vaccines for this disease.

For herpes simplex virus type 1 (HSV-1), a synthetic 16-mer corresponding to amino acid residues 8 to 23 of glycoprotein D was reported to react with anti-gpD monoclonal antibody known to neutralize both HSV-1 and HSV-2. Also, sera from animals immunized with the 16-mer (conjugated to protein carriers in complete Freund's adjuvant) reacted with native glycoprotein D and neutralized both HSV-1 and HSV-2 (Cohen et al., 1984). Because of these results, experiments are planned to assess the protective effect induced by this synthetic peptide.

The potential of synthetic peptides as vaccine candidates is actively being investigated for certain picornaviruses. Following the pioneering work on the immunization of livestock with the surface protein (and segments thereof) of type A FMD virus, isolated from both virions (Bachrach et al., 1975, 1979, 1982) and reprogrammed E. coli (Kleid et al., 1981), it was reported that one dose of an organically synthesized peptide 20 amino acids long corresponding to residues 141 through 160 of the surface protein of type O_1 virus coupled to a carrier protein evokes neutralizing antibody in cattle and guinea pigs and protects the guinea pigs against challenge with type O_1 FMD virus (Bittle et al., 1982). However, protection of the important natural hosts, cattle and swine, using the synthetic peptide approach remains to be demonstrated. While initial trials in cattle have been unsuccessful (Wilson, 1984), further work is expected to be productive because a vaccine containing a 13-kDa CNBr fragment composed of amino acid residues 55–179 derived from type A surface protein (24 kDa) protects both cattle and swine against challenge with homologous virus (Bachrach et al., 1979, 1982). Similarly, based on the demonstrations that low-level poliovirus neutralizing antibody can be obtained by immunizing rabbits and rats with type 1 poliovirus capsid protein VP_1 (Blondel et al., 1982; Chow and Baltimore, 1982), several small peptides corresponding to hydrophilic domains of VP_1 were synthesized (Emini et al., 1983). Five peptides reacted with poliovirus-neutralizing antibodies, but only one of these peptides and a peptide corresponding to a region in capsid protein VP_2 (Wimmer et al., 1984) elicited neutralizing antibodies when inoculated into rabbits (Emini et al., 1983). However, all of the VP_1-specific peptides—linked to BSA and emulsified in complete

Freund's adjuvant—primed and immune system of rabbits for a long-lasting, virus-neutralizing antibody response to a single inoculation with poliovirus. Consequently, work is underway to determine whether peptide-mediated priming can protect animals against *naturally* acquired infections. The capsid protein VP_2 of Coxsackie virus B3 has been shown to induce neutralizing antibodies (Beatrice et al., 1980); however, this finding apparently has not been followed up using synthetic peptides.

Progress is also being reported on the chemical synthesis of peptide vaccines for bacterial diseases, for example, diphtheria and cholera. A synthetic hexadecapeptide corresponding to amino acid residues 186–201 of the A chain of diphtheria toxin—covalently bonded to both synthetic muramyl dipeptide adjuvant and synthetic multichain poly-DL-alanine carrier—induced protective antitoxic immunity in guinea pigs. This vaccine appears to be the first completely synthetic peptide vaccine with built-in adjuvant and carrier, at least for diphtheria (Audibert et al., 1982). For cholera, two antibodies are known to protect animals and humans independently and synergistically against this disease, one being directed against *Vibrio cholerae* lipopolysaccharide and the other against cholera toxin (Holmgren and Svennerholm, 1982). Antibodies to the B subunit of the toxin are known to prevent the binding of toxin molecules to mucosal receptors. Consequently, several peptides ranging between 11 and 18 amino acid residues in length corresponding to regions of the 103 amino acid chain of the B subunit of *V. cholerae* have been synthesized and linked either to tetanus toxoid or to multichain poly-DL-alanine (Sela et al., 1984). These peptides are currently under test in rabbits for determination of their efficacy as vaccines against cholera.

B. Recombinant Virus Vaccines

Progress with protein vaccines for infectious diseases prepared by rDNA technology and chemical synthesis has stimulated several groups of investigators to construct and examine *live* recombinant viruses, most commonly vaccinia virus recombinants, carrying guest genes for the immunodominant proteins of other infectious agents. This approach appears to possess considerable practical potential. Only a small quantity of the recombinant virus is needed for vaccination because it replicates in the vaccinated animal, thereby expressing the foreign proteins encoded by the guest genes. Vaccinia virus possesses some advantages over other vectors—such as SV40, bovine papilloma virus, adenoviruses, and retroviruses—because of its large genome (187,000 base pairs) and wide host range. Also, unlike these alternative vectors, vaccinia virus has never been shown to transform cells or to be oncogenic. Experiments indicate that vaccinia virus can accommodate up to 25,000 base pairs of foreign DNA and still retain infectivity (Smith and Moss, 1983). Thus, it possesses the potential to serve as a vector for several guest genes in tandem and elicit immunity to several diseases concurrently. Experimental recombinant vaccinia vaccines have been reported for hepatitis B, herpes simplex, influenza, TGE of swine, and malaria. Insertion of the foreign genes is generally accomplished by site-directed homologous recombination (Mackett et al., 1984). Cells infected with vaccinia virus carrying the gene for HBsAg express and secrete this antigen in the form of 22-nm particles (Paoletti et al., 1984), and rabbits vaccinated with recombinant virus produce antibodies to HBsAg (Smith et al., 1983a; Paoletti et al., 1984). Similarly, the inoculation of rabbits with recombinant vaccinia virus expressing glycoprotein D of type 1 herpes simplex virus (HSV–gD) induces antibodies that react with authentic HSV–gD and neutralize HSV. Mice immunized with this recombinant virus are completely protected against challenge with lethal doses of HSV (Paoletti et al., 1984). Similarly, recombinant vaccinia viruses containing cloned hemagglutinin (HA) genes of influenza viruses elicit hemagglutination-inhibiting and influenza-virus-neutralizing antibodies in rabbits and hamsters (Panicali et al., 1983; Smith et al., 1983b). Hamsters vaccinated intradermally with recombinant virus produced antibody levels comparable with those obtained after primary infection with influenza virus, and the hamsters were protected against respiratory tract challenge by homologous virus (Smith et al., 1983b). A vaccinia virus recombinant that carries the gene for gp195 of porcine TGE virus is reported to stimulate neutralizing antibodies to TGE virus (Hu, et al., 1985).

Recombinant virus vaccines are also being developed for parasitic diseases. Cells infected with recombinant vaccinia virus containing the gene coding for the sporozoite antigen of the malaria parasite *Plasmodium knowlesi* have been shown to synthesize 53- and 45-kDa proteins reactive with monoclonal antibody specific for the repeating epitopes of the malarial protein. In addition, intradermal inoculation of rabbits with the infectious recombinant virus produced antibodies that bind to the sporozoites. While these initial results demonstrate the potential for producing a recombinant virus vaccine against malaria, it may be necessary to increase the expression of the sporozoite antigen by the recombinant virus and to add genes for antigens from additional life stages of the parasite (G. L. Smith *et al.*, 1984). Because of their exposure to the host immune system, merozoite surface antigens are considered important in stimulating protective immunity against malaria (Kilejan, 1980).

The aforementioned successes with experimental recombinant vaccinia virus vaccines, as well as the apparent eradication of smallpox from the world with the help of vaccinia virus, presages the possibility of using recombinant vaccinia viruses as *live* vaccines for the prevention of many important diseases of animals and humans. However, some questions regarding the safety of such vaccines remain to be addressed. Thus, although vaccinia virus is still used to vaccinate U.S. military recruits against smallpox, it is known to produce disseminated vaccinitis (and sometimes encephalitis) in about one in every 300,000 vaccines with a mortality of nearly 20% in those so affected (B. Moss, personal communication). Also, it is considered that recombinant vaccinia viruses could have adverse affects in cattle, which are natural hosts for the unmodified vector. Research is in progress to genetically engineer attenuated strains of vaccinia virus that will lessen these risks for animals and humans. However, if the adverse side effects occur principally in recipients having marked immunodeficiencies, this goal will be difficult if not impossible to achieve. Another concern for humans already vaccinated against smallpox is that the recombinant vaccinia virus may not replicate well enough to confer the desired immunity. Thus, it may be necessary to express the guest genes to very high levels or to use one or another of the alternate viral vectors mentioned above. For the latter approach, an SV40-based vector has been developed for the direct and efficient expression of the gene for HBsAg in permissive monkey cells. The HBsAg is assembled into and secreted as 22-nm particles indistinguishable from those formed naturally during human infection with HBV (Liu *et al.*, 1982). In addition, the *HBsAg* gene has been cloned and expressed in mouse cells using bovine papillomavirus as the vector (Denniston *et al.*, 1984).

C. Genetically Engineered Reassortants and Deletion Mutants

The ability of genetic engineering to manipulate genes allows for the removal of pathogenic genes from infectious agents without destroying their ability to propagate and express immunodominant epitopes. It is interesting that the NIH guidelines for biological confinement in rDNA research far exceed this degree of modification. They require that the bacterial hosts used in cloning experiments, generally strains of *E. coli*, be so modified as to be unable to colonize in the intestines of animals and humans.

Gene reassorting and deletion techniques are being applied to both viruses and bacteria. Recombinant HSV-1 × HSV-2 viruses and mutants lacking genes expressed early in infection are reduced in virulence for mice by intracerebral inoculation and induce protective immunity in the mice against challenge with 3000 LD_{50} of virulent virus (Roizman *et al.*, 1982). These and other attenuated herpesvirus mutants are being genetically engineered to minimize the chances of back-mutation to virulence and yet permit multiplication without loss of immunogenicity. Highly attenuated temperature-sensitive mutants of influenza virus or avian strains of the virus (that do not replicate efficiently in mammals) are being used with virulent wild-type virus to co-infect cell cultures. Some reassortants can be isolated that contain the six internal genes from the avirulent parental virus and the two genes for the surface proteins HA and NA of the wild-type virus. Humans immunized with such reassortants from temperature-sensitive mutants exhibit lower rates of infection and shed less virus than vaccinees who received inactivated influenza vaccine (Murphy *et al.*, 1982, 1984). In human trials, an avian–human influenza A reassortant virus had the immunogenicity of wild virus and was not transmissible between individuals. Similar reassortants are under development as vaccines for equine influenza (Brundage-Anguish *et al.*, 1982). The 11 genes of rotaviruses, which cause diarrheal diseases in young animals and humans, can also undergo reassortment in mixed infections. A reassortant with its surface antigen VP_7 gene from a human rotavirus and its other genes from bovine or rhesus rotaviruses has diminished growth characteristics in humans and is being examined for its immunizing potential (Greenberg *et al.*, 1984).

Deletion mutants of several bacteria have been engineered, and their potential usefulness as vaccines is being explored. Included in those studied are deletion mutants of *Salmonella, Shigella,* and *Vibrio cholerae*. A gal-E strain of *Salmonella typhi*, Ty21a (lacking UDPgalactose-4-empimerase activity and highly deficient in two additional enzyme activities as well), was able to proliferate long enough following oral administration to confer immunity against wild-type strains of *Salmonella typhi* (Germainier and Fürer, 1983). Similarly, mutant strains of *Salmonella* defective in aromatic biosynthesis (they require amino- and dihydroxybenzoate, which are not available in host tissues) given in two doses either intramuscularly or orally to calves resulted in the induction of resistance to oral challenge with more than

10^{11} organisms of a virulent UDC strain of *S. typhi* (B. P. Smith *et al.*, 1984).

A hybrid strain of *Salmonella typhi/Shigella sonnei* appears to have potential as a vaccine against both typhoid and dysentery. A plasmid encoding genes for *Shigella sonnei* transferred by conjugation to the Ty21a-attenuated strain of *Salmonella typhi* produces a hybrid bacterium which elicits antibodies in animals to antigens of both organisms (Tramont *et al.*, 1984).

Vibrio cholerae 01, subspecies *El Tor* has been manipulated by genetic techniques (Kaper *et al.*, 1984). After genes encoding the A and B subunits of the organism's toxin are deleted, the gene coding for the immunogenic B subunit is reintroduced by transformation with a plasmid. Nine of ten human volunteers vaccinated with this deletion mutant resisted oral challenge with one million virulent *El Tor Inaba* organisms, whereas seven of eight unvaccinated control volunteers contracted severe cases of cholera. The investigators suggest that "this is the first vaccine [presumably against cholera] to confer a degree of immunity equivalent to that provided by previous infection with the natural bacterium." However, the vaccine apparently needs further attenuation owing to residual, varying, mild diarrheas. While trials are underway to minimize this problem by reducing the vaccine dose to 10^3–10^4 organisms, it may be necessary to engineer self-destruction into the organism after a predetermined number of multiplications.

D. Antiidiotype Antibody Vaccines

However incredulous it may seem, antiidiotype antibodies have the potential to act as vaccines for animals and humans against infectious diseases. Animals modulate their response to a foreign antigen by the production of a cascade of idiotype, antiidiotype, antiantiidiotype, and higher antiidiotype antibodies. The antiparatope antibody is of particular importance. The paratope, which is the binding site in the crevice of the Fab of the antibody molecule, is the complement of a specific epitope on an antigen. Being foreign to the animal, the paratope raises antiparatope antibody, which has sites that are in the image of the epitope on the original inciting antigen. As now generally used, the terms antiidiotype and antiparatope appear to be synonymous. The advent of monoclonal antibody and rDNA technologies have made the development of antiidiotype antibody vaccines a realistic goal. Thus, antiidiotype antibodies can now be produced in quantity in hybridomas or by cloning and expression of DNA transcribed from antiidiotype antibody specific mRNA. Reports are beginning to appear on the development of antiidiotype antibody vaccines. For example, the infection of mice with antiidiotype antibody to hepatitis B surface antigen (HBsAg) primes an anamnestic-like response to subsequent injection with HBsAg (Kennedy et al., 1983). Moreover, the antibody induced by the antiidiotype antibody recognizes a group-specific epitope of HBsAg, indicating that antiidiotypes may be useful as vaccines or as primers for vaccines (Kennedy et al., 1984). Antiidiotype antibodies have been prepared against five monoclonal antibodies to rabies virus glycoprotein G. Two of the five antiidiotype antibodies injected into mice elicited specific virus-neutralizing antibody responses (Reagan et al., 1983). African trypanosomiasis in mice is a disease for which antiidiotype antibodies are reported to evoke a protective immunity (Sacks and Sher, 1983). These studies indicate that antiidiotype antibody research may give rise to useful vaccines.

VI. Conclusions

It is clear from this article and many other sources that a number of innovative and interconnected procedures are being developed for the production of a new generation of vaccines against human and animal diseases. The rapid advances being made are a result in large part from long ongoing investigations of infectious agents, particularly of viruses, at the molecular level coupled with the more recent introduction of rDNA and monoclonal antibody technologies. A thread linking all of the procedures is the use of purified or *in situ* immunodominant epitopes (or images thereof) free of constituents and genes that contribute to pathogenicity. All five of the general procedures described in this article should provide practical vaccines, some of which can be expected to help control heretofore intractable diseases, including cancer. These vaccines will have to be cost effective to satisfy users and safe and effective to gain the approval of regulatory agencies like the FDA and USDA. However, considerable developmental work needs to be done on the new vaccines, not only on immunogenic aspects, but also on perfecting adjuvants and carriers that will be acceptable to manufacturers, users, and regulators. Once the remaining obstacles are overcome, a large variety of vaccines should become available for use in humans and animals.

Acknowledgment

The author wishes to acknowledge the contribution to this review of Mr. Stephen E. Perlman, the librarian at the Plum Island Animal Disease Center, whose expertise in computer searches of scientific literature databases assisted greatly in the preparation of this chapter. In fact, the literature is so voluminous that many relevant reports could not be cited simply because of space limitations.

REFERENCES

Anderer, F. A. (1963). *Biochim. Biophys. Acta* **71,** 246 - 248.
Anfinsen, C. B., and Scheraga, H. A. (1975). *In* "Advances in Protein Chemistry" (C. B. Anfinsen, J. T. Edsall, and F. M. Richards, eds.), pp. 205–300. Academic Press, New York.
Appleyard, G., and Andrews, C. (1974). *J. Gen. Virol.* **23,** 197–200.
Arnon, R., Maron, E., Sela, M., and Anfinsen, C. B. (1971). *Proc. Natl. Acad. Sci. U.S.A.* **68,** 1450–1455.
Atassi, M. Z. (1980). *Mol. Cell. Biochem.* **32,** 21–44.
Atassi, M. Z., and Webster, R. G. (1983). *Proc. Natl. Acad. Sci. U.S.A.* **80,** 840–844.
Audibert, F., Jolivet, M., Chedid, L., Arnon, R., and Sela, M. (1982). *Proc. Natl. Acad. Sci. U.S.A.* **79,** 5042–5046.
Bachrach, H. L. (1977). *In* "Beltsville Symposium in Agricultural Research, I. Virology in Agriculture" (J. A. Romberger, ed.), pp. 3–32. Allenheld Osmun, Montclair, New Jersey.
Bachrach, H. L. (1978). *Adv. Virus Res.* **22,** 163–186.
Bachrach, H. L. (1982). *J. Am. Vet. Med. Assoc.* **181,** 992–999.
Bachrach, H. L., and Hess, W. R. (1973). *Biochem. Biophys. Res. Commun.* **55,** 141–149.
Bachrach, H. L., Swaney, J. B., and Vande Wande, G. F. (1973). *Virology* **52,** 520–528.
Bachrach, H. L., Moore, D. M., McKercher, P. D., and Polatnick, J. (1975). *J. Immunol.* **115,** 1636–1641.
Bachrach, H. L., Moore, D. M., McKercher, P. D., and Polatnick, J. (1978). *In* "Perspectives in Virology X" (M. Pollard, ed.), pp. 147–159. Raven, New York.
Bachrach, H. L., Morgan, D. O., and Moore, D. M., (1979). *Intervirology* **12,** 65–72.
Bachrach, H. L., Morgan, D. O., McKercher, P. D., Moore, D. M. and Robertson, B.H. (1982). *Vet. Microbiol.* **7,** 85–96.
Balachandran, N., Seth, P., and Mohapatra, L. N. (1980) *Infect. Immun.* **29,** 846–852.
Barré-Sinoussi, F., Chermann, J. C., Rey, F., Nugeyre, M. T. Chamaret, S., Gruest, J., Dauguet, C., Axler-Blin, C., Vézinet-Brun, F., Rouzioux, C., Rozenbaum, W., and Montagnier, L. (1983). *Science* **220,** 868–871.
Bastardo, J. W., McKimm-Breschkin, J. L., Sonza, S., Mercer, L. D., and Holmes, I. H. (1981). *Infect. Immun.* **34,** 641–647.
Baxby, D. (1982). *J. Gen. Virol.* **58,** 251–262.
Beatrice, S. T., Katze, M. G., Zajac, B. A., and Crowell, R. L. (1980). *Virology* **104,** 426–438.
Bellini, W. J., McFarlin, D. E., Silver, G. D., Mingioli, E. S., and McFarland, H. F. (1981). *Infect. Immun.* **32,** 1051–1057.
Bittle, J. L., Houghten, R. A., Alexander, H., Shinnick, T. M., Sutcliffe, J. G., Lerner, R. A., Rowlands, D. J., and Brown, F.(1982) *Nature (London)* **298,** 30–33.
Blondel, B., Crainic, R., and Horodinceanu, F. (1982). *C. R. Acad. Sci. Paris* **294,** 91–94.
Brundage-Anguish, L. J., Holmes, D. F., Hosier, N. T., Murphy, B. R., Massicott, J. G., Appleyard, G., and Coggins, L. (1982). *Am. J. Vet. Res.* **43,** 869–874.
Cappel, R., and Decuyper, F. (1976). *Arch. Virol.* **50,** 207–213.
Carlson, J., Maxwell, I., Maxwell, F., McNab, A., Rushlow, K., Mildbrand, M., Teramoto, Y., and Winston, S. (1984). *In* "Modern Approaches to Vaccines" (R. Chanock and R. Lerner, eds.), pp. 195–201. Cold Spring Harbor Lab., Cold Spring Harbor, New York.

Casas, R. (1981). Reports of PAHO Foot-and-Mouth Disease Center, Director Informations, 1980; 1st-half 1981; and Situation in Uruguay, 1979. Rio de Janeiro.
Chatterjee, N. K., Polatnick, J., and Bachrach, H. L. (1976). *J. Gen. Virol.* **32**, 383–394.
Chow, M., and Baltimore, D. (1982). *Proc. Natl. Acad. Sci. U.S.A.* **79**, 7518–7521.
Cohen, G. H., Dietzschold, B., Ponce de Leon, M., Long, D., Golub, E., Varrichio, A., Pereira, L., and Eisenberg, R. J. (1984). *J. Virol.* **49**, 102–108.
Compans, R. W., and Bishop, D. H. L., eds. (1983). *In* "Double-Stranded RNA Viruses." Elsevier, Amsterdam.
Cox, J. H., Dietzschold, B., Weiland, F., and Schneider, L. G. (1980). *Infect. Immun.* **30**, 572–577.
Dalsgaard, K., and Overby, E. (1976). *Acta Vet. Scand.* **17**, 465–474.
Davis, A. R., Nayak, D. P., Ueda, M., Hiti, A. L., Dowbenko, D., and Kleid, D. G. (1981). *Proc. Natl. Acad. Sci. U.S.A.* **78**, 5376–5380.
DeGraef, F. K., Krenn, B. E., and Klassen, P. (1984). *Infect Immun.* **43**, 508–514.
Denniston, K. J., Yoneyama, T., Hoyer, B., and Gerin, J. (1984). *Gene,* **32**, 357–368.
Dix, R. D., Pereira, L., and Baringer, J. R. (1981). *Infect Immun.* **34**, 192–199.
Dreesman, G. R., Hollinger, F. B., Sanchez, Y., Oefinger, P., and Melnick, J. L. (1981). *Infect. Immun.* **32**, 62–67.
Dreesman, G. R., Sanchez, Y., Ionescu-Matiu, I., Sparrow, J. T., Six, H. R., Peterson, D. L., Hollinger, F. B., and Molnick, J. L. (1982). *Nature (London)* **295**, 158–160.
Edman, J. C., Hallewell, R. A., Valenzuela, P., Goodman, H. M., and Rutter, W. J. (1981). *Nature (London)* **291**, 503–506.
Ellis, J., Ozaki, L. S., Gwadz, R. W., Cochrane, A. H., Nussenzweig, V., Nussenzweig, R. S., and Godson, G. N. (1983). *Nature (London)* **302**, 536–538.
Emini, E. A., Jameson, B. A., and Wimmer, E. (1983). *Nature (London)* **304**, 699–703.
Emtage, J. S., Tacon, W. C. A., Catlin, G.H., Jenkins, B., Perter, A. G., and Corey, N. H. (1980). *Nature (London)* **283**, 171–174.
FAO (1981). European Commission Report for the Control of Foot-and-Mouth Disease, 24th Session, FAO; and Outbreak, Isle of Wight, 1981.
Flores, J., Sereno, M., Kalica, A., Keith, J., Kapikian, A., and Chanock, R. (1984). *In* "Modern Approaches to Vaccines" (R. Chanock and R. Lerner, eds.), pp. 159–164. Cold Spring Harbor Lab., Cold Spring Harbor, New York.
Fox, G. M., Langley, D., and Hu, S. (1984). *In* "Modern Approaches to Vaccines" (R. Chanock and R. Lerner, eds.), p. 447. Cold Spring Harbor Lab., Cold Spring Harbor, New York.
Friedricks, W. H., and Grose, C. (1984). *J. Virol.* **49**, 992–996.
Gallo, R. C., Salahuddin, S. Z., Popovic, M., Shearer, G. M., Kaplan, M., Haynes, B. F., Palker, T. J., Redfield, R., Oleske, J., Safai, B., White, G., Foster, P., and Markham, P. D. (1984). *Science* **224**, 500–502.
Genet. Eng. News (1983). **3**, no. 3, p. 41.
Gentsch, J. R., Rozhon, E. J., Klimas, R. A., El Said, L. M., Shope, R. E., and Bishop, D. H. L. (1980). *Virology* **102**, 190–204.
Germainier, R., and Fürer, E. (1983). *Dev. Biol. Standard.* **53**, 3–7.
Gething, M. J., and Sambrook, J. (1981). *Nature (London)* **293**, 620–625.
Gething, M. J., and Sambrook, J. (1982). *Nature (London)* **300**, 598–603.
Ginsberg, H. S. (1975). *In* "Viral Immunology and Immunopathology" (A. L. Notkins, ed.), pp. 317–326. Academic Press, New York.
Gough, P. M., Ellis, C. H., Frank, C. J., and Johnson, C. J. (1983). *Antiviral Res.* **3**, 211–221.
Green, N., Alexander, H., Olson, A., Alexander, S., Shinnick, T. M., Sutcliffe, J. G., and Lerner, R. A. (1982). *Cell* **28**, 477–487.

Greenberg, H., Midthun, K., Wyatt, R., Flores, J., Hoshino, Y., Chanock, R., and Kapikian, A. (1984). *In* "Modern Approaches to Vaccines" (R. Chanock and R. Lerner, eds.), pp. 319–327. Cold Spring Harbor Lab., Cold Spring Harbor, New York.
Gupta, K. C., Morgan, E. M., Kitchingman, G., and Kingsbury, D. W. (1983). *J. Gen. Virol.* **64,** 1679–1688.
Gupta, P., Kashmiri, S. V. S., and Ferrer, J. F. (1984). *J. Virol.* **50,** 267–270.
Halstead, S. B. (1982). *Prog. Allergy* **31,** 301–364.
Heiland, I., and Gething, M. J. (1981). *Nature (London)* **292,** 851–852.
Heinz, F. X., Tuma, W., and Kunz, C. (1981). *Infect. Immun.* **33,** 250–277.
Hilleman, M. R., Buynak, E. B., McAleer, W. J., McLean, A. A., Provost, P. J., and Tytell, A. A. (1981). *In* "Perspectives in Virology XI" (M. Pollard, ed.), pp. 219–247. Liss, New York.
Hofshneider, P. H., Burgelt, E., Kauzmann, M., Mussgay, M., Franze, R., Ahl, R., Bohm, H., Strohmaier, K., Küpper, H., and Otto, B. (1981). *Munich Symp. Microbiol. Prod. Viral Dis.* pp. 105–113.
Holmgren, J., and Svennerholm, A-M. (1982) *Karger Gaz.* **44–45,** 9–11.
Hopp, T. P., and Woods, K. R. (1981). *Proc. Natl. Acad. Sci. U.S.A.* **78,** 3824–3828.
Hosaka, Y. (1980). *Infect. Immun.* **30,** 212–218.
Hu, S., Bruszewski, J., Boone, T., and Souza, L. (1984). *In* "Modern Approaches to Vaccines" (R. Chanock and R. Lerner, eds.), pp. 219–223. Cold Spring Harbor Lab., Cold Spring Harbor, New York.
Hu, S., Bruszewski, J., Smalling, R., and Browne, J. K. (1985). *Proc. Int. Symp. Immunobiol. Proteins Peptides 3rd,* pp. 63–82.
Huismans, H., and Erasmus, B. J. (1981). *Onderstepoort J. Vet. Res.* **48,** 51–58.
Huismans, H., van der Walt, N. T., Cloete, M., and Erasmus, B. J. (1983). *In* "Double-Stranded RNA Viruses" (R. W. Compans and D. H. L. Bishop, eds.), pp. 165–172. Elsevier, Amsterdam.
Ihle, J. N., Lee, J. C., Collins, J. J., Fischinger, P. J., Pazmino, N. H., Moenning, V., Schafer, W., Hamia, M. G., Jr., and Bolognesi, D. P. (1976). *Virology* **75,** 88–101.
ILRAD Reports (1983). Issue No. 2, pp. 1–2.
Issacson, R. E. (1981). *Proc. Int. Symp. Neonatal Diarrhea* **3,** 213–236.
Jennings, R., Smith, T. L., Spencer, R. C., Mellersh, A. M., Edey, D., Fenton, P., and Potter, C. W. (1984). *Vaccine* **1,** 75–80.
Joklik, W. K. (1981). *Microbiol. Rev.* **45,** 483–501.
Kaaden, O. R., and Dietzschold, B. (1974). *J. Gen. Virol.* **25,** 1–10.
Kaaden, O. R., Adam, K. H., and Strohmaier, K. (1977). *J. Gen. Virol.* **34,** 397–400.
Kaper, J. B., Lockman, H., Baldini, M. M., and Levine, M. M. (1984). *Nature (London)* **308,** 655–658.
Kashmiri, S. V. S., Mehdi, R., and Ferrer, J. F. (1984). *J. Virol.* **49,** 583–587.
Kennedy, R. C., Adler-Storthz, K., Henkel, R. D., Sanchez, Y., Melnick, J. L., and Dreesman, G. R. (1983). *Science* **221,** 853–855.
Kennedy, R. C., Melnick, J. L., and Dreesman, G. R. (1984). *Science* **223,** 930–931.
Kew, O. M., Nottay, B. K., Hatch, M. H., Nakano, J. H., and Obijeski, J. F. (1981). *J. Gen. Virol.* **56,** 337–347.
Kilejan, A. (1980). *Am. J. Trop. Med. Hyg.* **29**(Suppl.), 1125–1128.
Killen, H. M., and Dimmock, N. J. (1982). *J. Gen. Virol.* **62,** 297–311.
Kleid, D. G., Yansura, D., Small, B., Dowbenko, D., Moore, D. M., Grubman, M. J., McKercher, P. D., Morgan, D. O., Robertson, B. H., and Bachrach, H. L. (1981). *Science* **214,** 1125–1129.
Klenk, H.-D., Rott, R., Orlich, M., and Blödorn, J. (1975). *Virology* **68,** 426–439.

Langbeheim, H., Arnon, R., and Sela, M. (1976). *Proc. Natl. Acad. Sci. U.S.A.* **73,** 4636–4670.
Lasky, L. A., and Dowbenko, D. (1984). *DNA* **3,** 23–29.
Laub, O., Rall, L. B., Truett, M., Shaul, Y., Standring, D. N., Valenzuela, P., and Rutter, W. J. (1983). *J. Virol.* **48,** 271–280.
Lerner, R. A., Green, N., Alexander, H., Liu, F-T., Sutcliffe, J. G., and Shinnick, T. M. (1981). *Proc. Natl. Acad. Sci. U.S.A.* **78,** 3403–3407.
Letchworth, G. J., III, and Appleton, J. A. (1983). *Infect. Immun.* **39,** 208–212.
Lewis, M. G., Mathes, L. E., and Olsen, R. G. (1981). *Infect. Immun.* **34,** 888–894.
Liu, C-C., Yansura, D., and Levinson, A. D. (1982). *DNA* **1,** 213–221.
Lupton, H. W., and Reed, D. E. (1980). *Am. J. Vet. Res.* **41,** 383–390.
McAleer, W. J., Markus, H. Z., Wampler, D. E., Buynak, E. B., Miller, W. J., Weibel, R. E., McLean, A. A., and Hilleman, M. R. (1984). *Proc. Soc. Exp. Biol. Med.* **175,** 314–319.
Mackett, M., Smith, G. L., and Moss, B. (1982). *Proc. Natl. Acad. Sci. U.S.A.* **79,** 7415–7419.
Mackett, M., Smith, G. L., and Moss, B. (1984). *J. Virol.* **49,** 857–864.
Marx, J. L. (1982). *Science* **217,** 1021–1022.
Matheka, H-D., and Bachrach, H. L. (1975). *J. Virol.* **16,** 1248–1253.
Maxam, A. M., and Gilbert, W. (1977). *Proc. Natl. Acad. Sci. U.S.A.* **74,** 560–564.
Mayer, L. W., Aasted, B., Garon, C. F., and Bloom, M. E. (1983). *J. Virol.* **48,** 573–579.
Mayfield, J. E., Good, P. J., VanOort, H. J., Campbell, A. R., and Reed, D. E. (1983). *J. Virol.* **47,** 259–264.
Merz, D. C., Scheid, A., and Choppin, P. W. (1980). *J. Exp. Med.* **151,** 275–283.
Meyer, T. F. (1982). *Cell* **30,** 45–52.
Morein, B., Sundquist, B., and Hoglund, S. (1982). *Int. Conf. Comp. Virol., 4th* Abstr. S3-4, p. 87.
Morein, B., Sharp, M., Sundquist, B., and Simons, K. (1983). *J. Gen. Virol.* **64,** 1557–1569.
Morse, G. (1984). *Sci. News* **125,** 354.
Müller, G. M., Shapira, M., and Arnon, R. (1982). *Proc. Natl. Acad. Sci. U.S.A.* **79,** 569–573.
Murphy, B., Buckler-White, A., Tian, S.-F., Chanock, R., Clements, M., Maasab, H. F., and London W. (1984). *In* "Modern Approaches to Vaccines" (R. Chanock and R. Lerner, eds.), pp. 329–337. Cold Spring Harbor Lab., Cold Spring Harbor, New York.
Murphy, B. R., Sly, D. L., Tierney, E. L., Hosier, N. T., Massicot, J. D., London, W. T., Chanock, R. M., Webster, R. G., and Hinshaw, V. S. (1982). *Science* **218,** 1330–1332.
Nagai, Y., and Klenk, H. D. (1977). *Virology* **77,** 125–134.
Neurath, A. R., Kent, S. B. H., and Strick, N. (1984). *Science* **224,** 392–395.
Palmiter, R. D., Norstedt, G., Gelinas, R. E., Hammer, R. E., and Brinster, R. L. (1983). *Science* **222,** 809–814.
Panicali, D., Davis, S. W., Weinberg, R. L., and Paoletti, E. (1983). *Proc. Natl. Acad. Sci. U.S.A.* **80,** 5364–5368.
Paoletti, E., Lipinskas, B. R., Samsonoff, C., Mercer, S., and Panicali, D. (1984). *Proc. Natl. Acad. Sci. U.S.A.* **81,** 193–197.
Pilacinski, W. P., Glassman, D. L., Krzyzek, R. A., Sadowski, P. L., and Robbins, A. K. (1984). *Biotechnology* **2,** 356–360.
Platt, K. B. (1982). *Vet. Microbiol.* **7,** 515–534.
Qualtiere, L. F., Chase, R., and Pearson, G. R. (1982). *J. Immunol.* **129,** 814–818.
Ramsingh, A., and Leung, W. C. (1982). *Int. Conf. Comp. Virol., 4th* Abstr. S4-11, p. 105.

Reagan, K. J., Wunner, W. H., Wiktor, T. J., and Koprowski, H. (1983). *J. Virol.* **48,** 660–666.
Robbins, A. K., Enquist, L. W., and Watson, R. J. (1984a). *Abstr. Int. Herpesvirus Workshop, 9th,* Seattle.
Robbins, A. K., Weis, J. H., Enquist, L. W., and Watson, R. J. (1948b). *J. Mol. Appl. Genet.,* **2,** 485–496.
Roizman, B., Warren, J., Thuning, C. A., Fanshaw, M. S., Norrild, B., and Meignier, B. (1982). *Dev. Biol. Standard.* **52,** 287–304.
Rose, J. K., and Bergmann, J. E. (1982). *Cell* **30,** 753–762.
Rose, J. K., and Shafferman, A. (1981). *Proc. Natl. Acad. Sci. U.S.A.* **78,** 6670–6674.
Rozenblatt, S., Gesang, C., Lavie, V., and Neuman, F. S. (1982). *J. Virol.* **42,** 790–797.
Sacks, D. L., and Sher, A. (1983). *J. Immunol.* **131,** 1511–1515.
Salk, D., and Salk, J. (1984). *Vaccine* **1,** 58–74.
Schmidt, O. W., and Kenney, G. E. (1982). *Infect. Immun.* **35,** 515–522.
Scolnick, E. M., McLean, A. A., West, D. J., McAleer, W. J., Miller, W. J., and Buynak, E. B. (1984). *J. Am. Med. Assoc.* **251,** 2812–2815.
Sela, M., Jacob, C. O., and Arnon, R. (1984). *In* "Modern Approaches to Vaccines" (R. Chanock and R. Lerner, eds.), pp. 87–92. Cold Spring Harbor Lab., Cold Spring Harbor, New York.
Sherman, D. M., Acres, S. D., Sadowski, P. L., Springer, J. A., Bray, B., Raybould, T. J. G., and Muscoplat, C. C. (1983). *Infect. Immun.* **42,** 653–658.
Simons, K., Helenius, A., Morein, B., Balcorova, J., and Sharp, M. (1980). *In* "New Developments with Human and Veterinary Vaccines" (A. Mizraki, I. Hertman, and M. A. Klingberg, eds.), pp. 217–228. Liss, New York.
Simpson, R. W., McGinty, L., Simon, L., Smith, C. A., Godzeski, C. W., and Boyd, R. J. (1984). *Science* **223,** 1425–1428.
Smith, B. P., Reina-Guerra, M., Hoiseth, S. K., Stocker, B. A. D., and Habasha, F. (1984). *Am. J. Vet. Res.* **45,** 59–66.
Smith, G. L., and Moss B. (1983). *Gene* **25,** 21–28.
Smith, G. L., Mackett, M., and Moss, B. (1983a). *Nature (London)* **302,** 490–495.
Smith, G. L., Murphy, B. R., and Moss, B. (1983b). *Proc. Natl. Acad. Sci. U.S.A.* **80,** 7155–7159.
Smith, G.L., Godson, G. N., Nussenzweig, V., Nussenzweig, R. S., Barnwell, J., and Moss, B. (1984). *Science* **224,** 397–399.
Stamm, L. V., and Bassford, P. J., Jr. (1982). *DNA* **1,** 329–333.
Summers, J., and Mason, W. S. (1982). *Cell* **29,** 403–415.
Sutcliffe, J. G., Shinnick, T. M., Green, N., Liu, F.-T., Niman, H. L., and Lerner, R. A. (1980). *Nature (London)* **287,** 801–805.
Szmuness, W., Stevens, C. E., Harley, E. J., Zang, E. A., Alter, H. J., Taylor, P. E., Devera, A., Chen, G. T. S., and Keller, A. (1982). *N. Engl. J. Med.* **307,** 1481–1486.
Tramont, E. C., Chung, R., Berman, S., Keren, D., Kapfer, C., and Formal, S. B. (1984). *J. Infect. Dis.* **149,** 133–136.
Trevis, J., and Bertelsen, A. (1982). *Feedstuffs* **54**(5) 32–37.
Trudel, M., and Payment, P. (1982). *Int. Conf. Comp. Virol.* Abstr. S3–6, p. 88.
USDA (1983). Notes from the Director, No. 148. Beltsville, Maryland.
U.S. Dept. of Health, Education and Welfare (1976). *Morbid. Mortal. Weekly Rep.* **25,** 357–369.
Valenzuela, P., Medina, A., Rutter, W. J., Ammerer, G., and Hall, B. D. (1982). *Nature (London)* **298,** 347–350.

Walter, G., Scheidtmann, K.-H., Carbone, A., Laudano, A. P., and Doolittle, R. F. (1980). *Proc. Natl. Acad. Sci. U.S.A.* **77,** 5197–5200.

Walter Reed Army Inst. Research (1982a). *Rep. Div. Communicable Dis. Immunol.* **3–4,** 1–2.

Walter Reed Army Inst. Research (1982b). *Rep. Div. Biochem.* **3–4,** 4–5.

Watson, R. J., Weis, J. H., Salstrom, J. S., and Enquist, L. W. (1982). *Science* **218,** 381–384.

Wiley, D. C., Wilson, I. A., and Skehel, J. J. (1981). *Nature (London)* **289,** 373–378.

Wilson, T. (1984). *Biotechnology* **2,** 29–39.

Wimmer, E., Jameson, B. A., and Emini, E. A. (1984). *Nature (London)* **308,** 19.

Winter, A. J., Verstreate, D. R., Hall, C. E., Jacobson, R. H., Castleman, W. L., Meredith, M. P., and McLaughlin, C. A. (1983). *Infect. Immun.* **42,** 1159–1167.

Yelverton, E., Norton, S., Obijeski, J. F., and Goeddel, D. V. (1983). *Science* **219,** 614–620.

Yilma, T., Breeze, R. G., Ristow, S., Gorham, J. R., and Leib, S. R. (1985). *Proc. Int. Symp. Immunobiol. Proteins Peptides 3rd,* pp. 101–115.

Atherosclerosis: The Consequence of Infection with a Herpesvirus

CATHERINE G. FABRICANT

Department of Microbiology, New York State College of Veterinary Medicine, Cornell University, Ithaca, New York

I.   Introduction 39
II. Initial Experiments 42
     A. Experimental Design 42
     B. Serum Cholesterol Levels 42
     C. Marek's Disease: Index of MDV Infection 43
     D. Arterial Lesions 45
     E. MDV-Specific Antigens in Arteries 48
     F. Conclusions 51
III. Pathogenetic Mechanisms of MDV-Induced Atherosclerosis 52
     A. Pathogenesis Experiments 52
     B. Alteration of Arterial SMC Lipid Metabolism: A Major Mechanism in MDV Atherogenesis 56
     C. Conclusions 58
IV. Evidence of MDV Infection in Cells Comprising Arterial Lesions 59
V.   Immunization Protects against MDV-Induced Atherosclerosis 60
     A. Experimental Plan 60
     B. Results 60
     C. Conclusions 61
VI. Preliminary Evidence for a Herpesvirus Role in Human Atherosclerosis . 62
VII. Summary and Conclusions 63
     References 65

I. Introduction

Human atherosclerosis is distinguished by proliferation of smooth muscle cells (SMCs) with accumulations of cholesterol and cholesteryl esters forming plaques in arterial walls (Ross and Glomset, 1976; Pietilä and Nikkari, 1983). The flow of blood is restricted by plaques narrowing the lumen of arteries. Segments of the arterial tree which are frequently involved include the aorta as well as the coronary, cerebral, femoral, and iliac arteries (Ross and Glomset, 1973). Depending upon the location and extent of the arterial lesions, atherosclerosis may lead to heart attacks, stroke, or kidney failure (Zanchetti, 1984).

Our interest in atherosclerosis was stimulated by observations made in the course of studies on urinary obstruction in cats. In these studies we isolated a previously undescribed cell-associated feline herpesvirus (Fabricant and Gillespie, 1974). Various cell cultures infected with this virus were found to have appreciable intracellular and extracellular lipid and crystalline accumulations (Fabricant et al., 1973). Cholesterol crystals were identified as one of the crystalline accretions (Fabricant et al., 1973). These serendipitous observations led us to hypothesize a herpesvirus role in the pathogenesis of atherosclerosis (Fabricant et al., 1973; Fabricant, 1975). An almost heretical resistance to the unquestioned acceptance of current dogma urged an exploration of this hypothesis. Preliminary studies in Denmark of cell cultures initiated from human atherosclerotic specimens suggested that further studies were warranted. These cultures appeared to have cellular changes which resembled those induced by the feline herpesvirus in infected cell cultures (C. G. Fabricant, 1973, unpublished observations). In addition, a literature search supported the merit of investigating our hypothesis.

Although high risk factors in atherosclerosis have been recognized for many years, their relationship to the origin and development of the human arterial disease remains unclarified (Gordon et al., 1974; Castelli, 1984). Gordon et al. reported that serum cholesterol levels, blood pressure, smoking, obesity, and diabetes could not account for the increased incidence of atherosclerosis in Framingham, Massachusetts, compared with the incidences in Honolulu and Puerto Rico. These investigators suggested that other factors should be sought to explain these differences.

Other investigators have suggested that injury to the arterial wall initiates atherosclerotic lesions and that high serum cholesterol levels are secondary to such injury (Minick and Murphy, 1973; Harker et al., 1974; Ross and Harker, 1976). They reported that elevated serum cholesterol levels resulting from dietary intake appeared to accelerate or complicate preexisting arterial lesions. Various initiators of arterial injury have been cited. These include physical (Taylor, 1955), chemical (Walters, 1955), and immunologic factors (Minick and Murphy, 1973), as well as infections (Burch et al., 1973; Benditt and Benditt, 1973).

Prior to our studies only a few reports were made considering the role of viruses in human atherosclerosis. In 1973 Burch *et al.* suggested that viral infections may be associated with early atherosclerotic changes. Benditt and Benditt (also in 1973) reported that atheromatous plaques were monoclonal and might be due to the effects of chemical or viral mutagens.

Relative to our hypothesis, earlier reports on human cytomegalovirus (CMV) infections were of particular interest. However, these reports were not directly associated with atherosclerosis research. Intranuclear inclusions (indicating site of virus replication) were found in vascular endothelial cells of individuals with these herpesvirus infections (Haymaker *et al.*, 1954; Smith, 1959; Weller and Handshaw, 1962; Ward *et al.*, 1965). Since endothelial cells compose the single layer of cells lining the lumen of blood vessels, these reports were evidence that a human herpesvirus was capable of causing injury to cells of arterial walls. One report was of special interest: it described advanced atherosclerosis in the pulmonary arteries of a 4-year-old child dead of congenital CMV infection (McCracken *et al.*, 1967). In addition, herpesvirus infections in other animal species have been reported to cause vascular disease, for example, infections in cattle (Liggitt *et al.*, 1978) and horses (Crawford and Henson, 1973; McGuire *et al.*, 1974). Reports of human and animal infections with herpesviruses involving blood vessels strengthened our hypothesis.

The Paterson and Cottral report (1950) not only supported our hypothesis but suggested a method for testing it. They investigated the relationship of neurolymphomatosis (NL) to atherosclerosis in chickens. At that time, the etiologic agent of NL was unknown. Furthermore, no chicken flock was entirely free of this neoplastic disease (i.e., Marek's disease). However, these investigators inoculated chickens having a low incidence of NL with tracheal washings from chickens with a high NL incidence. They reported that the chickens inoculated with the tracheal washings had a significant increase in atherosclerosis compared to the uninoculated controls. Because NL was considered a neoplastic disease peculiar to chickens, Paterson concluded that their findings were not relevant to human atherosclerosis.

However, in 1967 Churchill and Biggs reported that the etiologic agent of Marek's disease (i.e., NL) was a herpesvirus. This finding raised the question, Did Marek's disease herpesvirus (MDV) cause atherosclerosis as well as the neoplastic lesions in chickens? If so, Paterson's conclusion merited reconsideration because humans are extensively infected with as many as five human herpesviruses (Nahmias *et al.*, 1981).

The Paterson–Cottral and Churchill–Biggs reports suggested the method to test our hypothesis of a herpesvirus role in atherogenesis. Other advances in avian medicine facilitated testing this hypothesis. Not only was a herpesvirus identified as the cause of NL, but cloned MDV strains of known virulence were available. Further, specific pathogen-free (SPF) chickens of known genetic susceptibility to infection with MDV had been bred and were available to us. These SPF chickens, maintained in isolation, were free of all known avian microbial pathogens and were regularly monitored for adventitious infections.

Our hypothesis was tested as described in this article.

II. Initial Experiments

A. Experimental Design

Our initial experiment was based on Paterson's (1950) experimental design. However, we used defined reagents which were unavailable to him. The experiment included four groups of cockerels from the SPF White Leghorn P-line of chickens maintained by the Department of Avian and Aquatic Animal Medicine at the New York State College of Veterinary Medicine, Cornell University (Fabricant et al., 1977, 1978; Minick et al., 1979). This genetically selected line of chickens is moderately susceptible to infection with MDV. Chickens in two of the groups were infected with 100 PFU of the cell-free, clone-purified, low-virulence CU-2 strain of MDV, which induces neural and gonadal tumors in susceptible chickens. The two infected groups (I and II) were housed in separate isolation units from the two uninfected groups (III and IV) of chickens (Fig. 1).

For the first 15 weeks, the four groups were fed a commercial diet containing 0.025% (w/w) cholesterol. Beginning with the sixteenth week, one infected and one uninfected group were fed a diet supplemented with 2% (w/w) cholesterol. The other infected group and uninfected group remained on the unsupplemented cholesterol-poor diet. At the end of 30 weeks the surviving chickens in the four groups were euthanized and examined for gross Marek's disease lesions as well as for gross and microscopic arterial lesions (Fig. 2).

B. Serum Cholesterol Levels

Serum cholesterol concentrations were determined on blood serums of all birds in the four-chicken groups prior to and after feeding cholesterol-supplemented diets (Fabricant et al., 1977, 1978; Minick et al.,

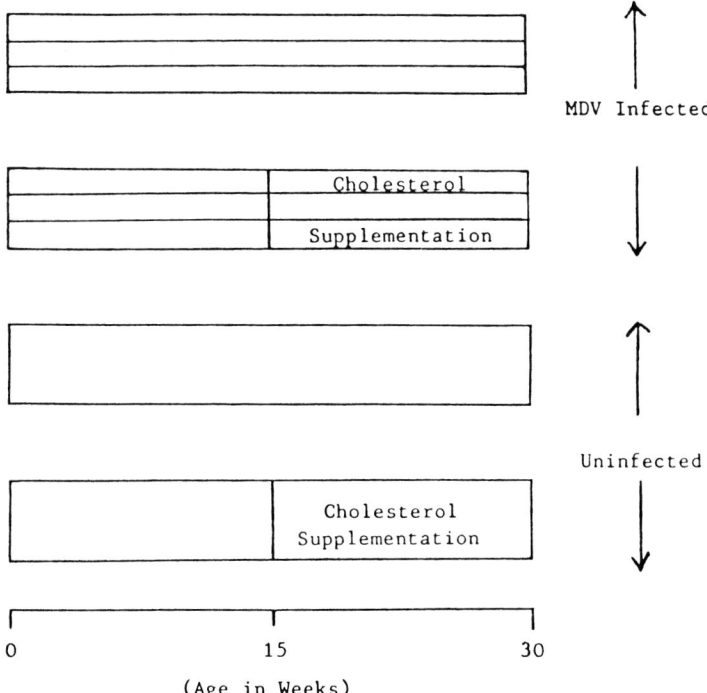

FIG. 1. Schematic design of experiments: SPF P-line cockerels inoculated at 2 days of age with a CU-2 strain of MDV. Unless otherwise specified, the chickens were fed a diet low in cholesterol.

1979). Before feeding the supplemented diets, birds in the four groups had serum cholesterol levels within the normal range (65–159 mg/100 ml; Table I). As expected, cholesterol supplementation elevated the serum cholesterol levels of the birds in both the MDV-infected and uninfected groups (Table I). Serum cholesterol levels of birds in the MDV-infected and uninfected groups maintained on the cholesterol-poor diet remained within the normal range (Table I). The almost identical serum cholesterol levels found in these two groups were evidence that MDV infection had no apparent effect on serum cholesterol levels.

C. Marek's Disease: Index of MDV Infection

Grossly visible neural and/or gonadal Marek's disease lesions as well as agar gel precipitin tests for MDV antibody were used as evidence of MDV infection (Fabricant *et al.*, 1977, 1978; Minick *et al.*,

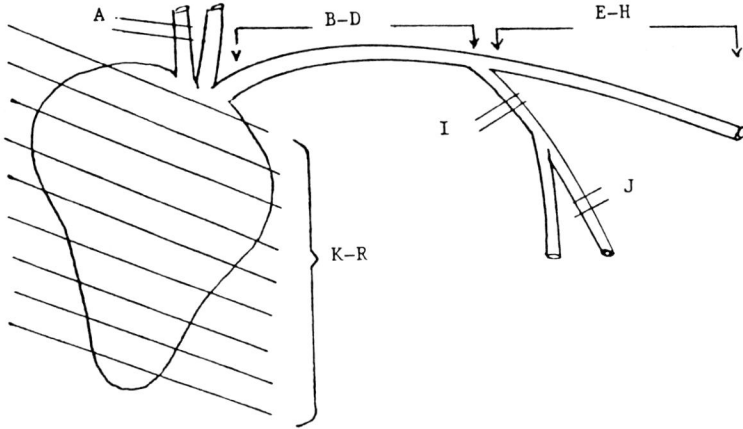

FIG. 2. Diagram of tissue specimens collected: A, brachiocephalic artery; B–D, proximal descending aorta; E–H, distal descending aorta; I, celiac artery; J, gastric artery; K–R heart sections.

1979). Serums of all birds in group III (uninfected) and group IV (uninfected with cholesterol supplementation) remained negative for MDV precipitin antibodies throughout the experimental period. However, 80% of MDV-inoculated group I and II birds were found to have developed MDV precipitin antibodies. The failure to detect these antibodies

TABLE I

SERUM CHOLESTEROL CONCENTRATIONS OF MDV-INFECTED AND UNINFECTED CHICKENS BEFORE AND AFTER FEEDING THE CHOLESTEROL SUPPLEMENT DIET

Experimental group	Predietary supplementation (1–15 weeks)	Postdietary supplementation (16–30 weeks)
Group I; MDV	136.9 ± 5.2[a] (N = 30)[b]	136.1 ± 6.1 (N = 28)
Group II: MDV plus cholesterol	133.7 ± 3.5 (N = 29)	460.6 ± 39.3 (N = 23)
Group III: untreated	—	137.0 ± 3.7 (N = 27)
Group IV: cholesterol	146.5 ± 15.4 (N = 11)	425.1 ± 29.9 (N = 23)

[a]Overall mean in mg/100 ml.
[b]N, Number of serum samples tested.

in 20% of the birds in these groups was not unexpected. In other experiments with this genetic line of chickens, the agar gel precipitin tests were shown to detect a similar percentage of MDV-infected chickens. However, 100% infection was demonstrated in P-line chickens in these experiments using more sensitive techniques, such as virus isolation (Calnek, 1972).

Infection with MDV in groups I and II was also demonstrated by a 30% mortality with grossly visible Marek's disease lesions. In addition when euthanized and examined at 7 months, 40.9% of the chickens in group I and 27.8% of the chickens in group II had grossly visible Marek's disease lesions, primarily involving peripheral nerves. However, none of the uninfected birds in groups III and IV had any evidence of Marek's disease lesions at any time during the experimental period (Fabricant *et al.*, 1977, 1978; Minick *et al.*, 1979).

D. ARTERIAL LESIONS

1. *Grossly Visible Lesions*

Grossly visible atherosclerotic lesions were seen only in virus-infected chickens of groups I and II (Fabricant *et al.*, 1977, 1978; Minick *et al.*, 1979). These lesions were found in coronary arteries, aortas, and major arterial branches (Fig. 3, Table II). The marked atherosclerotic change, in some instances, involved entire segments of major arteries and practically occluded the arterial lumens. Other grossly visible arterial lesions were observed as discrete plaques involving 1 to 2 mm of arterial segments. Grossly visible atherosclerotic lesions were not found in any chickens in the uninfected groups, including the hypercholesterolemic chickens of group IV (Table II).

2. *Microscopic Lesions*

Microscopically proliferative and fatty proliferative arterial lesions were frequently found in aortas and in coronary, gastric, mesenteric, and celiac arteries in MDV-infected group I and II birds (Fig. 4B–D; Fabricant *et al.*, 1977, 1978; Minick *et al.*, 1979). Many fatty proliferative arterial lesions, with intimal and medial foam cells, cholesterol clefts, extracellular lipid, and calcium deposits, had a marked resemblance to chronic human artherosclerosis (Figs. 4C and D). The proliferative lesions without fatty deposits resembled human arteriosclerosis. There appeared to be a synergy between virus infection and cholesterol dietary supplementation in this experiment. MDV-infected hypercholesterolemic birds seemed to have more arterial le-

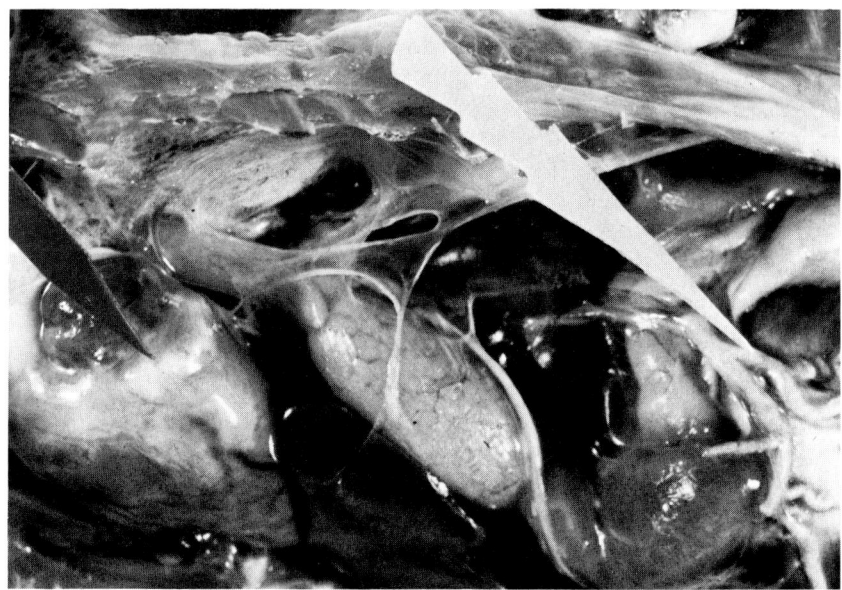

FIG. 3. Heart and abdominal viscera of an MDV-infected normocholesterolemic chicken. A grossly visible atherosclerotic change in coronary arteries is indicated by the black pointer. The white pointer indicates a grossly visible atherosclerotic change in gastric arteries on the gizzard. ×1.4

sions as well as more fatty proliferative arterial lesions. However, appreciable lipid accumulations were demonstrated by histochemical stain in arterial lesions of virus-infected normocholesterolemic birds. These microscopic arterial lesions were not found in corresponding arterial segments of uninfected normocholesterolemic group III birds or uninfected hypercholesterolemic group IV birds. A few microscopic, relatively acellular fatty lesions bearing little resemblance to human atherosclerosis were seen in some arteries, including small intracardial arteries of hypercholesterolemic group IV chickens (Fabricant et al., 1978; Minick et al., 1979).

Miscroscopic arterial lesions were found in the distal descending aortas of all four groups of chickens (Table II; Fabricant et al., 1978; Minick et al., 1979). These lesions have been described in pigeons and chickens (Clarkson et al., 1959, and Dauber, 1944, respectively) and are of unknown origin. The lesions in this segment appeared to be modified both by virus infection and cholesterol supplementation in this experiment (Table II).

TABLE II

NUMBER OF CHICKENS WITH GROSS AND MICROSCOPIC ARTERIAL LESIONS
(EXPERIMENT 1)

Treatment group	Grossly visible lesions		Microscopic lesions		
	Coronary arteries	Gastric and mesenteric arteries	Coronary arteries	Brachiocephalic arteries and proximal aorta	Gastric and mesenteric arteries	Distal aorta
Group I: MDV ($N = 22$)[a]	3	3	11	10	8	18
Group II: MDV plus cholesterol ($N = 19$)	4	4	17	14	16	14
Group III: untreated ($N = 24$)	0	0	1	1	0	6
Group IV: cholesterol ($N = 23$)	0	0	3	1	1	16

[a] N, Number of chickens necropsied at 7 months.

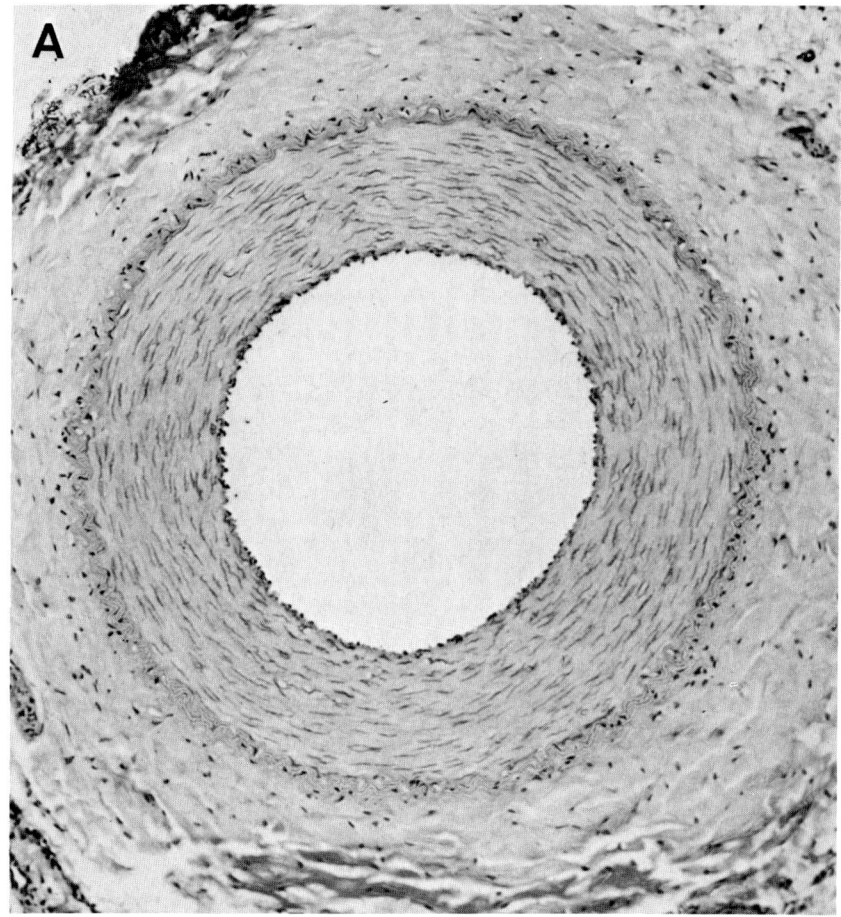

Fig. 4. (A) Normal artery from an uninfected normocholesterolemic chicken, included for comparative purposes. H & E, ×40. (B) Mesenteric artery from an MDV-infected normocholesterolemic chicken: note the intimal and medial proliferation with foam cells in both of these areas. H & E, ×63. (C) Occluded gastric artery from another MDV-infected normocholesterolemic chicken. Atheromatous changes with cholesterol clefts are clearly visible deep in the media. H & E, ×40. (D) Occluded coronary artery from an MDV-infected hypercholesterolemic chicken with atheromatous changes. H & E, ×40.

E. MDV-Specific Antigens in Arteries

Specific viral (MDV) internal antigens (VIAs) were found by immunofluorescence technique in medial layers of arteries in four infected birds. The VIA appeared to be located in a few arterial SMCs of the media (Fabricant et al., 1978; Minick et al., 1979).

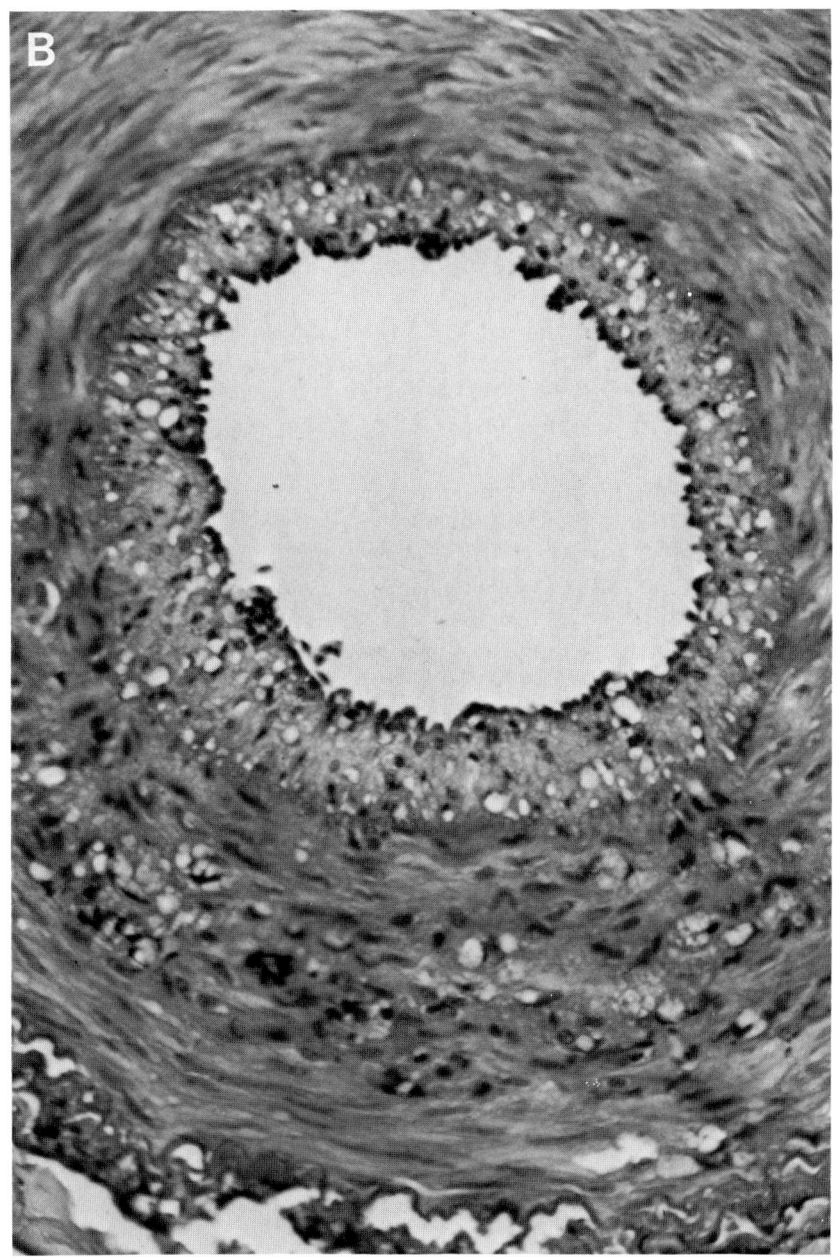

FIG. 4B.

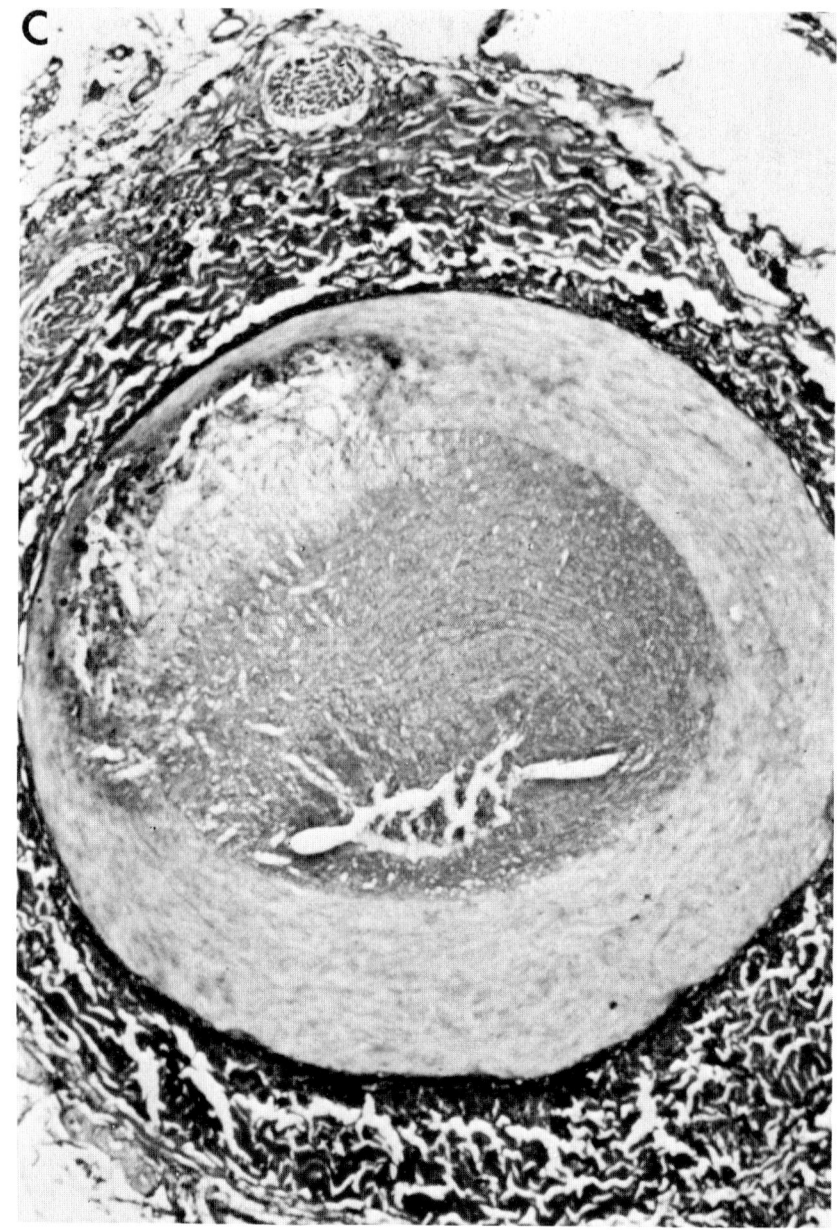

FIG. 4C. See legend on p. 48.

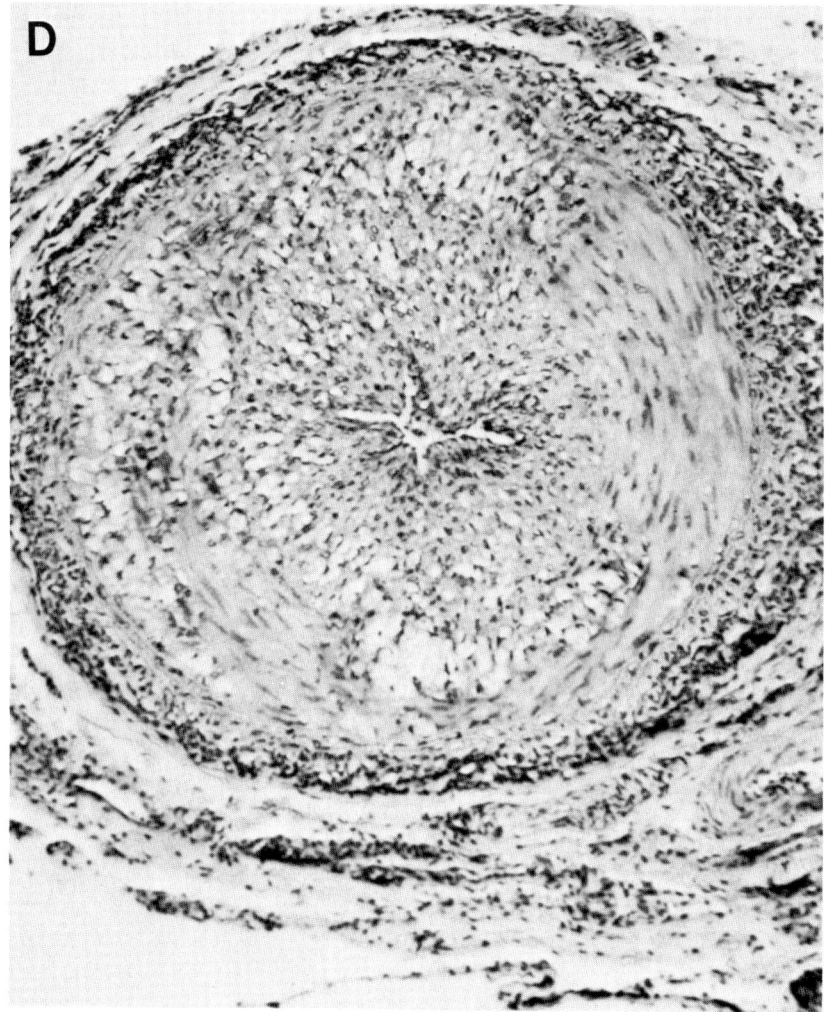

Fig. 4D. See legend on p. 48.

F. Conclusions

The results of our first experiments supported our hypothesis. Only MDV-infected SPF chickens developed atherosclerotic lesions. *These lesions did not develop in uninfected hypercholesterolemic SPF chickens.* It was of particular significance that *the herpesvirus induced atherosclerosis even in normocholesterolemic SPF-infected chickens.* There appeared to be a synergy between virus infection and hypercholesterolemia. This synergy was suggested by an apparent increase in the number of lesions as well as the number of fatty proliferative arterial lesions in MDV-infected hypercholesterolemic chickens. However, an appreciable number of fatty proliferative lesions were found in virus-infected normocholesterolemic chickens. This finding suggesting that the herpersvirus-infection-altered lipid metabolism of arterial cells was consistent with the observations leading to our hypothesis (Fabricant et al., 1973). Added evidence associating MDV infection with the atherosclerotic lesions was provided by specific VIAs found in medial SMCs adjacent to arterial lesions.

Further, the nature and distribution of the atherosclerotic lesions induced by MDV infection in chickens were strikingly like those of chronic human atherosclerosis. The potential significance of these findings to human atherosclerosis was apparent in view of the widespread, persistent human infections with herpesviruses (Nahmias et al., 1981).

III. Pathogenetic Mechanisms of MDV-Induced Atherosclerosis

A. Pathogenesis Experiments

Experiments designed similarly to the initial ones were performed to elucidate the pathogenesis of MDV-induced atherosclerosis (Fig. 1.; Fabricant et al., 1980b). In these experiments chickens from infected as well as uninfected groups were randomly selected and euthanized by cervical dislocation at 5, 10, 15, and 30 days after MDV infection and at monthly intervals thereafter for 7 months. As in the earlier experiments, all groups of chickens were initially fed a diet low in cholesterol. The infected groups were housed in separate isolation facilities from the uninfected groups. After 15 weeks half of the infected groups and half of the uninfected groups were placed on cholesterol-supplemented diets, while the corresponding groups remained on the low-cholesterol diet. Birds were examined both for grossly visible atherosclerotic lesions and Marek's disease lesions at necropsy. Tissues collected for histopathologic examinations included brains, as well as hearts and arterial segments (Fig. 2). In addition, portions of each collected arterial segment were reserved for electron microscopy and for immunofluorescent studies.

1. Gross Marek's Disease and Atherosclerotic Lesions

Gross Marek's disease lesions were not found in any uninfected normocholesterolemic or hypercholesterolemic chickens (Fabricant et al., 1980b). The earliest gross Marek's disease lesions in infected chickens were found beginning at 1 month of age. These lesions continued to be found in infected chickens thereafter during the 7-month experimental period (Table III).

Gross atherosclerotic lesions were seen only in MDV-infected birds, beginning at 3 months (Table III). These arterial lesions were found thereafter during the experimental period in chickens of normocholesterolemic and hypercholesterolemic infected groups (Table III). The gross arterial lesions found were similar in character and distribution to those described earlier. Gross atherosclerotic lesions were not found in cerebral arteries of either infected groups or uninfected groups of chickens examined (C. G. Fabricant, J. Fabricant, C. R. Minick, and M. M. Litrenta, 1979, unpublished data).

2. Microscopic Arterial Lesions

a. Infected Normocholesterolemic Chickens. Microscopic arterial lesions were found in infected normocholesterolemic chickens beginning at 1 month postinfection (Fabricant *et al.*, 1980b). These arterial lesions were found in brachiocephalic arteries and in the proximal descending aortal segments nearest the heart (Table IV). By 3 months an appreciable number of these infected normocholesterolemic chickens had microscopic lesions in all arterial segments examined (Table IV). At 7 months practically all the birds in this group had one or more microscopic arterial lesions in the arterial segments examined (Table IV; Fabricant *et al.*, 1980b).

b. Comparisons of Microscopic Arterial Lesions in Various Groups. Percentages of birds with microscopic arterial lesions in

TABLE III

Evolution of Gross Marek's Disease Lesions and Atherosclerotic Lesions in Chickens Infected with MDV at 2 Days of Age

		Number of chickens	
Age (months)	Number necropsied	With gross Marek's disease lesions	With gross atherosclerotic lesions
0–1	105	0	0
1–2	16	14	0
2–3	25	13	0
3–4	56	33	17
4–5	39	21	14
5–6	38	15	11
6–7	60	32	18
Totals	339	128 (38%)	60 (18%)

TABLE IV

PERCENTAGE OF CHICKENS WITH MICROSCOPIC LESIONS AND SEQUENCE OF EVOLUTION IN VARIOUS ARTERIAL SEGMENTS IN THE NORMOCHOLESTEROLEMIC GROUP INFECTED AT 2 DAYS OF AGE WITH MDV[a]

Age (months)	Brachiocephalic artery	Proximal descending aorta	Gastric artery	Celiac artery	Distal descending aorta
0–1	0	0	0	0	0
1	20	10	0	0	0
2	70	18	10	0	13
3	65	46	25	25	31
4	57	37	29	15	19
5	75	30	40	9	71
6	76	44	45	9	67
7	92	57	50	8	73

[a]Each percentage is based on examination of 10 to 15 birds.

groups of infected normocholesterolemic chickens were compared, beginning with the fourth month (1 month after cholesterol supplementation was begun; Fabricant et al., 1980b; Table V). Comparative 7-month data for the uninfected hypercholesterolemic group of chickens are also included in Table V.

Both infected groups of chickens had high incidences of microscopic lesions in proximal descending aortas and in brachiocephalic as well as gastric arteries (Table V). Results indicate that the infected hypercholesterolemic group of chickens had a somewhat higher incidence of these arterial lesions at 4, 5, and 6 months. However, this trend was not consistent, because at 7 months the infected normocholesterolemic group had higher incidences of microscopic lesions in these arterial beds (Table V). Both infected groups of chickens also had lesions in the celiac artery; however, the incidence of lesions in this segment was variable (Table V).

Uninfected hypercholesterolemic birds at 7 months had no lesions in the arterial beds where the infected groups of chickens had numerous lesions (Table V). This finding was added evidence that arterial lesions in proximal descending aortas and brachiocephalic, gastric, and celiac arteries were specifically associated with virus infection and provided confirmatory evidence that a cholesterol effect was secondary to the virus effect.

Chickens in the three groups, two infected and one uninfected, had a high incidence of lesions in the distal descending aortas (Table V).

TABLE V

PERCENTAGE OF CHICKENS WITH MICROSCOPIC ARTERIAL LESIONS:
COMPARISON OF THREE TREATMENT GROUPS[a]

Age (months)	Treatment group	Brachiocephalic artery	Proximal descending aorta	Gastric artery	Celiac artery	Distal descending aorta
4[b]	MDV[c]	57	37	29	15	19
	MDV plus cholesterol	75	45	35	0	32
5	MDV	75	30	40	9	71
	MDV plus cholesterol	88	48	54	25	46
6	MDV	76	44	45	9	67
	MDV plus cholesterol	100	74	38	17	74
7	MDV	92	57	50	8	73
	MDV plus cholesterol	70	50	36	13	51
	Uninfected plus cholesterol[d]	0	0	0	0	48

[a]Each percentage is based on examination of 10 to 15 birds.
[b]Comparisons start at 4 months because cholesterol supplementation began at 3 months.
[c]MDV inoculated at 2 days of age.
[d]Percentages for this group for other months are unavailable.

These lesions, as mentioned earlier, are of unknown origin. They were found as early as 2 months of age in infected normocholesterolemic chickens (Table IV). The percentage of birds with microscopic lesions in this aortal segment increased with age (Tables IV and V). From the available data, of the pathogenesis experiments, we cannot conclude that the incidence of arterial lesions in this segment was altered significantly either by virus infection or cholesterol supplementation.

Processing of the voluminous number of specimens generated in these experiments is incomplete; therefore, comparative data on microscopic arterial lesions in other arterial beds, including hearts and brains, are not yet available.

3. Evidence of MDV-Induced Arterial Injury

It was mentioned earlier that injury to arterial walls has been implicated in atherosclerosis. Perceptible injury induced by MDV was observed in a few arterial cells of some infected birds in the early experiments. This cellular injury was demonstrated by identification of specific VIAs in arterial SMCs. Since cells with these antigens are productively infected and expected to die (Roizman, 1972), VIAs were evidence of MDV injury to arterial SMCs.

In the pathogenesis experiments, arterial cell injury as indicated by specific VIAs was found as early as 1 month post-MDV infection (Table VI; Fabricant et al., 1980b). Thereafter, VIAs were detected throughout the time span of arterial lesion development (Table VI). These viral antigens were found only in a few cells in medial layers of arteries adjacent to arterial lesions. As in the early experiments, cells with VIAs appeared to be SMCs.

Arterial wall injury mediated by immunological means has been implicated in atherogenesis (Minick et al., 1966; Minick and Murphy, 1973; Minick, 1976). Whether immunological injury at the cellular level has a role in virus-induced atherosclerosis has not yet been established. However, extensive examination of arterial lesions of MDV-infected chickens by immunofluorescent techniques with IgG and C3 complement were done during the pathogenesis experiments. No significant deposition of immune complexes was found in any of the numerous specimens examined. It was concluded that this type of immunologic injury had a minor, if any, role in MDV-induced atherogenesis (J. Fabricant, C. G. Fabricant, M. M. Litrenta, C. R. Minick, and C. A. Becker, 1979, unpublished data; Fabricant et al., 1980b; J. Fabricant and C. G. Fabricant, 1985).

B. Alteration of Arterial SMC Lipid Metabolism: A Major Mechanism in MDV Atherogenesis

Appreciable accumulations of lipids, particularly cholesterol, were found in arterial lesions of MDV-infected normocholesterolemic chickens (Fabricant et al., 1978, 1980b; Minick et al., 1979). This finding was, as mentioned earlier, consistent with observations leading to our hypothesis of a herpesvirus role in artherogenesis. The lipid accumulations observed in atherosclerotic lesions of infected normocholesterolemic chickens led to a series of experiments to assess the effects of MDV infection on lipid metabolism of arterial SMCs (Fabricant et al., 1980a, 1981).

1. Cholesterol and Cholesteryl Ester Increased

In vitro morphometric, qualitative, and quantitative experiments were performed to determine whether MDV infection altered lipid metabolism of chicken arterial SMCs (C. G. Fabricant et al., 1981). For these experiments SMCs were derived from arterial segments of the

TABLE VI

Detection of MDV-Specific Viral Internal Antigens by Immunofluorescence

	Age (months)	Number of animals		Percentage positive
		Positive	Total tested	
Infected	0–1	0	40	0
	1–2	1	10	10
	2–3	3	10	30
	3–4	17	44	39
	4–5	8	38	21
	5–6	22	37	59
	7	20	49	41
Uninfected	7	0	29	0

same genetic P-line of SPF chickens used in the *in vivo* experiments (Fabricant *et al.*, 1980a, 1981). Lipid accumulations in SMC cultures infected with MDV were compared to lipids in uninfected SMC cultures and to lipids of SMC cultures infected with a second avian herpesvirus—turkey herpesvirus (HVT).

Morphometrically, MDV-infected cultures were found to have more cells with more lipid accumulations as compared to uninfected SMC cultures (Fabricant *et al.*, 1980a, 1981). Results of the quantitative and qualitative lipid analyses revealed that the total lipid content was significantly greater in MDV-infected cultures than in uninfected SMC cultures or SMC cultures infected with HVT (Table VII; Fabricant *et al.*, 1981). Cholesterol and cholesteryl ester increases accounted for the major total lipid increase in MDV-infected SMCs (Table VII). It is noteworthy that the saturated cholesteryl esters (myristic, palmitic, and stearic) represented the significant cholesteryl ester increase in MDV-infected SMCs (Fabricant *et al.*, 1981). Preliminary analyses of arterial specimens from experimental chickens suggested that MDV infection had the same effect on lipid metabolism *in vivo* (Fabricant *et al.*, 1981).

2. Mechanisms of Altered Lipid Metabolism

Increased lipoprotein uptake was suggested as leading to increased lipid accumulations in MDV-infected SMC cultures. However, the culture medium used in these studies was analyzed and found to have a minimal content of lipoprotein. In fact, the total lipid content of the medium was extremely low: 1.23 ± 0.07 µg/ml (Fabricant *et al.*, 1981). Since the culture medium *was not supplemented with lipids*, it was

TABLE VII

Total Lipid Content of Infected and Uninfected Arterial SMC Cultures[a]

	Uninfected (N = 10)	HVT infected (N = 10)	MDV infected (N = 10)
Cholesterol	1.00 ± 0.29[b]	2.78 ± 0.23[b]	4.81 ± 0.87[b]
Cholesteryl esters	0.73 ± 0.15[c]	0.64 ± 0.10[d]	4.94 ± 1.08[c,d]
Nonesterified fatty acids	1.39 ± 0.27[e]	2.49 ± 0.45	3.20 ± 0.42[e]
Triglycerides	1.00 ± 0.18	1.92 ± 0.35	2.74 ± 0.97
Phospholipids	0.44 ± 0.08[f]	0.93 ± 0.20[g]	1.97 ± 0.41[f,g]
Other	1.22 ± 0.21[h]	1.96 ± 0.37[i]	3.57 ± 1.04[h,i]
Total	5.78 ± 0.59[j]	10.72 ± 1.72[j]	21.24 ± 2.95[j]

[a]Measured as μg lipid/μg DNA ± SEM. Values with same letters are significantly different ($p < 0.05$).

considered unlikely that lipid uptake from the medium contributed to the significant changes in lipid metabolism of MDV-infected SMC cultures. On the other hand, changes in cellular enzymatic activity induced by MDV appeared likely to account, at least in part, for the lipid accumulation in SMCs infected with this herpesvirus. In other experiments, the cholesteryl ester synthetic activity of cholesterol acyltransferase (ACAT) was found to be almost seven times greater in MDV-infected SMC cultures than in uninfected control cultures (Fabricant *et al.*, 1983b; Hajjar *et al.*, 1985). In addition, acid cytosolic cholesteryl ester (ACEH) hydrolytic activity was found to be three times greater in uninfected SMC cultures than in the MDV-infected SMC cultures. It is likely that the alterations of ACAT and ACEH activity in SMCs induced by MDV infection may account for increased accumulations of cholesteryl esters *in vitro* and *in vivo*.

C. Conclusions

The results of the pathogenesis experiments were evidence that the findings of our initial experiments were reproducible. *Only MDV-infected SPF normocholesterolemic or hypercholesterolemic chickens developed atherosclerosis* (C. G. Fabricant *et al.*, 1981). The striking resemblance of the MDV-induced arterial lesions to human arterioatherosclerosis was also evident in the pathogenesis experiments.

In addition, these pathogenesis experiments established the sequential development of arterial lesions following MDV infection (Tables III and IV). Further, the results of these experiments unequivocally placed a cholesterol effect secondary to the herpesvirus effect because (1) arterial lesions were found in MDV-infected normocholesterolemic chickens 2 months before cholesterol supplementation began (Table III); (2) uninfected hypercholesterolemic chickens had no arterial lesions in arterial beds where infected chickens had numerous lesions (Table IV).

In addition, the results of these experiments firmly associated the herpesvirus infection with the arterial lesions. Specific MDV VIAs were found, beginning at 1 month after infection, throughout the span of arterial lesion development. This finding was evidence of herpesvirus injury to arterial cells and showed that the injury was persistent. Evidence that cells in arterial lesions are also infected with MDV will be presented later.

Injury mediated by immunologic factors at the humoral level was not found to be important in MDV atherogenesis, since significant deposition of immune complexes in arterial lesions was not detected (J. Fabricant, C. G. Fabricant, M. M. Litrenta, C. R. Minick, and C. A. Becker, 1979, unpublished data; J. Fabricant et al., 1981; J. Fabricant and C. G. Fabricant, 1985). Whether immunologic injury at the cellular level has a role in MDV atherogenesis will depend upon the results of future studies.

However, a major mechanism in the pathogenesis of MDV-induced atherosclerosis was found to be the alteration of arterial SMC lipid metabolism by MDV infection. Cholesterol and cholesteryl esters were found to specifically accumulate in SMC cultures infected with MDV. Preliminary analyses revealed similar accumulations *in vivo* (Fabricant et al., 1981). It is noteworthy that cholesterol and cholesteryl esters are the two principal lipids found to accumulate in human atherosclerotic plaques (Day and Wahlquist, 1970; Portman, 1970; Smith, 1974).

IV. Evidence of MDV Infection in Cells Comprising Arterial Lesions

The failure to identify MDV-specific VIAs in cells of arterial lesions was not unexpected. Although arterial cell injury may initiate arterial lesions, the evolution and progression of such lesions to plaque formation depend upon increased SMC proliferation. In spite of the fact that MDV is an oncogenic virus, we do not have evidence to demonstrate that increased SMC proliferation, either *in vitro* or *in vivo*, results from oncogenic transformation of SMCs. In *in vitro* studies, however, MDV infection was found to stimulate proliferation of chicken arterial SMCs (C. G. Fabricant, 1979, unpublished observations).

A similar MDV effect on SMCs *in vivo* was considered likely in viral atherogenesis after a collaborative study revealed that cells comprising the arterial lesions were latently infected. Evidence of latent infection was demonstrated by identification of the MDV genome in plaque SMCs by *in situ* DNA hybridization techniques (E. P. Benditt, 1982, personal communication; MDV probes were supplied by N. Ross, Houghton Research Station, England). A latent viral infection, unlike a productive one, is compatible with cell proliferation—a necessary adjunct for plaque formation.

V. Immunization Protects against MDV-Induced Atherosclerosis

A. EXPERIMENTAL PLAN

To prevent MDV-induced tumors, commercial chicken flocks have been successfully immunized with HVT for a number of years. It was therefore reasonable to test whether HVT immunization would also be efficacious in preventing MDV-induced atherosclerosis (J. Fabricant *et al.*, 1981; Fabricant *et al.*, 1983a).

An experiment using four groups of SPF, P-line chickens was performed (Table VIII). Group I was infected with MDV at 2 days of age, groups II and III were immunized with HVT at the same time, and group IV remained untreated. Two weeks after immunization, group II was challenged with MDV.

At 7 months of age the chickens in the four groups were euthanized by cervical dislocation and examined for grossly visible atherosclerotic lesions. At necropsy arterial segments were collected and examined for microscopic lesions.

B. RESULTS

Grossly visible arterial lesions were found only in group I chickens infected with MDV (Table VIII). In addition, of the chickens in this group with microscopic arterial lesions in the arterial segments that were examined 91% had lesions in proximal aorta–brachiocephalic artery and 66% had lesions in gastric–celiac arteries (Table VIII). In

TABLE VIII

The Incidence of Arterial Lesions in Various Groups of Chickens, Testing the Efficacy of HVT Immunization in Preventing MDV-Induced Atherosclerosis

Treatment groups	Grossly visible lesions	Microscopic lesions	
		Proximal aorta and brachiocephalic arteries	Gastric and celiac arteries
Group I + MDV	4/35[a] (11%)	32/35 (91%)	23/35 (66%)
Group II HVT + MDV	0/18	4/18 (22%)	1/18 (6%)
Group III + HVT	0/28	8/29 (28%)	2/28 (7%)
Group IV untreated	0/28	0/28	0/28

[a] Numerators, number of chickens with arterial lesions; denominator, number of chickens examined.

group II, immunized with HVT and challenged with MDV, the number of birds with microscopic arterial lesions was significantly reduced as compared to group I. Only 4 of 18 (22%) and 1 of 18 (6%) chickens in group II had lesions in the proximal aorta–brachiocephalic artery and gastric–celiac arteries, respectively (Table VIII). Further, in group III, immunized with HVT *but not challenged with MDV,* the number of birds with microscopic arterial lesions was not significantly different from that in group II. In group III, 8 of 28 (29%) and 2 of 28 (7%) chickens had lesions in the proximal aorta–brachiocephalic artery and in the gastric–celiac arteries, respectively (Table VIII). No microscopic arterial lesions were found in the untreated group IV chickens (Table VIII; J. Fabricant *et al.,* 1981; Fabricant *et al.,* 1983a).

C. Conclusions

The microscopic arterial lesions found in group III chickens inoculated with HVT only suggest that the vaccine may have had a low level of residual pathogenicity for the P-line chickens. The arterial lesions in group II may have been due to the same effect. However, there was a significantly marked reduction in the number of chickens with arterial lesions in group II, which was immunized and challenged with MDV, as compared to the number of chickens with these lesions, in group I, infected with MDV but not immunized (Table VIII). This finding was added evidence that MDV infection was specifically associated with the development of atherosclerotic lesions. Further, this finding was of great significance because immunization was found to protect against MDV-induced atherosclerosis as well as against MDV-induced tumors.

VI. Preliminary Evidence for a Herpesvirus Role in Human Atherosclerosis

Determining whether one or more of the human herpesviruses has a role in human atherosclerosis depends upon *amassing significant and convincing indirect evidence*. As mentioned earlier, there are five human herpesviruses, including herpes simplex type 1 (HSV-1) and type 2 (HSV-2), Varicella-Zoster (VZ), Epstein–Barr virus (EBV), and CMV (Nahmias et al., 1981). Once acquired, infections with these viruses persist for life, generally as latent infections without evidence of clinical disease.

Studies to gather evidence on the role of these viruses in atherosclerosis are underway in our laboratory and elsewhere. Barret et al. (1983) and Benditt et al. (1983) reported that evidence of HSV (type unknown) was found by in situ DNA hybridization techniques with viral probes in human aortal specimens. These investigators did not find evidence of either EBV or CMV in the specimens examined. They suggested that HSV infection might initiate and/or enhance the progression of some atherosclerotic plaques. On the other hand, Melnick et al. (1983) reported finding evidence of CMV antigens, but not HSV-1 or HSV-2 antigens, in cell cultures of human arterial specimens.

Studies in our laboratory concerning the effects of three human herpesviruses on human fetal arterial SMC cultures were recently completed. Results of these experiments indicated that HSV-1 and HSV-2 infections were lytic. However, CMV infections tended to be latent, induced cell proliferation and crystalline accumulations. It is significant to note that this crystalline material, when examined and compared with polarized light microscopy, was birefringent at the same degree of light polarization as a known cholesterol standard. These results suggest that CMV may have an atherogenic potential (C. G. Fabricant et al., 1985).

Although some evidence is accumulating which suggests herpesvirus role in human atherosclerosis, considerably more evidence will be needed to establish the definitive role of herpesviruses in this arterial disease.

VII. Summary and Conclusions

Infection with Marek's disease herpesvirus was demonstrated to cause atherosclerosis in SPF normocholesterolemic chickens. In addition, our experiments established that uninfected hypercholesterolemic SPF chickens do not develop this arterial disease. These reproducible results are especially significant because the MDV-induced arterial disease is similar to chronic human atherosclerosis.

These studies have provided significant evidence that the viral infection is specifically associated with the development of atherosclerosis because

1. The atherosclerotic lesions were induced only in MDV-infected chickens.
2. MDV-specific VIAs were found in medial SMCs during arterial lesion development.
3. MDV genome was found in cells comprising arterial plaques.
4. MDV infection altered the lipid metabolism of arterial SMCs, increasing accumulations of cholesterol and cholesteryl esters.
5. Immunization with HVT protected against MDV-induced atherosclerosis as well as MDV-induced tumors.

Not all of the mechanisms involved in the pathogenesis of MDV atherogenesis have been identified. However, three viral effects appear to have significant roles in the pathogenesis of the viral-induced arterial disease. These effects include

1. MDV-initiated injury to arterial SMCs. This viral effect is suggested by the foci of lymphocytic infiltration and evidence of specific VIAs found in medial layers of arteries. Injury to arterial cells has been suggested as the primary event in atherogenesis (Harker *et al.,* 1974; Ross and Glomset, 1976).

2. MDV stimulation of arterial SMC proliferation appears to be a second important effect. This viral effect was suggested by the proliferative and fatty proliferative arterial lesions in MDV-infected normocholesterolemic chickens. In addition, this effect was also suggested by our (unpublished) observations of increased proliferation of MDV-infected SMC cultures. Further, other MDV-infected cells have been reported to have increased proliferative rates (Smith and Calnek, 1974). Finally, since MDV genome was identified in SMCs in arterial plaques, (E. P. Benditt, 1982, personal communication; Benditt *et al.,* 1983), it is reasonable to suggest that this latent infection may result in increased proliferation of these cells.

3. MDV alteration of SMC lipid metabolism is a third major viral mechanism in the pathogensis of MDV atherogenesis. This viral mechanism was demonstrated by increased lipid accumulations, particularly cholesterol and cholesteryl esters, in arterial SMCs infected with MDV *in vitro* and *in vivo*. As mentioned earlier, other investigators have reported that cholesterol and cholesteryl esters are the principal lipids founds in human atherosclerotic plaques (Day and Wahlquist, 1970; Portman, 1970; and Smith, 1974).

The establishment of a herpesvirus (MDV) as the etiologic agent of atherosclerosis in a pathogen-free normocholesterolemic animal model (chickens) is of great importance to other models of atherosclerosis research. Infections with herpesviruses frequently occur in animal models used in this research (McKercher, 1973; Barahona *et al.*, 1974). Since herpesvirus infections in animals may be without clinical signs of disease and/or latent infections, cell cultures derived from these animals may be infected also. Therefore, results obtained from studies utilizing microbially undefined models may be difficult to evaluate. Additionally, such results may be subject to question.

Further, our findings have introduced important new concepts in the pathogenesis of atherosclerosis—a disease long considered of degenerative or metabolic origin. These concepts are a primary herpesvirus etiology and a herpesvirus induced alteration of arterial smooth muscle cell lipid metabolism.

In summary, the results of our studies have direct relevance to human atherosclerosis because (1) the arterial lesions resulting from infection with MDV of an SPF animal model closely resemble those found in chronic human atherosclerosis, (2) these results are reproducible in repeated experiments, and (3) humans are known to be widely and persistently infected with as many as five herpesviruses. Finally, our studies suggest that establishment of a causal relationship between herpesvirus(es) and human atherosclerosis may eventually lead to preventive therapy. In the future, use of vaccines and/or antiviral agents may prevent cardiovascular disease—a major cause of human death.

Acknowledgments

The author acknowledges the close collaboration on all these studies with Dr. Julius Fabricant from the Department of Avian and Aquatic Animal Medicine at the New York State College of Veterinary Medicine, Cornell University, Ithaca, New York. We acknowledge that pathological examinations of animal arterial specimens were done in the Department of Pathology of the Cornell Medical Center–New York Hospital, New York,

New York by Doctors Maria Litrenta and C. Richard Minick. In addition, Doctor David P. Hajjar, also from the Department of Pathology at the Cornell Medical Center, has our sincere acknowledgments for performing the quantitative and qualitative analyses of lipids in arterial SMCs *in vitro* and *in vivo*. In addition, he has been the principal investigator elucidating the enzymatic activities altered by MDV infection causing cholesteryl ester accumulations *in vitro* and *in vivo*. We also wish to acknowledge that Dr. K. A. Schat of the Department of Avian and Aquatic Animal Medicine at the New York State College of Veterinary Medicine assisted us in determining CMV stimulation of human SMC proliferation. Sincere thanks are also due to Doctor Julius Fabricant for his critical review of this manuscript and to Kathryn Freese for her patience in typing it. These studies were supported in part by grants from the Heart, Lung and Blood Institute of the National Institutes of Health.

References

Barahona, H., Melendez, L., and Melnick, J. (1974). *Intervirology* **3**, 175–192.
Barrett, T. B., McDougall, J. K., and Benditt, E. P. (1983) *Fed. Proc., Fed. Am. Soc. Exp. Biol.* **42**, 501.
Benditt, E. P., and Benditt, J. M. (1973). *Proc. Natl. Acad. Sci. U.S.A.* **70**, 1753–1756.
Benditt, E. P., Barrett, T. B., and McDougall, J. K. (1983). *Proc. Natl. Acad. Sci. U.S.A.* **80**, 6386–6389.
Burch, G. E., Harb, J. M., Hiramoto, Y., and Shewey, L. (1973). *Am. Heart J.* **86**, 523–534.
Calnek, B. W. (1972). In "Oncogenesis and Herpesviruses" (P. M. Biggs, G. deThé, and L. N. Payne, eds.), pp. 129–136. Elsevier, Amsterdam.
Castelli, W. P. (1984). *Am. J. Med.* **76(A)**, 4–12.
Churchill, A. E., and Biggs, P. M. (1967). *Nature (London)* **215**, 528–530.
Clarkson, T. B., Prichard, R. W., Netsky, M. G., and Lofland, H. B. (1959). *Arch. Pathol.* **68**, 143–147.
Crawford, P. B., and Henson, J. B. (1973). *Proc. Conf. Equine Infect. Dis., 3rd, Paris* pp. 282–302.
Dauber, D. V. (1944). *Arch. Pathol.* **38**, 46–51.
Day, A. J., and Wahlquist, M. L. (1970). *Exp. Mol. Pathol.* **13**, 199–216.
Fabricant, C. G. (1975). *Artery* **1**, 361.
Fabricant, C. G., and Fabricant, J. (1985). In Proc. Int. Symp. Murek's Disease" (B. W. Calnek and J. L. Spencer, eds.), pp. 391–407. Am. Assoc. Avian Pathol. Inc.
Fabricant, C. G., and Gillespie, J. H. (1974). *Infect. Immun.* **9**, 460–466.
Fabricant, C. G., Krook. L., and Gillespie, J. H. (1973). *Science* **181**, 566–567.
Fabricant, C. G., Fabricant, J., Litrenta, M. M., and Minick, C. R. (1977). *Circulation* **56** *(Suppl. 3)*, 144.
Fabricant, C.G., Fabricant, J., Litrenta, M. M., and Minick, C. R. (1978). *J. Exp. Med.* **148**, 335–340.
Fabricant, C. G., Fabricant, J., Litrenta, M. M., and Minick, C. R. (1980a). In "Resistance and Immunity to Marek's Disease" (P. M. Biggs, ed.), pp. 146–155. Commission of the European Communities, Brussels, Luxembourg.
Fabricant, C. G., Fabricant, J., Minick, C. R., and Litrenta, M. M. (1980b). In "Viruses in Naturally Occurring Cancers" (M. Essex, G. Todaro, and H. Zür Hausen, eds.), Vol. **7(B)**, pp. 1251–1258. Cold Spring Harbor Lab., Cold Spring Harbor New York.
Fabricant, C. G., Hajjar, D. P., Minick, C. R., and Fabricant, J. (1981). *Am. J. Pathol.* **105**, 176–184.

Fabricant, C. G., Fabricant, J., Minick, C. R., and Litrenta, M. M. (1983a). *Fed. Proc., Fed. Am. Soc. Exp. Biol.* **42,** 2476–2479.

Fabricant, C. G., Hajjar, D. P., Minick, C. R., and Fabricant, J. (1983b). *Fed. Proc., Fed. Am. Soc. Exp. Biol.* **43,** 501.

Fabricant, J., and Fabricant, C. G. (1985). *In* "Proc. Int. Symp. Murek's Disease" (B. W. Calnek and J. L. Spencer, eds.), pp. 408–417. Am. Assoc. Avian Pathol. Inc.

Fabricant, J., Fabricant, C. G., Litrenta, M. M., and Minick, C. R. (1981). *Fed. Proc., Fed. Am. Soc. Exp. Biol.* **40,** 335.

Gordon, T., Garcia-Palmieri, M. R., Kagan, A., Kannel, W. B., and Schiffman, J. (1974). *J. Chron. Dis.* **27,** 329–344.

Hajjar, D. P., Falcone, D. J., Fabricant, C. G., and Fabricant, J. (1985). *J. Biol. Chem.* **260,** 6124–6128.

Harker, L. A., Slichter, S. J., Scott, C. R., and Ross, R. (1974). *N. Engl. J. Med.* **291,** 537–543.

Haymaker, W., Girdany, B. R., Stephens, J., Lillie, R. D., and Fetterman, G. H. (1954). *J. Neuropathol. Exp. Neurol.* **13,** 562–586.

Liggitt, H. D., DeMartini, J. C., McChesney, A. E., Pierson, R. E., and Storz, J. (1978). *Am. J. Vet. Res.* **39,** 1249–1257.

McCracken, J. H., Shinfield, H. R., Coff, K., Rausen, R., Dische, R., and Eichenwald, H. F. (1967). *Am. J. Dis. Child.* **117,** 522–537.

McKercher, D. G. (1973). *In* "The Herpsviruses" (A. S. Kaplan, ed.), pp. 428–493. Academic Press, New York.

McGuire, T. C., Crawford, T. B., and Henson, J. B. (1974). *Am. J. Vet. Res.* **35,** 181–185.

Melnick, J. L., Driesman, G. R., McCollum, C. H., Petrie, B. L., Burek, J., and DeBakey, M. E. (1983). *Lancet* **2,** 644–647.

Minick, C. R. (1976). *Ann. N.Y. Acad. Sci.* **275,** 210–227.

Minick, C. R., and Murphy, G. E. (1973). *Am. J. Pathol.* **73,** 265–300.

Minick, C. R., Murphy, G. E., and Campbell, W. G., Jr. (1966). *J. Exp. Med.* **124,** 635–652.

Minick, C. R., Fabricant, C. G., Fabricant, J., and Litrenta, M. M. (1979). *Am. J. Pathol.* **96,** 673–706.

Nahmias, A. J., Dowdle, W. R., and Schinazi, eds. (1981). "The Human Herpesvirus." Elsevier, Amsterdam.

Paterson, J. C., and Cottral, G. E. (1950). *Arch. Pathol.* **49,** 699–709.

Pietilä, K., and Nikkari, T. (1983). *Med. Biol.* **61,** 31–44.

Portman, O. W. (1970). *Adv. Lipid Res.* **8,** 41–114.

Roizman, B. (1972). *In* "Oncogenesis and Herpesviruses" (P. M. Biggs, G. deThé, and L. N. Payne, eds.), pp. 1–17. Elsevier, Amsterdam.

Ross, R., and Glomset, J. A. (1973). *Science* **180,** 1332–1339.

Ross, R., and Glomset, J. A. (1976). *N. Engl. J. Med.* **295,** 369–377.

Ross, R., and Harker, L. A. (1976). *Science* **193,** 1094–1100.

Smith, E. B. (1974). *Adv. Lipid Res.* **12,** 1–49.

Smith, M. G. (1959). *Prog. Med. Virol.* **2,** 171–202.

Smith, M. W., and Calnek, B. W. (1974). *Avian Pathol.* **3,** 229–246.

Taylor, C. B. (1955). *In* "Symposium on Atherosclerosis," pp. 74–90. National Academy of Sciences, Washington, D.C.

Ward, P. H., Lindsay, J. R., and Warner, N. E. (1965). *Laryngoscope* **75,** 628–638.

Waters, L. L. (1955). *In* "Symposium on Atherosclerosis," pp. 91–98. National Academy of Sciences, Washington, D.C.

Weller, T. H., and Hanshaw, J. B. (1962). *N. Engl. J. Med.* **266,** 1233–1244.

Zanchetti, A. (1984). *Am. J. Med.* **76(A),** 1–3.

The Ontogeny and Microenvironment of the Avian Thymus and Bursa of Fabricius: Contribution of Specialized Cells to the Avian Immune Response

BRUCE GLICK

*Poultry Science Department, Mississippi State University
Mississippi State, Mississippi*

I.	Introduction	67
II.	Bursal Ontogeny and Microenvironment	68
III.	Nonbursal Site for Immunoglobulin Synthesis	73
IV.	Identifying the Nonbursal Site and Associated Cells	76
V.	The Role of the Avian Thymus	82
VI.	The Multipotential Stem Cell	82
VII.	Thymic Ontogeny	83
VIII.	The Thymic Microenvironment	84
	References	87

I. Introduction

The chicken has contributed unequivocally to our understanding of the immune response. Conceptualization of the division of labor among lymphocytes supervened following experiments with the bursa of Fabricius and the avian thymus. These experiments helped establish the T and B cell concept in which T cells, derived from the thymus, controlled cell-mediated immunity and B cells, derived from the bursa of Fabricius or equivalent sites, controlled humoral immunity. During the past two decades, the T and B cell concept has matured to include interactions of T cells, B cells, and accessory cells for most humoral immune responses (Thorbecke *et al.,* 1972; Glick, 1982), the necessity of histocompatibility in these cellular interactions, identification of subpopulations in the repertoire of T cells, and the role of lymphokines in the immune response. In this review I will identify research that supplies answers or questions concerning the ontogeny, microenvironment, and function of the bursa and thymus.

II. Bursal Ontogeny and Microenvironment

The observation in the mid-1950s that removal of the bursa of Fabricius markedly impaired or eliminated antibody production led to the concept that B cell ontogeny was dependent on a functioning bursa (Glick, 1983). While we were responsible for this initial observation, we were also responsible for the perception that bursaless birds were capable of immunoglobulin (Ig, viz. IgM) synthesis and for the thesis that alternative sites exist for B cell ontogeny (Lerner et al., 1971; Subba Rao et al., 1978). Others have verified and extended these considerations to include the presence of IgG and B cells in chicks in ovo bursectomized before 70 hr of embryonic development (Fitzimmons et al., 1973; Jankovic et al., 1977; Eerola et al., 1983a). Now, it is our contention that B cell ontogeny within the bursa is dependent on the presence of a specialized cell we have named the secretory cell and that the precursor of this cell homes to the bursal epithelium, where it is responsible for bud formation, B stem cell attraction, and B cell differentiation. The precursor secretory cell at other sites, e.g., spleen, may interact with B stem cells and, under the influence of a cytokine from the bursa secretory cell, fully differentiate into the periellipsoid white pulp cell, ellipsoid-associated cell (EAC), interdigitating dendritic cell within the T-dependent region of the spleen, and follicular dendritic cell of the germinal center (Glick and Olah, 1984). Before emphasizing the immune response role of the bursa, an assessment of its ontogeny and microenvironment is necessary.

The bursa of Fabricius is a dorsal diverticulum of the proctadael region of the cloaca (Fig. 1). The numerous bursal plicae (Fig. 2a and b) each reveal 800–1200 follicles (Olah and Glick, 1978a) covered by a specialized follicle-associated epithelium which is pinocytotic (Bockman and Cooper, 1972). The follicle-associated epithelium may be differentiated from the interfollicular epithelium by its shorter microvilli (Fig. 3a and b), the absence of mucoid cells, and the association of its basement membrane with the corticomedullary border. The latter is formed by epithelial cells which divide the bursa into a vascular cortex containing lymphoblasts, lymphocytes, macrophages, and plas-

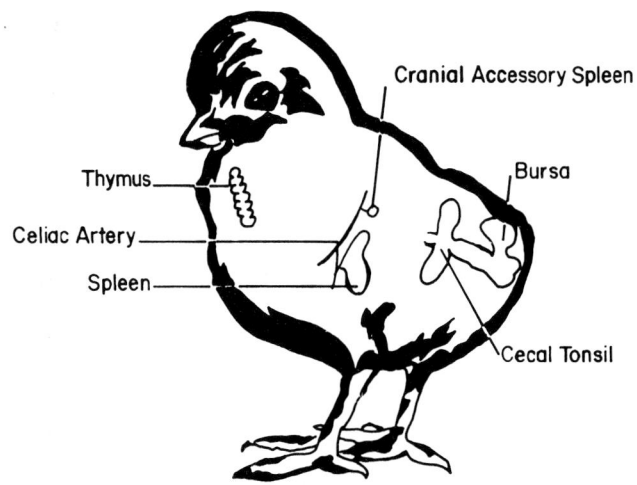

FIG. 1. Central lymphomyeloid tissues, thymus, bursa of Fabricius, and several peripheral lymphoid tissues of the chicken. (From Glick, 1970.)

ma cells and a medulla which contains reticular cells and fibers in addition to the same cells identified in the cortex (Glick, 1983).

The blood-borne progenitor-cell origin for the bursal (B) lymphocytes has been well documented (Jaffe and Fechheimer, 1966; Moore and Owen, 1965, 1966, 1967; LeDouarin and Jotereau, 1973a,b, 1975; LeDouarin et al., 1975; Houssaint et al., 1976; See reviews by Glick, 1977, 1983). The origin of the blood-borne stem cell appears to be intraembryonic rather than yolk sac in origin (Dieterlen-Lievre et al., 1976; Lasilla et al., 1978, 1979, 1980; Martin et al., 1979; Toivanen et al., 1979; Beaupain et al., 1979). Before the establishment of circulation, <14 somite stage, a quail-area pelucida (embryo) replaced that of a chick to form a yolk sac (chick) embryo chimera (Martin et al., 1978). The nuclear characteristics of the developing lymphocytes resembled those of the quail, and, therefore, were of intraembryonic origin. Since quail-type erythropoietic cells appeared in the yolk sac by day 13 of embryonic development, one could conclude that intraembryonic cells are highly mobile. Further work by Martin et al. (1979) with IgG allotypes confirmed the intraembryonic origin of the lymphocyte. When these mesodermal cells were transferred from 7-day embryos, i.e., before bursal colonization (LeDouarin et al., 1975), to cyclophosphamide-treated immunosuppressed embryos, reconstitution of the developing chicks' B cell system occurred (Lasilla et al., 1979).

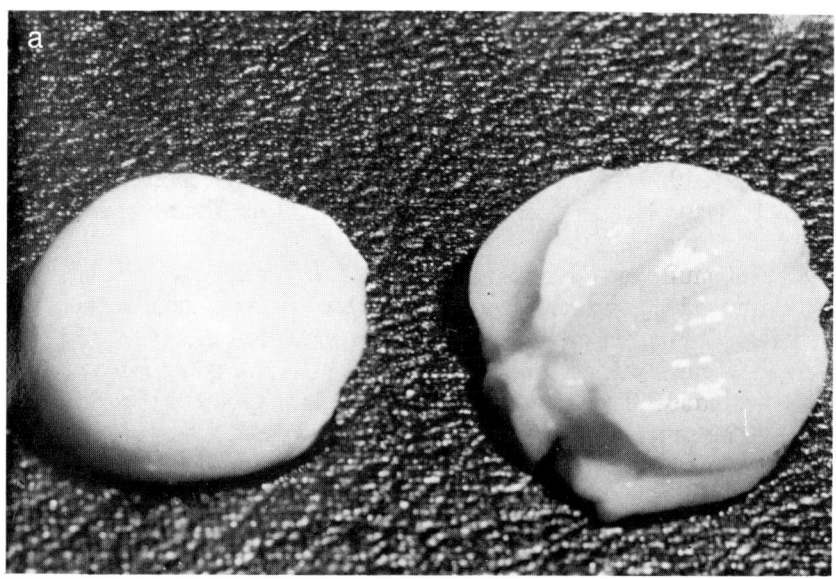

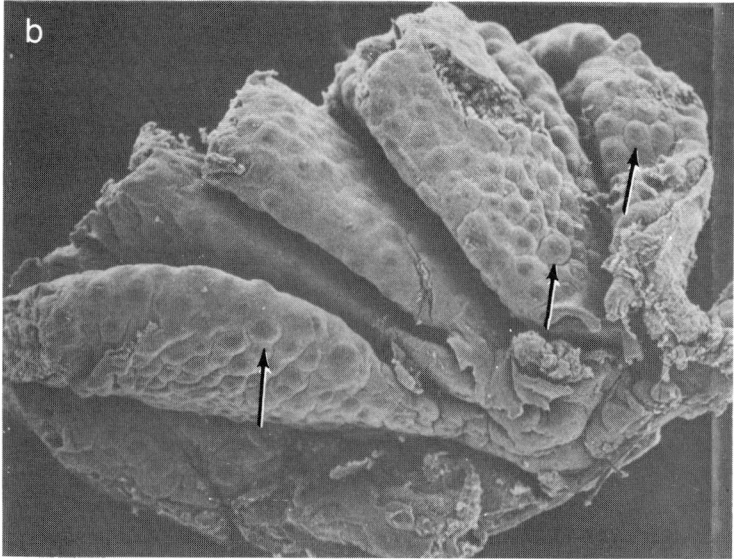

FIG. 2. (a) Bursae of Fabricius from a 2-week-old chicken. The bursa on the right has been everted to show the plicae. (From Glick, 1964.) (b) A scanning electron micrograph of the bursal plicae from a 2-day chick. Each raised area (arrow) is a projecting follicle. ×35.

The bursa of cyclophosphamide-treated embryos is devoid of lymphocytes but resembles the normal bursa in other cytoarchitectural features. This would suggest that a cellular or soluble component of the bursa may be contributing to B cell differentiation. While evidence for a soluble bursal factor has been advanced (Glick, 1960; St. Pierre and Ackerman, 1966; Jankovic and Leskowitz, 1965), the identification of a specific factor has only recently been discussed (Brand et al., 1976; Goldstein et al., 1977).

The low number of B cells in the bone marrow at hatch was markedly increased by incubation with a bursal extract termed "bursapoietin." Precursors of BU-1$^+$ cells were identified in the nonlymphoid population from the bursa and bone marrow of 14 to 21-day embryos subsequent to incubation with bursapoietin (Brand et al., 1983). The source of the bursapoietin-like molecule may be the alymphoid cells of the bursa (Eerola et al., 1982). These researchers evaluated the ability of alymphoid cells and soluble factors to affect the appearance of B-L (Ia$^+$) antigens, which are analogous to Ia$^+$ antigens of mammals (Briles et al., 1982; Ewert and Cooper, 1978; Ziegler and Pink, 1976). Immunoprecipitated [^{35}S]methionine-labeled B-L antigens possessed polypeptides of $29-32 \times 10^3$ Da, and thus showed a similarity to Ia antigen of mouse (Jalkanen et al., 1983a). Cells were collected from the mesenchyme of 7- or 9-day-old embryos by Eerola et al. (1982, 1983a) and then separated by sedimentation through a linear human serum albumin gradient. Five cellular fractions were collected, with fraction 1 possessing the smallest cell and the other fractions revealing the larger cells. Alymphoid bursal epithelium (BE) was effected by culturing bursal fragments from day-old chicks for 7 days. Supernatants collected from the BE were referred to as bursal-epithelium-conditioned medium (BECM). The incubation of BE or BECM with the five cellular fractions markedly stimulated the appearance of B-L antigens on the cells from fractions 1 and 5. BECM was more effective in differentiating fraction 1 cells than was BE. The low percentage of fraction 1 cells to the total, their lack of DNA activity, and the DNA activity and larger size of the cells in the other rapidly sedimenting fractions suggested that these cell populations represented different maturational stages of cells within the same lineage.

That the B-L antigen was present on a small percentage of the cells in each of the five fractions suggests that cellular interactions or necessary cytokines are active prior to 9 days of embryonic development. The active factor(s) may be dependent upon the presence of secretory cells, which we know to be cyclophosphamide resistant (Olah and Glick, 1978b) and which may be resistant to the cell-culturing tech-

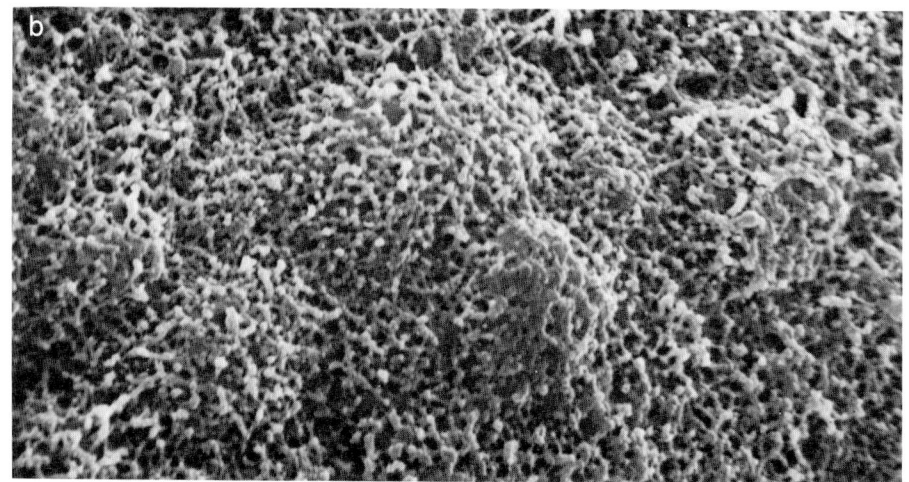

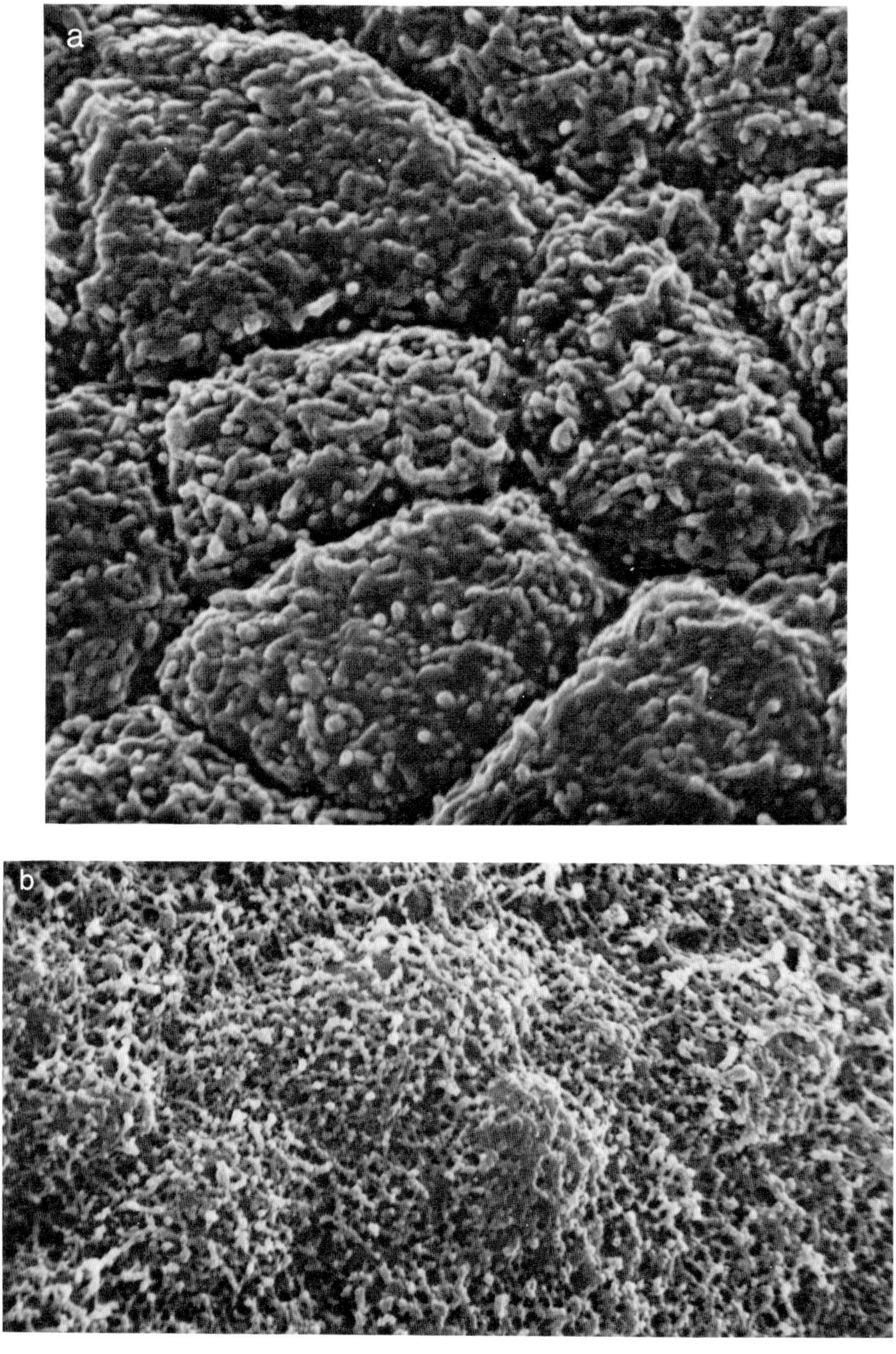

nique employed by Eerola et al. (1983a). Eerola et al. (1983b) envisioned events in the bursal microenvironment to include induction of a primitive cell type following cellular interaction and then the release by the undivided "primitive cell" of a soluble factor which acts on a more mature cell. Our thesis (Glick and Olah, 1984), to be described later, suggests that a precursor secretory cell would enter the BE and then develop into a secretory cell. The precursor secretory cell would then be the inducible primitive cell and the secretory cell responsible for the humoral factor.

III. Nonbursal Site for Immunoglobulin Synthesis

The available microenvironmental evidence might suggest that B cell differentiation and hence Ig and antibody synthesis is an obligate role of the bursa. Immunoglobulin and antibody suppression subsequent to at-hatch bursectomy and the initial synthesis of IgM and IgG in the bursa appeared to support an obligate role for the bursa (see review by Glick, 1983). Several subsequent reports appeared in which secondary and/or tertiary injections of at-hatch bursectomized birds led to antibody production. Perhaps, B cell release occurred prior to hatching and, therefore, at-hatch bursectomy was too late to effect a complete bursectomy. The demonstration that the bursa could be rendered alymphoid or could be eliminated with hormones prior to 12 days of incubation allowed one to more completely evaluate the bursa's role in humoral immunity (Meyer et al., 1959; Glick and Sadler, 1961; Warner and Burnet, 1961). Our method of dipping 3-day-old fertile eggs into testosterone propionate solutions (2 g%) eliminated the bursa in 80% of the hatched chicks. More dramatic was the ability of these birds to produce excessive quantities of IgM, especially in the presence of multiple injections of antigen (Fig. 4) (Lerner et al., 1971; Subba Rao et al., 1978). Also, these birds produced antibody to the specific antigen. Our results coupled with those of others led us to propose the thesis that "other sites in the chicken were capable of conditioning or supplying immunocompetent cells" (Glick, 1968; Lerner et al., 1971; Subba Rao et al., 1978). This concept of a bursa-independent pathway found

FIG. 3. (a) A scanning electron micrograph of the follicle-associated epithelium (FAE) which covers the bursal follicle. The FAE cells possess short microvilli and reveal a polygonal shape. ×5278. (b) A scanning electron micrograph of the interfollicular epithelium. The cell borders are obscured by the numerous microvilli. ×4328.

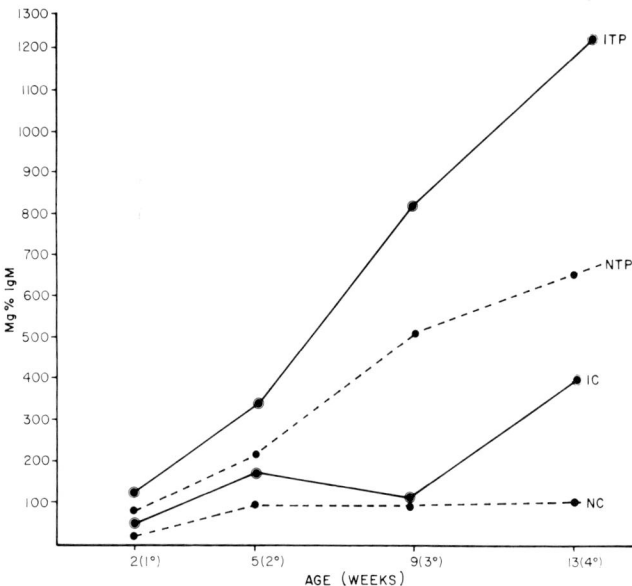

FIG. 4. A comparison of the IgM levels of bursaless chicks hatched from testosterone propionate-treated (ITP) eggs and control (NC) chicks subsequent to no immunization (NTP) or immunization (IC) with sheep red blood cells at 1, 4, 8, and 12 weeks of age. (From Subba Rao et al., 1978.)

support in the *in ovo* bursectomies first performed by Fitzimmons et al. (1973) and then by Jankovic et al. (1975) and finally from the laboratory of Auli and Paavo Toivanen. The latter group followed the procedure developed by Fitzimmons and Jankovic and surgically removed the bursa from 60-hr embryos (Granfors et al., 1982; Eerola et al., 1983a; Jalkanen et al., 1983b). Three intraperitoneal injections of nine different antigens revealed the *in ovo* bursectomized birds to be defective in their ability to make specific antibody (Granfors et al., 1982). Yet, these same birds were capable of synthesizing IgM, IgG, and IgA. The data were interpreted to suggest that the bursal microenvironment might be necessary for activation of the V gene repertoire. Subsequent to a 7-day culture in the presence of pokeweed mitogen, dextran sulfate, or anti-μ serum, peripheral blood or spleen cells from 10-day-old *in ovo* bursectomized birds produced significantly less of all three Ig isotypes than did control birds (Eerola et al., 1983a). However, by 10 weeks of age, the cultured cells from the bursectomized birds yielded comparable amounts of the three isotypes. Dextran sulfate stimulated an excessive increase in the peripheral levels of IgM in bursectomized birds, but the IgG levels were similar for bursectomized and control birds. These data led to the conclusion that the switch from IgM to IgG was not dependent on the presence of the bursa. Phytohemagglutinin and pokeweed mitogen markedly stimulated the peripheral blood and spleen cells from both control and bursectomized birds, as evidenced by DNA synthesis (Eerola et al., 1983a). While bone marrow cells of controls appeared to respond to PHA with a stimulation index of 7.9, the 1.3 index for bursectomized bone marrow cells would suggest minimal or no stimulation. Dextran sulfate did not stimulate peripheral blood or splenic cells of control or bursectomized birds but showed a slight stimulation of bone marrow cells. Anti-μ and anti-γ sera stimulated splenic and bone marrow cells from both control and bursectomized birds. These data confirmed that dextran sulfate is mitogenic for immature chicken cells but not mature ones and also demonstrated that dextran sulfate is capable of stimulating Ig secretion of mature cells but not immature ones. The conclusion that bursaless birds possess a B cell system was, therefore, inescapable (Eerola et al., 1983a). In ovo bursectomized birds lacked natural antibodies to phosphorylcholine, fecal bacteria, rabbit red blood cells, major histocompatibility complex antigens, and autoantibodies to liver, kidney, and thyroids (Jalkanen et al., 1983b). The results from these three papers support the authors' contention that the bursa is necessary for antibody production but not for immunoglobulin production or isotype switch. The presence of excessive quantities of IgM in these experiments, as well as our experiments, would suggest either external stimulation of the bursaless birds or interference with their homeostatic mechanism. We concluded, based on pathogen-free studies and infusing of IgG, that the excessive IgM levels in bursaless birds would be, in part, explained on the basis of viral action and the reduced level of IgG which acts as a negative feedback regulator of IgM (Subba Rao et al., 1978). Even though Toivanen and co-workers utilized nine different antigens and screened for the appearance of several natural antibodies, one would have to consider only the numerous environmental antigens to suggest that the IgM in their bursaless birds may reflect antibodies to those antigens. While the level of serum IgG reported by Jalkanen et al. (1983a,b) in in ovo bursectomized birds was markedly reduced, another report from the same laboratory revealed a variable influence in in ovo bursectomy on plasma IgG (Granfors et al., 1982). Therefore, the generally lower IgG levels of bursaless birds might influence homeostasis and contribute to the high IgM values.

•

IV. Identifying the Nonbursal Site and Associated Cells

It is now apparent that bursaless birds have an alternate pathway for B cell differentiation. Whether B cells resulting from this pathway are fully competent or need the bursal environment for attainment of the full repertoire of V chains has been debated. Our laboratory has recently proposed a thesis which attempts to identify the alternate pathway and would help explain the presence of B cells and Ig synthesis and the possible inability of antibody synthesis in bursaless birds (Glick and Olah, 1984).

Following the technique of Lerman and Weidanz (1970), we were able to produce a few agammaglobulinemic birds by injecting cyclophosphamide (Cy) immediately after hatching (Glick, 1971). Further studies with *in ovo* administration of Cy identified it to be highly effective in eliminating a primary antibody response but not in eliminating Ig synthesis (Glick, 1981, and unpublished). These results directed our attention to the fine structure of both central and peripheral immune tissue in normal, Cy-treated, and antigen-stimulated growing chickens. Cyclophosphamide injections of 7-week-old chickens led to the elimination of bursal lymphocytes and the revelation of a new cell termed the "secretory cell" (Olah and Glick, 1978b; Olah *et al.*, 1979). Secretory cells were 12–15 μm in diameter with a round or ovoid nucleus which contained numerous nucleoli (Fig. 5). The abundant cytoplasm possessed a well-developed Golgi apparatus, ergastoplasmic reticulum, and at least one long process containing variable numbers of dense granules (0.2 to 0.6 μm in diameter). The empty space within the bursal medulla apparently created by Cy elimination of lymphocytes was filled with a heavily stained substance (Fig. 6). Also, the intercellular substance appeared on the membrane of secretory cells, but not other cells.

Since these cell types had not been previously identified, the possibility arose that they had differentiated in the presence of Cy. However, the bursa of untreated birds revealed the secretory cell. This suggested that the secretory cell was a normal constituent of the bursa's cell pool and like B cells was capable of cellular expansion. The observation that the secretory cells from untreated birds possessed more cytoplasmic granules than after Cy treatment and that their membrane occasionally revealed a densely stained substance reinforced our belief that they were responsible for a secretory product and that the product was the intercellular substance observed subsequent to Cy treatment. We theorized that the products of the secretory cell

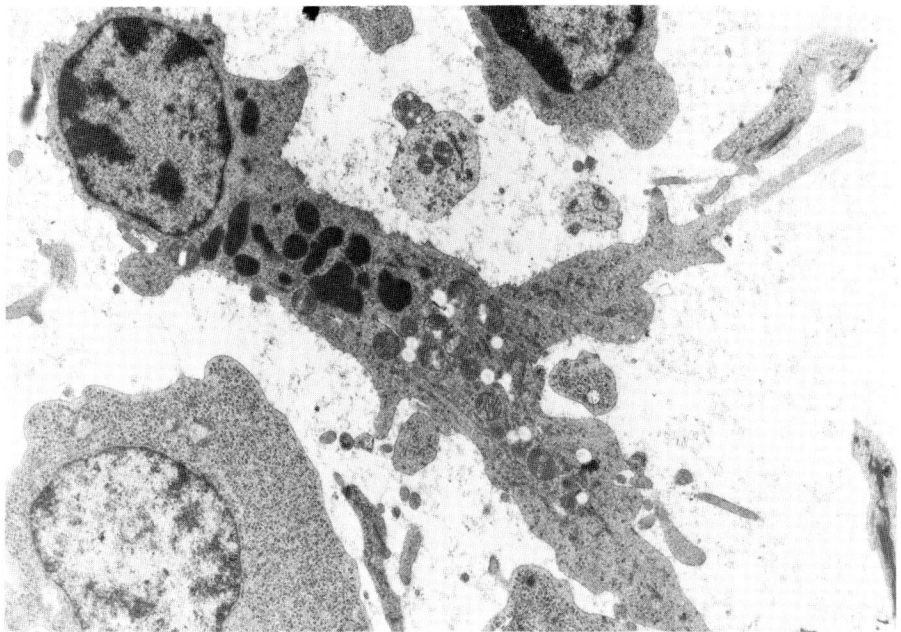

FIG. 5. The secretory cell possesses one or more cell processes. One process contains numerous membrane-bound granules. The heterochromatic nucleus may contain 1–3 nucleoli. ×6375.

contributed to the special microenvironment of the bursa and were responsible for, in part, attraction and B cell differentiation.

The presence of a cell resembling the bursal secretory cell in the germinal center of the spleen and caecal tonsil (Olah and Glick, 1979) raised further questions concerning the cell's function and origin. A detailed anatomical study of the spleen has suggested that the splenic secretory cell was the culmination of a cell transformation beginning with the cells of the periellipsoid white pulp (Olah and Glick, 1982). We have identified in the chicken's spleen an EAC that satisfies some but not all of the characteristics delineated for classical mammalian dendritic cells (Steinman and Nussenzweig, 1980) (Figs. 7–10). An avian splenic dendritic cell was first identified by White and co-workers (White, 1963; White et al., 1970, 1975). The immediate progenitor of the EACs appears to be the cells of the periellipsoid white pulp. There is extensive mitotic activity of the latter cells in the vicinity of the EAC, while mitosis of the EACs had not been evident. In animals injected with carbon, the carbon is bound not only by the EACs but also by the mitotic cells in close proximity to the EACs. Following binding

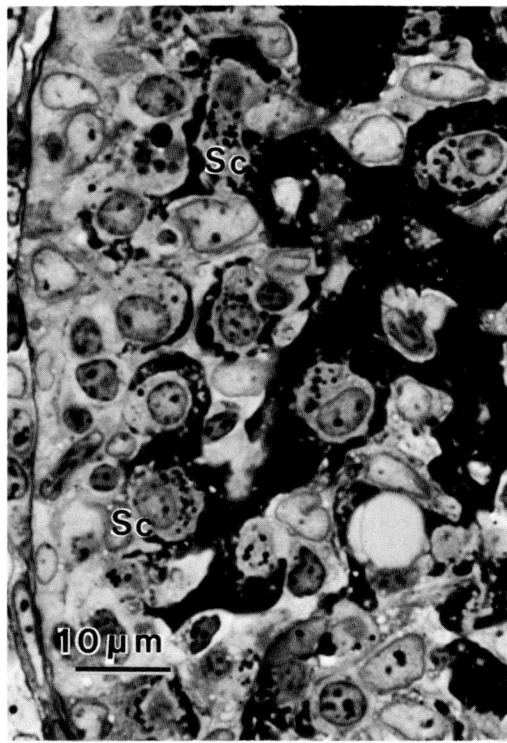

FIG. 6 Secretory cells (Sc) located at the corticomedullary border of follicles from untreated birds are amplified following the injection of cyclophosphamide. (From Olah et al., 1979.)

of soluble or particulate substances, the EACs phagocytose these substances and then migrate to the red pulp and the T-dependent and B-dependent (germinal centers) regions of the periarteriolar lymphatic sheath. Once the EAC is a part of the germinal center, it morphologically resembles the bursal secretory cell. The secretory cell, like the EAC, is dendritic but it is not phagocytic. The secretory cell of the germinal center may be analogous to the mammalian follicular dendritic cell. Therefore, the source of the germinal center's secretory cell appears to be the EAC. We have proposed that the ultimate source of splenic and bursal secretory cells is a common precursor secretory cell (Glick and Olah, 1984). The precursor secretory cell would enter the bursal epithelium of embryos, where it would induce bud formation and create a microenvironment conducive to the attraction of the precursor B cell (Fig. 11). The latter cell, under the influence of the se-

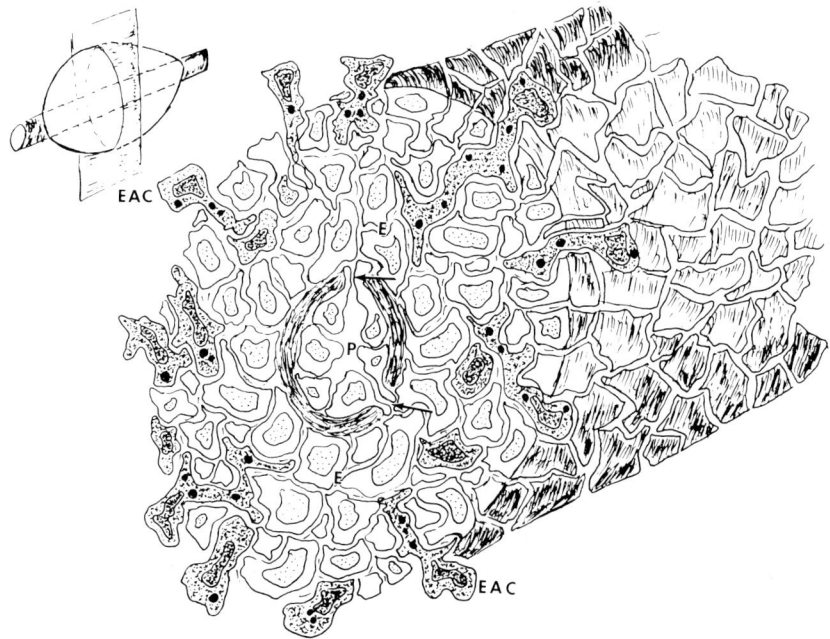

FIG. 7. A survey picture of the ellipsoid region. A few ellipsoid-associated cells (EAC) may occur inside the ellipsoid (E), but the majority are located on its surface. The processes of the EAC are inserted into the ellipsoid. P, penicilliform capillary; arrow, stomata which allow the escape of immunogens from the vascular system. (From Olah and Glick, 1982.)

cretory cell and the special microenvironment of the bursa, would differentiate from a cytoplasmic (c) μ^- surface (s) μ^- large stem cell to a $c\mu^+s\mu^+$ cell identified in the bursal follicle of 13-day embryos (Kincade and Cooper, 1971; Grossi et al., 1977). While bursal initiation or removal suppresses humoral immunity, it does not eliminate immunoglobulin synthesis or B cell differentiation (Glick, 1983). In order to explain these results, we suggest that the precursor secretory cell of the spleen may interact with the precursor B cell and induce partial B cell differentiation. Thus, the presence of precursor secretory cells in the spleen would explain the presence of B cells in in ovo bursectomized birds (Fitzimmons et al., 1973; Jankovic et al., 1975, 1976, 1977). However, the deficiency of the bursectomized birds to mount a normal humoral response would suggest that the bursa exerts a positive feedback on the spleen. Such does appear to be the case with respect to the periellipsoid white pulp. Bursectomy markedly inhibits the normal histological development of the periellipsoid white pulp.

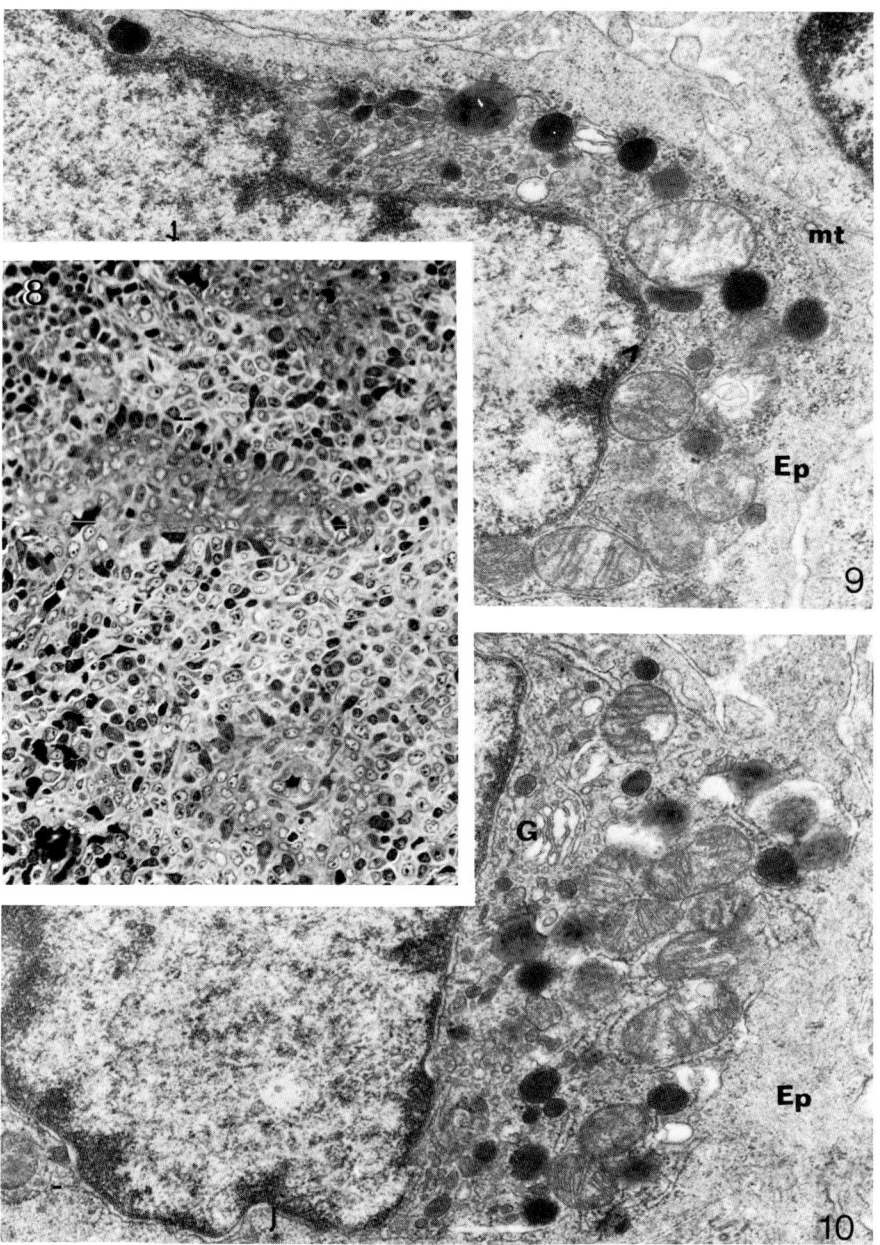

FIG. 8. Embroidering the penicilliform capillaries are the darkly stained ellipsoid-associated cells ×350. (From Olah and Glick, 1982.)

FIGS. 9 and 10. The membrane-bound granules originating from the Golgi (G) region are numerous and smaller than the mitochondria. Ep, ectoplasm; mt, microtubules. ×25,840.

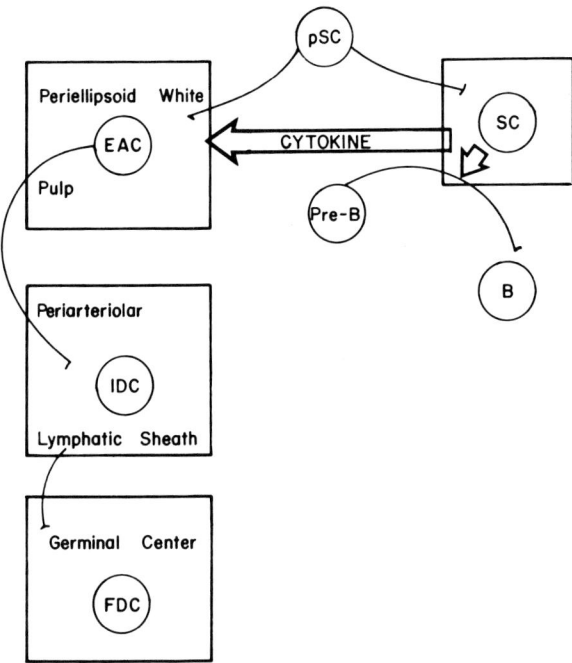

FIG. 11. This scheme identifies a precursor secretory cell (pSC) which homes to the periellipsoid white pulp of the spleen and bursal epithelium. Within the bursa, bud formation and B cell differentiation are dependent on the pSC, which differentiates into a secretory cell (SC). Maturation of cells in the PWP, e.g., the pSC, is dependent on a cytokine released by the bursal SC. The heavy arrow shows action of a putative cytokine. Pre-B, precursor B cell; B, differentiated B cell; EAC, ellipsoid-associated cell; IDC, interdigitating dendritic cell; FCD, follicular dendritic cell, similar in morphology to SC. See text for further discussion. (From Glick and Olah, 1984.)

The secretory cell appears to release a periellipsoid white pulp differentiating factor (cytokine). Therefore, in the absence of the bursa, such a cytokine would be missing.

The events leading to secretory cell differentiation may be used to develop a unifying concept to explain humoral immunity at the tissue level. Antigen substances enter the ellipsoid of the spleen through the stomata of the mid-penicilliform capillaries (Olah and Glick, 1982). Within a few minutes the EACs bind antigen to their surface. Then, the EACs migrate through the white pulp to the red pulp and the cellular region encompassing the central artery. The EACs also appear capable of entering the systemic circulation. Following the iv injection of horseradish peroxidase, large numbers of horseradish-peroxidase-positive mononuclear cells were observed in the blood coincident with the loss of EACs from the ellipsoid (Olah *et al.*, 1984). The circulating EACs would function as an effective vehicle for the transmission of antigenic messages. When the EACs enter the periarteriolar lymphatic sheath, they may be seen as interdigitating dendritic cells and follicular dendritic cells which relate to germinal center formation and B cell differentiation. The follicular dendritic cells are morphologically similar to secretory cells. Thus, the secretory cell of the spleen is the culmination of a series of cellular transformations made possible by the activation of the periellipsoid white pulp by the bursa of Fabricius (Glick and Olah, 1984).

V. The Role of the Avian Thymus

While it is desirable to formulate a theory based on the existing data, one should be aware that in time a modification of the theory will be necessary. Such has been the history of the dissociation concept of the immune response, in which humoral immunity was considered to be controlled by the bursa of Fabricius and cell-mediated immunity by the thymus. Warner and co-workers were responsible for the dissociation theory (Warner and Szenberg, 1962; Warner *et al.*, 1962; Szenberg and Warner, 1962). In their studies, chicks hatched from eggs injected on day 12 of incubation with testosterone propionate failed to produce antibody to several antigens but rejected skin grafts. However, 10% of these chicks exhibited a delayed homograft response. These chickens had experienced a marked reduction in the thymic cortex. From these data and others, Warner and co-workers suggested the dissociation of the immune response. However, a reduced antibody response in thymectomized birds suggested that the thymus was involved in humoral immunity (Cooper *et al.*, 1966; Graetzer *et al.*, 1963). Synergism between T and B cells was indicated (Rouse and Warner, 1972; Ivanyi and Salerno, 1971; Jacobs *et al.*, 1972) when antibody synthesis to a hapten-carrier conjugate was found to be dependent on the presence of the T cell, which acted as the carrier-specific cell (McArthur *et al.*, 1972; Weinbaum *et al.*, 1973).

VI. The Multipotential Stem Cell

While the T cell and B cell may originate from a multipotential stem cell (Moore and Owen, 1966; LeDouarin *et al.*, 1977), the cell that enters the thymic and bursal microenvironment may be precommitted to a pre-T or pre-B cell, respectively (Weber and Foglia, 1980; Weber and Mausner, 1977; Weber and Alexander, 1978; Weber, 1982). Chromosomally marked bone marrow cells of normal 14-day-old embryos (14 DE) or *in ovo* bursectomized embryos were transferred to irradiated recipients of the same age (14 DE). Donor cells identified in the thymus and bursa of recipients were characterized as functional T and B cells. On the other hand, chromosomally marked bone marrow cells from 2 DE normal or *in ovo* bursectomized birds transferred to irradiated 14 DE failed to populate the bursa but appeared in the marrow and thymus, where they were responsive to phytohemagglutinin and concanavalin A. Furthermore, while chromosomally marked bone marrow cells of 15 DE populated both the bursa and thymus of irradiated embryos, their ability to reconstitute the B cell pool of irradiated embryos was abrogated following 24–48 hr of cell culture. Since cells in culture retained their ability to proliferate into T cells, Weber reemphasized his previous conclusion that the bursa and thymus are not seeded by a multipotential stem cell but by cells "differentiated to the level of a committed pre-T or pre-B cell" (Weber, 1982). These observations are supported by the experiments of Boyd *et al.* (1983a,b). They reported that bursal and thymic reticuloepithelial cell monolayers were capable of inducing B and T cell differentiation of embryonic bone marrow or spleen but not bone marrow from posthatched chicks. There appeared to be a precommitment of cells in the embryonic bursa and thymus to B and T, respectively, since cells in these respective tissues were not influenced by exposure to the reciprocal reticuloepithelial monolayer.

If committed pre-T or pre-B cells exist outside the respective environments of the thymus and bursa, then one should not be surprised to find T and B cells present in thymusless and bursaless birds. Our original observation of a nonbursal site for B cell differentiation and the later observation that B cells are present in these birds (see Section III) would strengthen the concept of a pre-B cell. The target cell of the precursor secretory cell and secretory cell would then be the pre-B cell. It is my perception that the precursor secretory cell or similar cells in peripheral lymphoid tissue may act on pre-T cells, leading to the differentiation of T cells in thymusless birds.

VII. Thymic Ontogeny

LeDouarin and her co-workers, taking advantage of the nuclear differences between the quail (LeDouarin, 1973a,b) lymphocyte (one large clump of heterochromatic DNA and small masses attached to the nuclear membrane) and chick lymphocyte (numerous small peripheral clumps of chromatin in the nucleus), grafted presumptive thymic endoderm from different ages of quail and chicks into the somatopleure of the reciprocal 3 DE and determined that the time of colonization of the quail thymus and chick thymus was 5–6 and 6.5–8 days, respectively (LeDouarin et al., 1976; LeDouarin and Jotereau, 1975). The first wave of lymphocyte precursor cells enter the quail thymus at 6 days of embryonic development and lasts 24 hr (Jotereau and LeDouarin, 1982). The cyclic nature of lymphoid precursor cell seeding of thymus was demonstrated by chimeric experiments. Quail thymic grafts from 7 to 9 DE to the somatopleure of 3-day chick embryos failed to reveal lymphocytes of host origin when they remained in the host for the equivalent of 11 days of embryonic development. However, if extended an additional day, chick lymphoid precursor cells were observed. Therefore, the second wave of lymphoid precursor cells begins in 11 DE and appears to be complete within 24 hr since thymi from 12 or 13 DE implanted into chick embryos did not receive lymphoid precursor cells from the host. A third influx of cells into the thymus occurred in 17 DE.

VIII. The Thymic Microenvironment

The embryonic thymus also exhibits a rhythmicity when one follows ontogeny of cellular size and morphology. The large lymphoid cell (10 μm) of 11 DE decreased to 8 μm in 13 DE and declined to 5.5 μm between 15 and 16 DE (Sugimoto et al., 1977a). A contributory event leading to the appearance of small lymphocytes by day 13 is the presence of cytoplasmic processes which pinch off from the cell. This is not unusual to observe, since it has been recorded during spermiogenesis. Paralleling the appearance of small lymphocytes (13 DE) was the abrupt appearance of an embryonic T antigen in about 60% of the cells. The periods between 12 and 13 and 15 and 16 DE may reflect two waves of stimulation emanating within the microenvironment of the thymus. The significance of these waves of differentiation may originate from the reticuloepithelial cells, which contribute the soluble factors necessary for cell differentiation. Morphological evidence for the soluble factor was offered by Sugimoto et al. (1977b). Electron-lucent vacuoles and dense bodies were present in the epithelium of the thymic cortex of 12 and 13 DE. During this time, some vacuoles contained dense material. The density of the material within the inclusion vacuoles appeared to decrease after its entrance into the vacuoles. The lower density might reflect loss into cytoplasm or loss external to the cell. These events related to the appearance of small lymphocytes with T antigen in 12 to 13 DE. The authors suggested that the precursor of the thymus humoral factor may reside in the dense bodies and require activation by a proteolytic enzyme.

A second type of reticuloepithelial cell identified in the medulla lacked electron-lucent vacuoles but contained cysts with dense material. A second medullary epithelial cell possessed dense granules. These cells were referred to as secretory cells by the author. Lymphoid cells have been observed in the thymus of as early as 9 to 10 DE (Yasuda *et al.*, 1980). Their movement was characterized by the formation of an organelle-free hyaline process, which produced a bilobed appearance of the cell. The release of these products to the exterior suggests a similarity to the secretory cell of the bursa medulla. The authors concluded that lymphoid cell differentiation is first under the influence of the cortical reticuloepithelial cells, which affect the appearance of T antigen, and then the medullary epithelium contributes to the differentiation of the immunocompetent cell. Hakanson *et al.* (1974) identified in the thymus of posthatched chicks two cells which resembled endocrine cells. Both cells possessed granules. One cell contained 5-hydroxytryptamine and stained with argentaffin, chromaffin, and argyrophil. The other displayed the potential to store L-dopa and stained with argyrophil. Based on their fine structure and histochemistry, these cells resembled cells which synthesize polypeptide hormones. Thus, an endocrine function might be attributed to the thymic cells. It should be emphasized that Sherman and Auerbach (1966) and Peterson and Good (1966) had previously demonstrated differences in the size of thymic cells in embryos and Sherman and Auerbach (1966) had emphasized that a cellular difference exists among the thymic lobes. Since Sugimoto *et al.* (1977a,b) failed to identify the lobes used (possibly all lobes were used), one would be interested if the changes they noted would occur at different rates in the different lobes.

After hatch, a size-distribution analysis of thymocytes revealed three subpopulations of cells (Droege *et al.*, 1974). Cell type III was the largest, the fastest electrophoretically, and the lightest in density. Since it was the sole representative in 1-month-old adults, it may be responsible for the graft-versus-host reaction. Also, since cell types II and III were absent in neonatal chicks, the suppressor T cell may be their cell type I.

That the differentiation of thymic lymphocytes may reflect enzymatic changes was suggested by Sugimoto and Bollum (1979). Terminal deoxynucleotidyltransferase (Tdt) was absent from the thymus of 10 DE, appeared in 12 DE, and increased steadily between 13 and 15 and 16 and 19 DE. Paralleling the appearance and increase in Tdt was a decline in thymic cell size. The initial positive cells in 12 DE ranged between 7 and 7.5 μm, while the negative cells were 9 μm. By day 20 the majority of T cells were 6 μm or less. The declining cell size may reflect the rapid DNA cycling of thymic cells in 14 to 20 DE. We have demonstrated with cell-flow cytometry that the thymic cell has a greater percentage of cells in S phase than does the bursa in 15 DE (Glick *et al.*, 1984). The small thymic cells may be more receptive than the larger ones to signals from the thymus' microenvironment (reticuloepithelium and medullary epithelium), which would be responsible for activating the genomic loci coding for Tdt. Terminal deoxynucleotidyltransferase may be necessary to activate the major histocompatibility complex and hence the incorporation into the cells' membrane of antigenic products coded for by the B-F and B-L loci, which represent the chicken's major histocompatibility complex (Briles *et al.*, 1982). The appearance of Tdt correlated with the second inflow of cells to the thymus (Rouget and Penit, 1980). Are the Tdt cells the colonizing cells? Do the Tdt cells exert control over Tdt synthesis of host cells and/or transformation of cells to small lymphocytes? Further evidence that enzymatic changes may influence or relate to thymocyte maturation may be derived from the experiments with DNA ligase (David and Vinson, 1979; David *et al.*, 1980, 1981). DNA ligase I (185,000 Da) and DNA ligase II (85,000 Da) may be important in cell replication and DNA repair, respectively (David and Vinson, 1979). The heavy DNA ligase (8.25) is prominent in the embryo, disappears at the time of hatch, and is replaced by the lighter DNA ligase (6.25). The presence of 8.25 DNA ligase I and two populations of thymic cells (7.5 and 5.0 μm) were markedly altered in 16 DE receiving dexamethesone (David *et al.*, 1980). Within 2 days these embryos possessed only cells of 5 μm and DNA ligase II (6.25). Similar results were observed with hydrocortisone. All of the cells of the dexamethesone-treated embryos were T-Ag$^+$, while the T-Ag$^+$ cells of the control embryos were restricted to the 25% of the cells which were 5 μm. Therefore, the corticosteroids advanced the appearance of 6.2 DNA ligase, which appeared to be correlated with the size of the cell and acquisition of T antigen. These data suggest that 6.25 DNA ligase may be an indicator of thymic maturation.

Interleukin 2 (IL-2) with T cell growth potential has been isolated from chicken spleens exposed to concanavalin A (Schauenstein *et al.*, 1982; Schnetzler *et al.*, 1983). Splenic blast cells proliferate in the presence of avian IL-2 but not in the presence of murine T cell growth factor (Schauenstein et al., 1982). Avian lymphocytes cultured in the presence of IL-2 were maintained for several weeks (Schnetzler et al., 1983). These researchers identified two biologically active peaks by gel filtration in the ranges of 19,500 to 21,000 and 9,000 to 11,000 Da. Resting T cells (G_0) are activated by two signals, one for a lectin or antigen and the other for IL-1 (Klaus and Hawrylowicz, 1984). Without the presence of IL-2, the cell may be arrested in G_1. Therefore, avian IL-2 should allow one to maintain T cells in culture and assist studies concerning the transition of G_1 to S. Isolating the avian cell producing IL-2 would identify the avian T helper cells. This would allow one to raise antibody to T helper cells and eventually to other subpopulations of T cells.

Acknowledgments

Sincere appreciation is extended to Mrs. Janice Orr for typing the manuscript, Doris Thompson (MT, ASCP) for laboratory assistance, NIH for decades of research support, USDA for special research grant 84-CRSR-2-2435, and Mississippi Agricultural and Forestry Experiment Station (Journal article number 5862).

References

Beaupain, D., Martin, C., and Dieterlen-Lievre, F. (1979). *Blood* **53**, 212.
Bockman, D. E., and Cooper, M. D. (1973). *Am. J. Anat.* **136**, 455–478.
Boyd, R. L., Ward, H. A., and Muller, H. K. (1983a). *J. Reticuloendothel. Soc.* **34**, 371–382.
Boyd, R. L., Ward, H. A., and Muller, H. K. (1983b). *J. Reticuloendothel. Soc.* **34**, 383–393.
Brand, A., Gilmour, D. G., and Goldstein, G. (1976). *Science* **193**, 319–321.
Brand, A., Galton, J., and Gilmour, D. G. (1983). *Eur. J. Immunol.* **13**, 319–321.
Briles, W. E., Bumstead, N., Ewert, D. L., Gilmour, D. G., Gogusev, J., Hala, K., Koch, C., Longenecker, B. M., Nordskog, A. W., Pink, J. R. L., Shierman, L. W., Simonsen, M., Toivanen, O., and Wick, G. (1982). *Immunogenetics* **15**, 441–446.
Cooper, M. D., Peterson, R. D. A., South, M. A., and Good, R. A. (1966). *J. Exp. Med.* **123**, 73–103.
David, J. C., and Vinson, D. (1979). *Exp. Cell Res.* **119**, 69–74.
David, J. C., Vinson, D., and Fedecka-Bruner, B. (1980). *Exp. Cell Res.* **130**, 137–146.
David, J. C., Fedecka-Bruner, B., Mishal, Z., Vinson, D., and Rosenfeld, C. (1981). *Eur. J. Immunol.* **11**, 593–596.
Dieterlen-Lievre, T. D., Beaufain, D., and Martin, S. (1976). *Ann. Immunol. (Paris)* **127**, 857–863.
Droege, W., Zucker, R., and Hannig, K. (1974). *Cell. Immunol.* **12**, 186–193.
Eerola, E., Lassila, O., Gilmour, D. G., and Toivanen, A. (1982). *J. Immunol.* **128**, 2652–2655.
Eerola, E., Jalkanen, S., Granfors, K., and Toivanen, A. (1983a). *J. Immunol.* **131**, 120–124.

Eerola, E., Lassila, O., Gilmour, D. G., and Toivanen, A. (1983b). *Scand. J. Immunol.* **18,** 175–183.
Ewert, D. L., and Cooper, M. D. (1978). *Immunogenetics* **7,** 521–535.
Fitzimmons, R. C., Garrod, E. M., and Garnett, I. (1973). *Cell. Immunol.* **9,** 377–383.
Glick, B. (1960). *Poultry Sci.* **39,** 1097–1101.
Glick, B. (1964). *In* "The Thymus in Immunobiology" (R. A. Good and A. E. Gabrielsen, eds.), pp. 343–358. Harper and Row, New York.
Glick, B. (1968). *Proc. Soc. Exp. Biol. Med.* **127,** 1054–1057.
Glick, B. (1970). *BioScience* **20,** 602–604.
Glick, B. (1971). *Transplantation* **11,** 433–439.
Glick, B. (1977). *Int. Rev. Cytol.* **48,** 345–402.
Glick, B. (1981). *Fed. Proc.* **49,** 1102.
Glick, B. (1982). *In* "The Reticuloendothelial System: Phylogeny and Ontogeny" (N. Cohen and M. M. Siegel, eds.), Vol. 3, pp. 509–540. Plenum, New York.
Glick, B. (1983). *In* "Avian Biology" (D. S. Farner, J. R. King, and K. C. Parker, eds.), Vol. VII, pp. 443–500. Academic Press, New York.
Glick, B., and Olah, I. (1984). *Immunol. Today* **15,** 162–165.
Glick, B., and Sadler, C. R. (1961). *Poultry Sci.* **40,** 185–189.
Glick, G., LaVia, M. F., and Koger, B. (1984). *Poultry Sci.* **64.**
Goldstein, G., Scheid, M., Boyse, M. E., Brand, A., and Gilmour, D. G. (1977). *Cold Spring Harbor Symp. Quant. Biol.* **41,** 5–8.
Graetzer, M. A., Wolfe, H. R., Aspinall, O. L., and Meyer, R. K. (1963). *J. Immunol.* **90,** 878–887.
Granfors, K., Martin, C., Lassila, O., Suvitaival, R., Toivanen, A., and Toivanen, P. (1982). *Clin. Immunol. Immunopathol.* **23,** 459–469.
Grossi, C. E., Lydyard, P. M., and Cooper, M. D. (1977). *J. Immunol.* **119,** 749–756.
Hakanson, W., Larsson, L.-I., and Sundler, F. (1974). *Histochemistry* **39,** 25–34.
Houssaint, F., Belo, M., and LeDouarin, N. (1976). *Dev. Biol.* **53,** 250–264.
Ivanyi, J., and Salerno, A. (1971). *Eur. J. Immunol.* **1,** 227–230.
Jacobs, R. P., Blaese, R. M., and Oppehheim, J. S. (1972). *J. Immunol.* **109,** 324–333.
Jaffe, W. P., and Fechheimer, N. S. (1966). *Nature (London)* **212,** 92.
Jalkanen, S., Granfors, K., Jalkanen, M., and Toivanen, P. (1983a). *J. Immunol.* **130,** 2038–2041.
Jalkanen, S., Granfors, K., Jalkanen, M., and Toivanen, P. (1983b). *Cell. Immunol.* **80,** 367–373.
Jankociv, B. D., and Leskowitz, S. (1965). *Proc. Soc. Exp. Biol. Med.* **118,** 1164–1166.
Jankovic, B. D., Knezevic, A., Isakovic, K., Mitrovic, K., Markovic, M. G., and Rascevic, M. (1975). *Eur. J. Immunol.* **5,** 655–659.
Jankovic, B. D., Isakovic, K., Markovic, B. M., Rascevic, M., and Knezevic, Z. (1976). *Exp. Hematol. (Copenhagen)* **4,** 246–255.
Jankovic, B. D., Isakovic, K., Markovic, B. M., and Rascevic, M. (1977). *Immunology* **32,** 689–699.
Jotereau, F. V., and LeDouarin, N. M. (1982). *J. Immunol.* **129,** 1869–1877.
Kincade, P. W., and Cooper, M. D. (1971). *J. Immunol.* **106,** 371–382.
Klaus, G. G. R., and Hawrylowicz, C. M. (1984). *Immunol. Today* **5,** 15–19.
Lassila, O., Eskola, J., Toivanen, P., Martin, C., and Dieterlen-Lievre, F. (1978). *Nature (London)* **272,** 353–354.
Lassila, O., Eskola, J., and Toivanen, P. (1979). *J. Immunol.* **123,** 2091–2094.
Lassila, O., Eskola, J., Toivanen, P., and Dieterlen-Lievre, F. (1980). *Scand. J. Immunol.* **11,** 445–448.

LeDouarin, N. M. (1973a). *Exp. Cell Res.* **77,** 459–468.
LeDouarin, N. M. (1973b). *Dev. Biol.* **30,** 217–222.
LeDouarin, N. M., and Jotereau, F. V. (1973a). *C. R. Hebd. Seances Acad. Sci. Ser. D* **276,** 629–632.
LeDouarin, N. M., and Jotereau, F. V. (1973b). *Nature (London) New Biol.* **246,** 25–27.
LeDouarin, N. M., and Jotereau, F. B. (1975). *J. Exp. Med.* **142,** 17–40.
LeDouarin, N. M., Jotereau, F. V., and Houssaint, E. (1975). *Proc. Natl. Acad. Sci. U.S.A.* **72,** 2701–2705.
LeDouarin, N. M., Jotereau, F. V., and Houssaint, E. (1976). In "Phylogeny of Thymus and Bone Marrow-Bursa Cells" (R. K. Wright and E. L. Cooper, eds.), pp. 217–226. Elsevier, Amsterdam.
LeDouarin, N. M., Houssaint, E., and Jotereau, F. V. (1977). In "Avian Immunology" (A. A. Bendict, ed.), pp. 29–37. Plenum, New York.
Lerman, S. P., and Weidanz, W. D. (1970). *J. Immunol.* **105,** 614–619.
Lerner, K. G., Glick, B., and McDuffie, F. C. (1971). *J. Immunol.* **107,** 493–511.
McArthur, W. P., Gilmour, D. G., and Thorbecke, J. G. (1972). *Cell. Immunol.* **8,** 103–111.
Martin, C., Beaupain, D., and Dieterlen-Lievre, F. (1978). *Cell Differ.* **7,** 115–130.
Martin, C., Lassila, O., Nurmi, T., Eskola, J., Dieterlen-Lievre, F., and Toivanen, P. (1979). *Scand. J. Immunol.* **10,** 333–338.
Meyer, R. K., Rao, M. A., and Aspinall, R. L. (1959). *Endocrinology* **64,** 890–898.
Moore, M. A. S., and Owen, J. J. T. (1965). *Nature (London)* **208,** 989–990.
Moore, M. A. S., and Owen, J. J. T. (1966). *Dev. Biol.* **14,** 40–51.
Moore, M. A. S., and Owen, J. J. T. (1967). *Lancet* **2,** 658–659.
Olah, I., and Glick, B. (1978a). *Poultry Sci.* **57,** 1445–1450.
Olah, I., and Glick, B. (1978b). *Experientia* **34,** 1642–1643.
Olah, I., and Glick, B. (1979). *Poultry Sci.* **58,** 195–210.
Olah, I., and Glick, B. (1982). *Am. J. Anat.* **165,** 445–480.
Olah, I., Glick, B., McCorkle, F., and Stinson, R. (1979). *Dev. Comp. Immunol.* **3,** 101–115.
Olah, I., Glick, B., and Taylor, R. L., Jr. (1984). *J. Leuk. Biol.* **35,** 501–510.
Petersen, R. D. A., and Good, R. A. (1966). *Blood* **26,** 269–281.
Rouget, P., and Penit, C. (1980). *Cell Differ.* **9,** 329–337.
Rouse, B. T., and Warner, N. L. (1972). *Nature (London) New Biol.* **236,** 79–80.
Schauenstein, K., Globerson, A., and Wick, B. (1982). *Dev. Comp. Immunol.* **6,** 533–540.
Schnetzler, M., Oomen, A., Nowak, J. S., and Franklin, R. M. (1983). *Eur. J. Immunol.* **13,** 560–566.
Sherman, J., and Auerbach, R. (1966). *Blood* **27,** 371–379.
Steinman, R. M., and Nussenzweig, M. C. (1980). *Immunol. Rev.* **53,** 127–147.
St. Pierre, R. L., and Ackerman, G. A. (1966). *Proc. Soc. Exp. Biol. Med.* **122,** 1280–1284.
Subba Rao, D. S. V., McDuffie, F. C., and Glick, B. (1978). *J. Immunol.* **120,** 783–787.
Sugimoto, M., and Bollum, F. J. (1979). *J. Immunol.* **122,** 392–397.
Sugimoti, M., Yasuda, T., and Egashira, Y. (1977a). *Dev. Biol.* **56,** 281–292.
Sugimoto, M., Yasuda, T., and Egashira, Y. (1977b). *Dev. Biol.* **56,** 293–305.
Szenberg, A., and Warner, N. L. (1962). *Nature (London)* **194,** 146–147.
Thorbecke, G.-J., Palladino, M. A., and Lerman, S. P. (1972). *Contemp. Top. Immunobiol.* **9,** 91–107.
Toivanen, P., Lassila, O., Martin, C., Dieterlen-Lievre, F., Nurmi, T., and Eskola, J. (1979). *Folia Biol. (Prague)* **25,** 299–300.
Warner, N. L., and Burnet, F. M. (1961). *Aust. J. Biol. Sci.* **13,** 380–387.

Warner, N. L., and Szenberg, A. (1962). *Nature (London)* **96,** 784.
Warner, N. L., Szenberg, A., and Burnet, F. M. (1962). *Aust. J. Exp. Biol. Med. Sci.* **40,** 373–388.
Weber, W. T. (1982). *In* "In vivo Immunology" (P. Nieuwenhuis, A. A. van den Broek, and M. G. Hanna, Jr., eds.), Vol. 149, pp. 119–126. Plenum Press, New York.
Weber, W. T., and Alexander, J. E. (1978). *J. Immunol.* **121,** 653–657.
Weber, W. T., and Foglia, L. M. (1980). *Cell. Immunol.* **52,** 89–94.
Weber, W. T., and Mausner, R. (1977). *In* "Avian Immunology" (A. A. Benedict, ed.), pp. 47–59. Plenum, New York.
Weinbaum, F. I., Gilmour, D. G., and Thorbecke, J. G. (1973). *J. Immunol.* **110,** 1434–1436.
White, R. G. (1963). *In* "Ciba Foundation Study Group No. 16. The Immunologically Competent Cells" (G. E. W. Wolstenholme and J. K. Knight, eds.), pp. 6–16. Churchill, London.
White, R. G., French, F. I., and Stark, J. M. (1970). *J. Med. Microbiol.* **3,** 65–83.
White, R. G., Henderson, D. G., Eslami, M. G., and Nielsen, K. H. (1975). *Immunology* **28,** 1–21.
Yasuda, T., Sugimoto, M., and Egashira, Y. (1980). *Thymus* **2,** 5–18.
Ziegler, A., and Pink, J. R. L. (1976). *J. Biol. Chem.* **251,** 5391–5396.

Neutrophilic Leukocyte Structure and Function in Domestic Animals

T. A. BERTRAM[1]

National Animal Disease Center, Ames, Iowa

I.	Introduction	91
II.	Neutrophil Morphology	92
	A. Neutrophil Nucleus	92
	B. Neutrophil Granules	92
	C. Neutrophil Cytoplasmic Organelles Other Than Granules	102
	D. Neutrophil Membranes	102
III.	Neutrophil Metabolism and Antimicrobial Systems	103
	A. Oxygen-Dependent Mechanisms	104
	B. Oxygen-Independent Mechanisms	106
IV.	Neutrophil Migration and Activation	110
V.	Phagocytosis and Degranulation	114
VI.	Granulocytopoiesis	116
VII.	Neutrophils of the Circulating Blood (Neutrophil Heterogeneity)	117
VIII.	Neutrophil Function in Inflammatory and Immunologic Processes	118
IX.	Summary	121
	References	122

I. Introduction

The neutrophilic leukocyte is a short-lived cell which serves as a first line of defense in inflammation. Because neutrophils are mobile, they can migrate rapidly through vessel walls to release stored granules which contain several microbicidal systems. Release of granule components aids neutrophil migration through tissue spaces (chemotaxis) and can cause increased vascular permeability and tissue necrosis.

---

[1]Present address: Department of Veterinary Pathobiology, College of Veterinary Medicine, University of Illinois, Urbana, Illinois.

The purpose of this article is to discuss the structure and function of the neutrophilic leukocyte, emphasizing species differences where possible, and to discuss some recent advances relating to the neutrophil's role in host defense and inflammation.

II. Neutrophil Morphology

A. Neutrophil Nucleus

Species differences in neutrophilic leukocyte morphology can be seen at the light microscopic level. Mature equine neutrophils have a distinctly multilobulated nucleus, whereas there is only a slight indentation separating nuclear lobes in mature neutrophils from dogs and cats. Bovine neutrophil granules are faintly visible, in contrast to the indistinguishable granules of neutrophils from other domestic animals. Species differences in nucleus and granule morphology are much more evident at the ultrastructural and morphometric level (see Figs. 1, 2, and 3 and Table I).

Ultrastructurally, the mature neutrophil nucleus appears as separate nuclear lobes (a sectioning artifact) and is primarily composed of heterochromatin, seldom containing a nucleolus (Figs. 1, 2, and 3). The neutrophil nucleus is unlike most other nucleated eukaryotic cells because of its size, shape, and low number of nuclear pores (Baggiolini, 1980). Nuclear segmentation was once thought to facilitate neutrophil migration through blood vessel walls and connective tissue spaces. Nuclear segmentation is defective in the Pelger–Huet anomaly of Basenji dogs, yet random migration and chemotaxis are not affected (Latimer and Prasse, 1982). The Pelger–Huet anomaly of foxhounds is associated with defective chemotaxis, but this is not a result of abnormal nuclear lobulation (Parmely et al., 1982). These diseases indicate that nuclear segmentation is not a requirement for normal chemotaxis of neutrophils.

Neutrophils can conduct some functions without a nucleus. Neutrophil fragments with or without nuclear remnants ("pseudoplatelets") may represent the final stages of neutrophil maturation and nuclear segmentation (Hanker and Giammara, 1983). Neutrophil pseudoplatelets may augment the inflammatory response by releasing neutrophil enzymes into areas not readily accessible by intact neutrophils (see Section VIII).

B. Neutrophil Granules

Two types of neutrophilic leukocyte granules can be differentiated using peroxidase staining procedures (Graham and Karnovsky, 1966):

the peroxidase-positive azurophil or primary granules and the peroxidase-negative specific or secondary granule (Figs. 1 and 2). A problem of nomenclature becomes evident when discussing neutrophil granules. Primary granules are not primary lysosomes (membrane-bound structures that contain acid hydrolase) and secondary granules are not secondary lysosomes (phagocytic, pinocytotic, or autophagocytic vacuoles which contain acid hydrolases as a result of fusion with a primary lysosome). Furthermore, secondary granules do not originate from primary granules as was once believed (MacGregor, 1980).

Azurophil granules vary in size and shape among the domestic animals (Figs. 1, 2, and 3). In humans and horses these granules can be round or ellipsoidal with a crystalloid structure along their major axis (Fig. 4; Bertram and Coignoul, 1982). Both the round and crystalloid primary granules contain peroxidase (Baggiolini, 1980; Baggiolini *et al.*, 1974; Baintain *et al.*, 1971). Secondary granules have a variable size and shape in the same species and in different species of domestic animals (Figs. 1, 2, and 3). Distinction between granules is not always absolute and there may be more than two major granule populations in the human (Beard and Novikoff, 1968), rabbit (Spicer and Hardin, 1969), bovine (Gennaro *et al.*, 1983a; Baggiolini *et al.*, 1985), sheep (Baggiolini *et al.*, 1985), goat (Baggiolini *et al.*, 1985), equine (Bertram and Coignoul, 1982), and canine (O'Donnell and Anderson, 1982) neutrophil.

Azurophil granule function is characterized more completely than specific granule function. Azurophil granules contain microbicidal elements (myeloperoxidase and lysozyme) and digestive enzymes (acid hydrolases and neutral proteases). These enzymes, which function in concert with membrane-bound and cytoplasmic enzymes, are active in killing and digesting phagocytized microbes and when released will cause tissue damage (Goldstein, 1976). Primary granules also contain cationic proteins (Zeya and Spitznagel, 1966; Odeburg and Olsson, 1975; Drazin and Lehrer, 1977; Weiss *et al.*, 1978a) and other nonlysosomal enzymes. Two subpopulations of primary granules have been demonstrated in the rabbit. The two forms are similar in composition except that one contains lactoferrin and the other contains a unique iron-binding protein (Parmely *et al.*, 1982). The presence of acid hydrolase in primary granules is similar to DeDuve's original description of lysosomes found in other tissues (DeDuve and Wattiqux, 1966), but designating azurophil granules as lysosomes has been questioned. The problem is exemplified in the human, where lysosomal hydrolases were demonstrated in primary granules (making them lysosomes) but quantitatively this enzyme was only a minor constituent of the overall granule composition (Baggiolini, 1980).

Specific granules contain antimicrobial factors and microbicidal en-

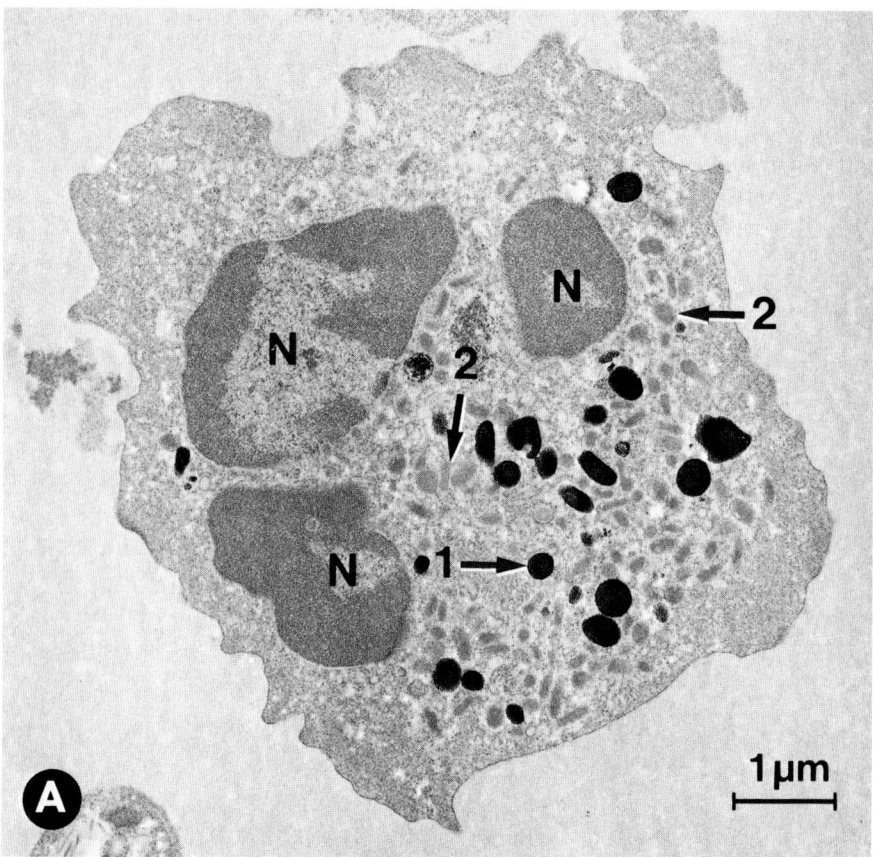

Fig. 1. Peripheral blood neutrophilic leukocyte: (A) equine neutrophil myeloperoxidase, unstained; (B) porcine neutrophil. Uranyl acetate and lead citrate stains were used. M, Mitochondria; 1, primary granules; 2, secondary granules; N, nucleus. Blood was collected into EDTA and buffy coat samples fixed with 2.5% glutaraldehyde in cacodylate buffer. Primary granules were stained to test for the presence of myeloperoxidase using H_2O_2 and diaminobenzidine.

zymes. Specific granules have been shown to contain lactoferrin and approximately 66% of the neutrophil's lysozyme (Spitznagel et al., 1974). Secondary granules have a strong nonspecific alkaline phosphatase activity but no acid phosphatase activity (Wetzel et al., 1963, 1967b) and thus are not lysosomes (if lysosomes are defined as being rich in acid hydrolases).

Human neutrophils have one primary granule for every two secondary granules (Baintain, 1977). In humans the total neutrophil granule

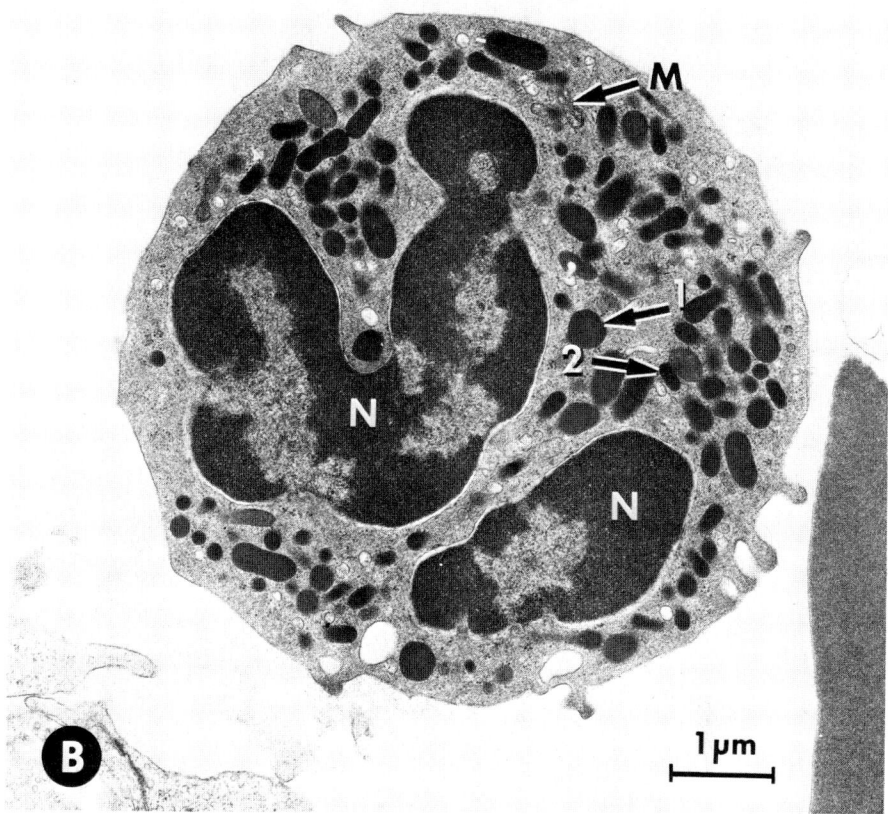

FIG. 1B.

volume is divided equally between primary and secondary granules because secondary granules are approximately 50% smaller than primary granules (Hoffstein and Weissmann, 1975). The percentage of neutrophil volume occupied by granules in various domestic animals is shown in Table I. Secondary granules make up a majority of the granule volume in mature equine neutrophils (Bertram and Coignoul, 1982).

Morphometric results for horses (Table I) differ from previously reported results (Bertram and Coignoul, 1982). Areas of the neutrophil and nucleus are 16 to 20% smaller than those previously reported. This discrepancy is the result of sampling differences between the two studies. Data for Table 1 were collected from all neutrophil profiles regardless of the presence or absence of nuclear profiles. Bertram and Coignoul (1982) collected data only from neutrophils which contained

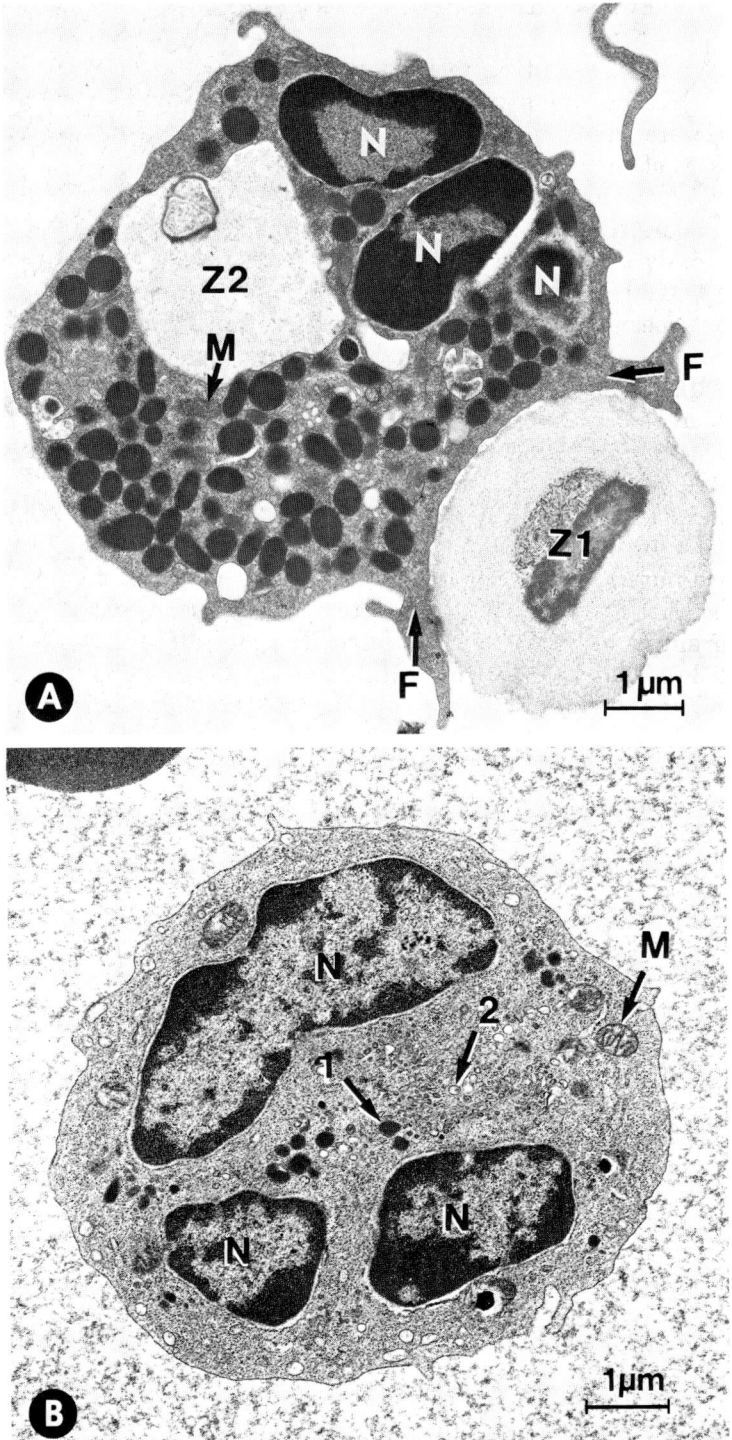

nuclear profiles resulting in a larger average cell area and average nuclear area but the same neutrophil granule volume. These results demonstrate the fact that granules are randomly distributed in the cytoplasm of resting neutrophils and the need for clearly designating sampling protocol in morphometric studies.

Morphometric results (Table I) indicate bovine neutrophils have a considerably larger cell granule volume than neutrophils of other domestic animals. Correlation of enzyme concentration in granules from different species has not been evaluated, although bovine and ovine neutrophils do have reduced myeloperoxidase and lysozyme activity (Table II). If the granule enzyme concentration were the same, cattle would have a marked increase in neutrophil-associated microbicidal enzymes compared to other domestic animals. If the enzyme concentration in bovine neutrophil granules were less than that of other species, then the total neutrophil enzyme concentration would be similar between the various species.

Cattle have a potent antimicrobial system which is distinct from other species. Two bactericidal proteins have been demonstrated in large granules (a third granule form) of bovine neutrophils (Gennaro *et al.*, 1983a). These proteins have different molecular weights and bactericidal activities. The high-molecular-weight protein is more active against Gram-negative bacteria, and the low-molecular-weight protein is more effective in killing Gram-positive bacteria. On the basis of *in vitro* antibacterial potency, these proteins are comparable to oxygen-dependent killing mechanisms (see Section III,A). This potent oxygen-independent antimicrobial activity is exclusively located in large granules (Gennaro *et al.*, 1983a,b). Using biochemical and morphological procedures these granules were shown to possess lactoferrin, but lack peroxidase, lysosomal hydrolases, and metalloproteases. This third granule type has also been reported in other ruminants (Gennaro *et al.*, 1983a,b; Baggiolini *et al.*, 1985). It has a round profile

FIG. 2. Peripheral blood neutrophilic leukocyte. (A) Bovine neutrophil and opsonized zymosan. The organelle free zone (F) near zymosan particle Z1 is an area of microfilament polymerization and pseudopodia formation. Degranulation can occur before phagosome formation is complete, resulting in extracellular release of granule enzymes. Primary and secondary granules are closely apposed to ingested zymosan particle Z2. Uranyl acetate and lead citrate stains were used. (B) Ovine neutrophil. Myeloperoxidase, uranyl acetate, and lead citrate stains were used. M = mitochondria, 1 = primary granules, 2 = secondary granules, N = nucleus. Blood was collected into EDTA and buffy coat samples fixed with 2.5% glutaraldehyde in cacodylate buffer. Primary granules were stained to test for the presence of myeloperoxidase using H_2O_2 and diaminobenzidine.

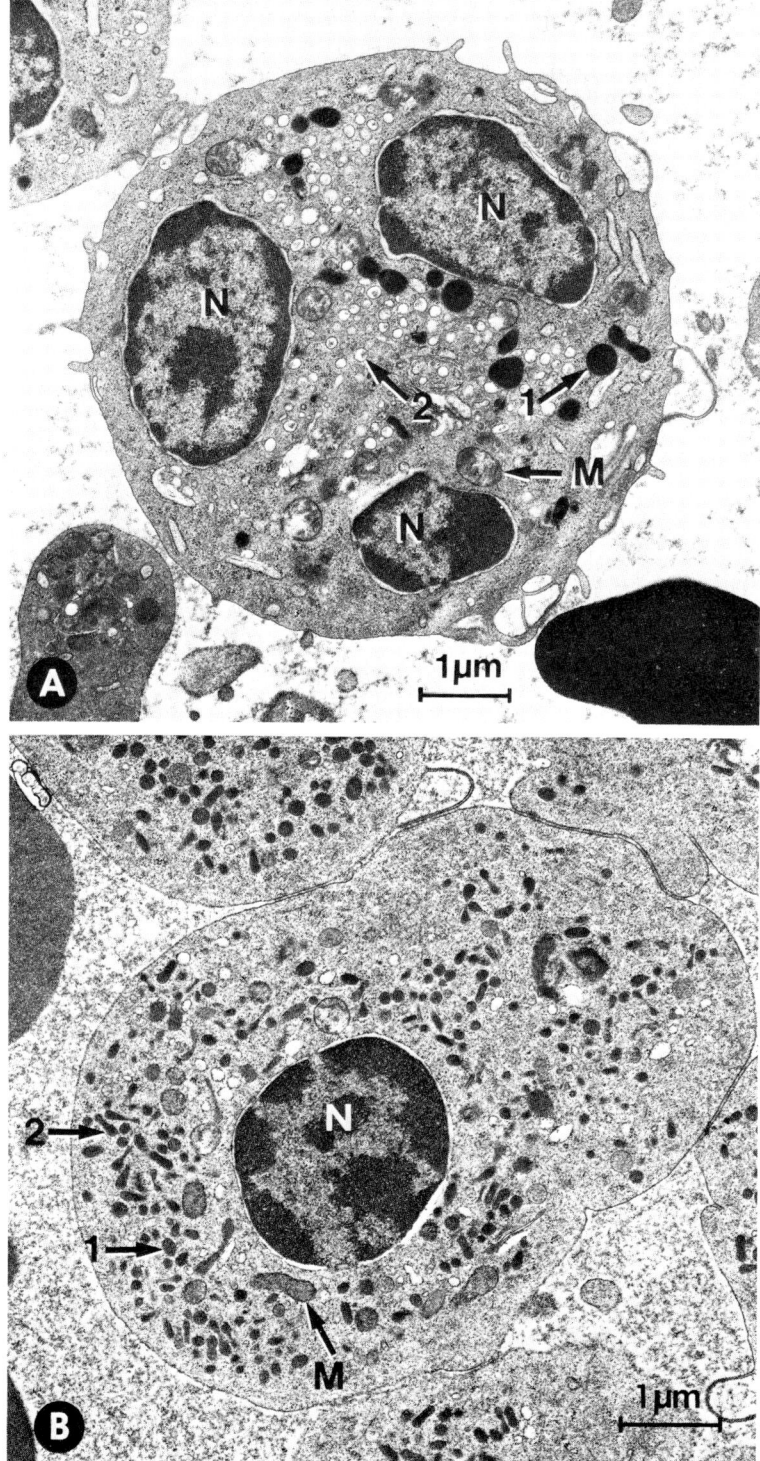

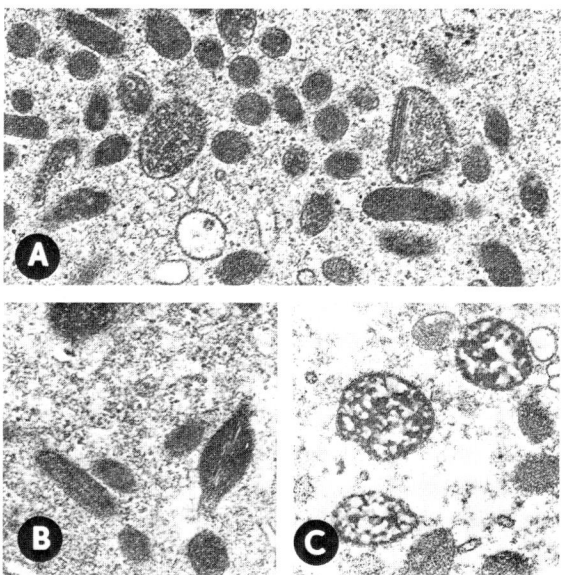

FIG. 4. Equine peripheral blood neutrophilic leukocyte granules. A flocculent granule which may be in the process of enzyme release (C) and a tertiary granule forms (A and B) with crystalline structures near granule membrane (A) and in a central location (B). Granules with crystalloid structures similar to those in (A) and (B) have been demonstrated in acute monoblastic leukemia in humans (Kim et al., 1982).

with a sharply defined membrane and a uniformly pale electron density and may be a unique characteristic of ruminant neutrophils (Baggiolini et al., 1985). The large granule of ruminant neutrophils does not likely correspond to the tertiary granule of rabbit and human neutrophils.

Other granule "types" have been proposed by various investigators. Their classification methods have been based on morphological and/or biochemical criteria. These classification systems cannot be extended beyond the species being studied. A third granule type has been seen in segmented rabbit heterophils (approximately 300 nm at the greatest length) and in human peripheral blood neutrophils (Spicer and Hard-

FIG. 3. Peripheral blood neutrophilic leukocyte: (A) Canine neutrophil stained with peroxidase, uranyl acetate, and lead citrate; (B) feline neutrophil stained with uranyl acetate and lead citrate. M = mitochondria, 1 = primary granules, 2 = secondary granules, N = nucleus. Blood was collected into EDTA and buffy coat samples fixed with 2.5% glutaraldehyde in cacodylate buffer. Primary granules were stained to test for the presence of myeloperoxidase using H_2O_2 and diaminobenzidine.

TABLE I

MORPHOMETRIC ANALYSIS OF PERIPHERAL BLOOD NEUTROPHILS OF VARIOUS DOMESTIC ANIMALS[a]

Species	Number of animals	Granule area (μm^2)	Mitochondria area (μm^2)	Neutrophil area (μm^2)	Nucleus area (μm^2)	Granule volume[b]
Equine	3	3.64 ± 0.3	1.0 ± 0.3	33.60 ± 0.9	4.06 ± 0.2	11.0
Porcine	2	4.83 ± 0.9	0.9 ± 0.2	33.96 ± 1.0	4.11 ± 0.4	14.0
Bovine	4	7.94 ± 0.2	1.7 ± 0.3	36.10 ± 2.6	6.00 ± 0.4	21.9
Canine	2	3.61 ± 0.3	1.0 ± 0.2	31.91 ± 1.2	4.61 ± 0.3	11.3
Feline	1	4.90 ± 0.4	0.5 ± 0.1	32.59 ± 3.0	5.36 ± 0.8	15.0

[a]Blood was collected into EDTA and buffy coat samples fixed with 2.5% glutaraldehyde in cacodylate buffer. The analysis was conducted as previously described by Bertram and Coignoul (1982).
[b]Percentage of neutrophil volume.

in, 1969; Zucker-Franklin, 1968). These granules have been called tertiary granules since they appear late in cell development (Wetzel et al., 1967a). Tertiary granules are electron lucent when seen in neutrophils fixed in glutaraldehyde but have a moderate density in cells fixed in Dalton's chromic–osmium solution. Acid phosphatase activity and acid mucosubstances have been demonstrated in these granules (Hardin et al., 1968). These granules have been shown to contain about 50% of the total neutrophil content of cathepsin D and B, protease 3 (Baggiolini et al., 1978), and plasminogen activator (Bretz, 1978).

Using ultrastructural and cytochemical techniques, several granule forms have been demonstrated in the equine neutrophil (Fig. 4). The number of these granule forms can be affected by using different isolation techniques (Bertram and Coignoul, 1982) or by viral infection (Coignoul et al., 1984a). The possibility that these forms relate to reduced neutrophil cytotoxicity has also been proposed (Coignoul et al., 1984b). These granules may represent the earliest stage of neutrophil activation leading to degranulation. Changes in granule morphology during degranulation also occur with mast cells.

Neutrophils with toxic granules are seen in tissue from infectious processes or after the administration of endotoxin (Horn et al., 1964; Horn et al., 1965). These are primary granules which have a uniquely high affinity for Romanowsky stains, resulting in a very intense staining pattern (McCall et al., 1969). The staining character of toxic granules is due to the high amount of sulfated mucosubstances present in

TABLE II

ENZYME ACTIVITY IN BLOOD NEUTROPHILS OF DOMESTIC ANIMALS[a]

Species	β-Glucuronidase	Arylsulphatase	Myeloperoxidase	Lysozyme	Alkaline phosphatase	Acid phosphatase
Equine	++	+	++	++	+++	++
Porcine	+	++	++	+	+++	++
Bovine	+	+++	+	−	++	+
Ovine	++	+	+	−	++	+
Canine	+	NR	+++	+	+	NR
Feline	+++	NR	+	−	−	NR

[a] Based on approximately 5×10^6 cells. Neutrophils in all species have nonspecific esterase, glycogen, and sudanophilic granules (Jain, 1967, 1968, 1970a,b). +++, high enzyme activity; ++, moderate enzyme activity; +, low enzyme activity; −, no detectable enzyme activity; NR, not reported. Data from Chibber and Castle (1983), Healy (1982), and Raush and Moore (1975).

the granule. Bone marrow release of immature neutrophils with mucosaccharide-rich primary granules probably explains the presence of these neutrophil granules after LPS administration (Horn and Spicer, 1964, 1965).

C. Neutrophil Cytoplasmic Organelles Other Than Granules

Subcellular structures other than granules are scarce in circulating neutrophilic leukocytes, indicating the high degree of differentiation of mature neutrophils. A narrow rim of cytoplasm around the periphery of the neutrophil is generally free of organelles and inclusions (glycogen, lipid, etc.) but is rich in cytoskeletal proteins (see Sections IV and V). Areas of opacity in the neutrophil cytoplasm are the result of glycogen extraction by staining in block with uranyl acetate (Baggiolini, 1980). This artifact may not be seen in each of the domestic animals, since the amount of neutrophil glycogen varies markedly between various species (Figs. 1, 2, and 3; Jain, 1969).

The ultrastructural morphology of cytoplasmic organelles in neutrophils isolated from the various domestic animals has been extensively studied (Bertram and Coignoul, 1982; Sonoda and Kobayashi, 1966, 1970a,b; Yamada and Sonoda, 1970). Neutrophils have a centrally located Golgi apparatus with limited amounts of smooth endoplasmic reticulum but a distinct perinuclear membrane. Structure and function of the cytocavitary network has gone unnoticed by most investigators studying neutrophils. With the introduction of morphometric techniques and cell-surface antigen markers, the role of the cytocavitary network in mature neutrophils may be evaluated.

D. Neutrophil Membranes

Neutrophilic leukocyte plasma and granule membranes differ from those of other eukaryotic cells (Baggiolini, 1980; Baggiolini *et al.*, 1976). Freeze-fracture procedures have demonstrated that granule membranes have a higher intramembrane particle density with higher numbers of intramembrane particles on the E fracture face (inner or exoplasmic leaflet) than the P fracture face (outer or protoplasmic leaflet). The neutrophil plasma membrane is rich in intramembrane particles but the particle density on the P face is similar to the E face of granule membranes. Intracellular membrane fusion in neutrophils occurs, as with other mammalian secretory cells, through the interaction of protein-depleted areas of involved membranes. Particle distribution in the granule membrane may have a role in the fusion of granules with phagocytic vacuoles since both granule and cytoplasmic membrane particle distribution is controlled by cytoskeletal elements (Amherdt et al., 1978).

Enzymes in neutrophil membranes vary among domestic animals. A membrane-associated acid aryl phosphatase (not lysosomal acid phosphatase) (Baggiolini et al., 1970a, 1976) that is likely to be identical to a previously isolated phosphatase (Woodin and Wieneke, 1970a,b) is stimulated by staphylococcal leukocidin. Stimulation of this enzyme occurs under the same conditions which allow leukocidin to exert its cytotoxic action (Woodin and Weineke, 1970b). Alkaline phosphatase has also been found to be associated with neutrophil membranes. In human neutrophils this is an exclusively membrane-associated enzyme. In most animals, except monkeys (Rausch and Canonico, 1975), the bulk of the alkaline phosphatase is in the secondary granules (Baggiolini, 1972). The enzyme location within the secondary granules may be restricted to the membrane of these granules. This has been demonstrated in rabbits (Bretz and Baggiolini, 1974), rats, and guinea pigs (Baggiolini, 1980).

Superoxide-anion-producing enzymes may also be membrane bound. In neutrophils stimulated by phorbal myristic acetate (PMA) or opsonized zymosan, superoxide anion is produced at the surface of the neutrophil (Briggs et al., 1975; Goldstein et al., 1977; Root and Metcalf, 1977) and is associated with the membrane fraction when the cell is disrupted (Dewald et al., 1979). This enzyme has a significant role in neutrophil oxidative metabolism (see Section III).

A 5'-nucleotidase (DePierre and Karnovsky, 1974a,b) and a Mg-dependent ATPase (Harlan et al., 1977; Smolen and Weissman, 1978) have also been demonstrated to exist on neutrophil membranes. Both can be used as neutrophil plasma membrane markers, but their functional significance has not been established.

III. Neutrophil Metabolism and Antimicrobial Systems

Neutrophilic leukocyte antimicrobial systems can be classified into oxygen-dependent and oxygen-independent systems. Both systems are contained in the neutrophil's granules and act in concert with membrane and cytoplasmic enzymes. These same systems are associated with neutrophil-induced tissue damage (see Section VIII).

The oxygen-dependent system directly or indirectly involves

glucose-6-phosphate dehydrogenase (hexose monophosphate shunt, HMP), NADPH-flavoprotein oxidase, superoxide dismutase, and myeloperoxidase (Fig. 5). These enzymes lead to the consumption of oxygen and the production of superoxide anion, hydrogen peroxide, HOCl, hydroxyl radical, and singlet oxygen (Klebanoff and Clark, 1978). The oxygen-independent system is more diverse and is composed of various factors, including acid pH, lysozyme, cationic proteins, lactoferrin, vitamin B_{12} binding protein, and acid hydrolases. Which, or what, combination of the various systems is actually involved with the killing of a given type of microbe or tissue damage is controversial; very likely all participate to some degree with varying efficacy.

A. OXYGEN-DEPENDENT MECHANISMS

Neutrophilic leukocytes produce various oxidizing agents, by reduction of molecular oxygen (O_2), in a process called the *respiratory burst*.

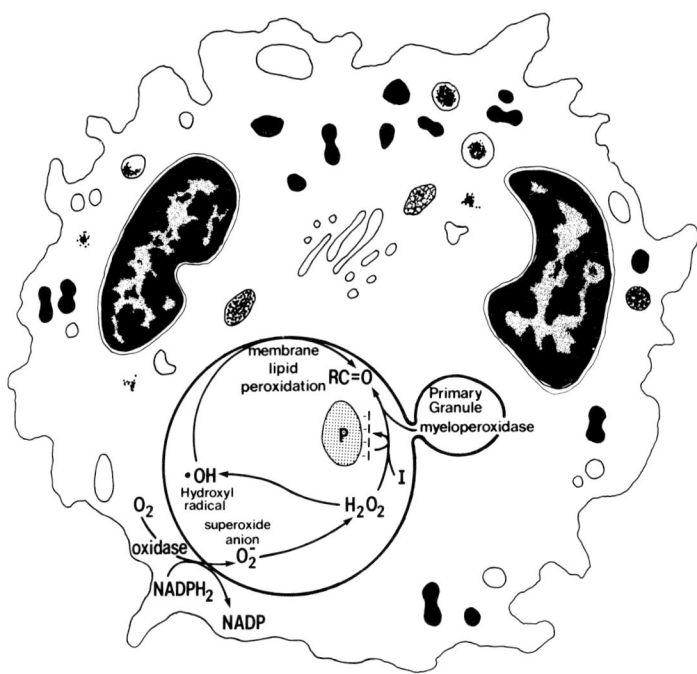

FIG. 5. Schematic diagram of neutrophil phagocytosis, degranulation, and oxidative metabolism. P is an ingested particle; the oxidase enzyme is membrane bound. Active oxygen radicals can also be released into the extracellular space. Oxidase is an NADPH-preferring flavoprotein oxidase.

The respiratory burst includes an increased usage of glucose via the HMP and the generation of reactive oxygen-derived free radicals and their metabolic products (Root and Cohen, 1981; Fantane and Ward, 1982; Sbarra and Karnovsky, 1969). Various aspects of the respiratory burst can be measured in the laboratory. They include increased oxygen consumption, increased fixation of inorganic halides to proteins (halogenation) (Roth and Kaeberle, 1981), generation of light (chemiluminescence), increased reduction of a dye (nitroblue tetrazolium reduction) (Root and Cohen, 1981; Fantane and Ward, 1982), and cytochrome reduction by superoxide anion.

The respiratory burst is a change from the low O_2 metabolism of unstimulated neutrophils (Karnovsky, 1968) to the increased O_2 utilization of stimulated neutrophils (Bachner and Johnston, 1971; Sbarra and Karnovsky, 1969). The increase is accompanied by increases in superoxide anion (O_2^-) (Klebanoff et al., 1977; Root and Metcalf, 1977), hydrogen peroxide (H_2O_2) production (Root and Metcalf, 1977), and glucose oxidation via the HMP (Sbarra and Karnovsky, 1969). The onset of O_2^- generation is preceded by membrane depolarization, which occurs at the same time as degranulation and is associated with changes in the intraneutrophilic cAMP concentration (Korchack and Weissman, 1978).

The basis of the respiratory burst is the activation of a membrane-bound flavoprotein oxidase, which catalyses the following reaction (Gabig and Babior, 1981): $2O_2 + NADPH \rightarrow 2O_2^- + NADP$. The dismutation of O_2^- to H_2O_2 occurs spontaneously or is catalyzed by superoxide dismutase (SOD). SOD is not limited to neutrophils and the concentration of SOD in neutrophils is approximately 10% of that found in the erythrocyte (Gabig and Babior, 1981). NADP availability is increased by the membrane-bound flavoprotein oxidase and the glutathione peroxidase–glutathione reductase system (Voetman et al., 1980). This increased availability of NADP increases HMP activity.

Several other oxygen-derived metabolites have been identified and are associated with neutrophil activation. These reactive derivatives include the hydroxyl radical OH· (Tauber and Babior, 1977; Weiss et al., 1978b; Repine et al., 1979; Rosen and Klebanoff, 1979), singlet oxygen ($^1O_2$) (Allen et al., 1972; Cheson et al., 1976; Anderson et al., 1977; Rosen and Klebanoff, 1977), and hypochlorous acid (HOCl) (Agner, 1972; Harrison and Schultz, 1976). Hydroxyl radicals can be formed by interaction of O_2^- and H_2O_2 in the presence of an oxidized trace metal (the Fenton reaction) (Fee and Valentine, 1977; Haber and Weiss, 1934), direct reduction of H_2O_2 by O_2^-, which also yields O_2 and OH· (the classic Haber–Weiss reaction) (Haber and Weiss, 1934;

Weinstein and Bielski, 1979), and the reaction of O_2^- with hydroperoxides of lipid peroxidation (Babior, 1978). The latter two reactions are either too slow to be physiologically significant (classical Haber–Weiss) or are simply amplification methods of the Fenton reaction which first require lipid oxidation. Which, if any, of these mechanisms is significant *in vivo* is uncertain. Singlet oxygen (delta and sigma forms) can be formed when molecular oxygen absorbs energy, causing one of its two unpaired electrons to reverse its spin direction (Wasserman and Murray, 1979), or as a result of the interaction of H_2O_2 with HOCl (Rosen and Klebanoff, 1977; Piatt and O'Brien, 1979). The latter method has only been demonstrated *in vitro* and may not occur under physiological conditions (Held and Hurst, 1978).

Hypochlorous acid is formed by a reaction combining myeloperoxidase with H_2O_2 to form an enzyme–substrate complex which oxidizes halides (probably chloride in biological systems) to form toxic products (Held and Hurst, 1978; Harrison and Schultz, 1976). Neutrophil-derived N-chloroamines react with chemotactic peptides and plasma protease inhibitors, allowing local and systemic regulation of inflammatory events (Weiss *et al.*, 1983).

The biological significance of the above information must be related to neutrophil structure and function (tissue injury, phagocytosis, and intracellular killing). Much of the information has been generated using *in vitro* systems and there is frequently a lack of *in vivo* correlations. Several naturally occurring neutrophil enzyme defects do support many of the conclusions drawn from *in vitro* data. Although the oxygen-dependent mechanisms are important in the neutrophil's antimicrobial armamentarium (Babior, 1978) and abnormalities in this system can have serious consequences (e.g., chronic granulomatous disease), the neutrophil has potent oxygen-independent mechanisms as well. The chicken heterophil, lacking myeloperoxidase, is a natural example of the ability of neutrophils to function without the myeloperoxidase–H_2O_2–halide antimicrobial mechanism (Brune and Spitznagel, 1973; Pennial and Spitznagel, 1975).

B. Oxygen-Independent Mechanisms

The presence of oxygen-independent killing mechanisms is well established (Klebanoff and Clark, 1978; see Section II,B). These mechanisms should probably not be thought of as being anaerobically dependent, since many of these mechanisms very likely function in the presence or absence of oxygen. In the laboratory complete removal of O_2 by using N_2 may not be an adequate test of anaerobic killing potential, since an intracellular source of H_2O_2 or other oxygen metabolites may persist. Thus, some *in vitro* test methods indicate only that various neutrophil antimicrobial systems can function after removal of O_2.

Hydrogen ion concentration in the phagosome increases rapidly after phagocytosis (Jacques and Baintain, 1978; Mandell, 1970; Jensen and Baintain, 1973). The lowest pH attainable in the phagocytic vacuole varies with animal species but ranges from 3.0 to 6.0 (Mandell, 1970; Jensen and Baintain, 1973). The increase in hydrogen ion concentration is likely the result of lactate produced during glycolysis, which occurs during phagocytosis (Kakinuma, 1970). Maintenance of this low pH occurs by several possible mechanisms, including an energy-dependent proton pump, equilibrium across a semipermeable membrane, or a mechanism using carbonic anhydrase (Reijngoud and Tager, 1977; Cline, 1973).

The low phagosome pH level may be microbicidal (organic acids and lipophilic acids) or microbiostatic depending on the sensitivity of the microbe to hydrogen ions (Freese *et al.*, 1973). Microbicidal substances such as cationic proteins have a pH optimum at seven or above (Spitznagel, 1977; Odeburg and Olsson, 1975; Drazin and Lehrer, 1977), whereas enzymes considered to have a digestive role (hydrolases) function best at an acid pH. Acid pH also facilitates the function of some antimicrobial enzyme systems (e.g., the MPO–H_2O_2–halide system, acid hydrolases, and lysozyme) (Root and Cohen, 1981).

Lysozyme, a cationic protein that attacks β1,4-glycosidic bonds (Baggiolini, 1972) in bacterial cell walls, is found in both the primary and secondary granules of some animal neutrophils (Table II). Lysozyme requires other neutrophilic and nonneutrophilic antimicrobial factors to induce microbial killing (Root and Cohen, 1981), or possibly digestion of already killed and phagocytized bacteria (Klebanoff, 1975a,b). In cattle, whose neutrophils naturally have small amounts of lysozyme, the contribution of this enzyme to the overall killing and digestive functions of the neutrophil is probably very small.

Various antimicrobial cationic proteins have been isolated from neutrophils (Odeburg and Olsson, 1975; Drazin and Lehrer, 1977; Weiss *et al.*, 1978a,b; Lehrer, 1972; Lehrer *et al.*, 1975). These proteins are isolated using a dilute acid and are present in the primary granules of human neutrophils (Ohlsson *et al.*, 1977; Spitznagel *et al.*, 1974). Some cationic proteins have phospholipase- and chymotrypsin-like activity (Weiss and Elsbach, 1977; Elsbach, 1980; Drazin and Lehrer, 1977). Enzymatic activity is not necessary for these proteins to have antimicrobial activity (Odeburg and Olsson, 1976). Cationic proteins can be inhibited by heparin or by the addition of calcium or magnesium to the *in vitro* medium (Odeburg and Olsson, 1976; Weiss *et al.*, 1975; Efrati *et al.*, 1976) and all are active at a neutral pH. The more cationic these are, the more potent the bacteriocidal action (Welsh and Spitznagel, 1971). Cationic proteins must bind to the organism in order to be bactericidal (Spitznagel, 1977). These proteins impair microbial replicative ability without altering bacterial structure (Odeburg and Olsson, 1976) and most likely act with other antimicrobial mechanisms (Spitznagel, 1977). Cationic proteins may enhance or augment the killing effects of the myeloperoxidase–H_2O_2–halide system (Rest *et al.*, 1978a).

Some cationic proteins are effective against Gram-negative bacteria but not against Gram-positive organisms (Weiss *et al.*, 1975). A possible explanation for this selectivity is that the binding site for these proteins is the lipopolysaccharide portion of the bacterial membrane (Weiss *et al.*, 1980). Cationic proteins also play a role in the degradation of cartilage proteoglycans and the cleavage of complements with production of chemotactic factors (protease-related activity) as well as increasing vascular permeability and cytotoxicity (nonenzymatic activity of these proteins) (Klebanoff and Clark, 1978).

Hydrolases probably act only after the microbe has been killed. A direct killing role may be ascribed to lysozyme, arginase, and glycosidases (Gabig and Babior, 1981; Rest *et al.*, 1978b; Bretz and Baggiolini, 1974).

Neutral and acid proteases, generally associated with azurophil granules, have been demonstrated in several species (Klebanoff and Clark, 1978). Proteases are associated with the breakdown of extracellular connective tissue components. The neutral pH of the extracellular environment suggests acid proteases have their most optimal function in exudates (Goldstein, 1976). Proteases are involved in the production of kinin-like mediators (leukokinins from serum proteins) (Greenbaum, 1972), the alteration of vascular permeability (possibly mediated by leukokinin) (Chang *et al.*, 1972; Greenbaum, 1972), and the digestion of various types of collagen, cartilage, and elastin (Klebanoff and Clark, 1978).

Connective tissue destruction is attributed to the specific enzymes elastase, collagenase, and chymotrypsin-like protease. These enzymes also have a role in the production of certain complement fragments (Ward and Hill, 1970; Goldstein and Weissman, 1974), in the generation of chemotactic factors (Tynelius-Bratthall and Lindhe, 1974; Ward and Zvaifler, 1970), and in the fibrinolytic system (Plow and Edington, 1975). Control of these potent tissue-damaging enzymes is found in serum as α_1-antitrypsin, an α_2-macroglobulin (Barrett, 1974; Venge and Olsson, 1975).

Neutrophil proteases may play a role in immune system control. Neutrophil neutral proteases, elastase, and chymotrypsin-like protease (cathepsin G) can act as a B cell mitogen but do not have a direct effect on T cells (Vischer et al., 1976; Yachnin and Richman, 1982). Neutrophils have been shown to enhance phytohemagglutinin-induced T cell stimulation, but the enzymes mediating this activation have not been identified (Nakamura et al., 1976). Neutrophil protease activity may enhance lymphocyte T and B responses to antigens.

The term "cathepsin" is often used for intracellular proteases which generally have optimal activity at an acid pH. There are seven different neutrophil cathepsins (A through G), with cathepsin G being used synonymously with chymotrypsin-like protease (Klebanoff and Clark, 1978).

Lactoferrin has been isolated from specific granules of several species (Baggiolini et al., 1970b; Green et al., 1971; Pryzwansky et al., 1978; Spitznagel et al., 1974). Like transferrin and apolactoferrin (Arnold et al., 1977), lactoferrin has antimicrobial activity. Lactoferrin, antibody (Bullen et al., 1972), and possibly lysozyme function in concert to exert antimicrobial activity, although this has not been demonstrated directly. Binding of iron to lactoferrin results in enhanced generation of the antimicrobial hydroxyl radicals (from the interaction of superoxide anion and hydrogen peroxide) in granulocytes (Ambruso and Johnston, 1981). Lactoferrin-deficient neutrophils have a reduced ability to kill phagocytized E. coli (Spitznagel, 1977). This suggests lactoferrin has an important function in the killing of some microbes. Lactoferrin also contributes to the control of neutrophil migration and oxygen-radical production. Lactoferrin increases granulocyte adherence and aggregation (Oseas et al., 1981) and reduces cell surface charges (makes them less negative) (Boxer et al., 1982).

Oxygen-dependent and oxygen-independent mechanisms have a partial (some more than others) role in neutrophil antimicrobial and tissue-damaging functions. The contribution or importance of each mechanism varies with the species of animal, type of tissue, type of organism, and the presence or absence of oxygen, antibody, and complement. Even the absence of a major antimicrobial system is compatible with life. Chicken and goose heterophils normally lack myeloperoxidase (Brune et al., 1972; Rausch and Moore, 1975), normal bovine, monkey, sheep, and goat neutrophils have little or no lysozyme (Rausch and Moore, 1975), and rabbit heterophils are especially rich in cationic proteins (Zeya and Spitznagel, 1971) but have low concentrations of other antimicrobial enzymes (Rausch and Moore, 1975). There are reported cases of normal rhesus monkeys lacking lysozyme and lactoferrin (Rausch et al., 1974) and reports of resistance to bacterial diseases in animals which have various neutrophil dysfunctions.

IV. Neutrophil Migration and Activation

Neutrophilic leukocytes adhere to the endothelium and exit from the blood in a random manner, not related to cell age. After the neutrophil has left the blood it probably remains in the tissue, although some studies suggest neutrophils may reenter the blood circulation (Vincent et al., 1974).

In inflammatory states neutrophil adherence to endothelium is influenced by and depends upon various chemotactic factors which cause calcium influx into the neutrophil (O'Flaherty et al., 1978), promote microtubular polymerization (Schneier et al., 1977; Boxer et al., 1978), reduce the net negative surface charge of the neutrophil (MacGregor et al., 1974; Gallin et al., 1975; Hoover et al., 1978), and increase the intracellular cyclic GMP and decrease the intracellular cyclic AMP (MacGregor, 1976; Boxer et al., 1976). Although the precise role of neutrophil membrane glycoproteins is not established, they likely augment endothelial cell adherence to endothelial cells (Beatty et al., 1984). Platelet activating factor (acetyl–glycerol–ether–phosphorylcholine) and thromboxane A_2 (Spagnuolo et al., 1980) promote neutrophil adherence (Valone and Goetzl, 1983). Some chemoattractants also cause degranulation of secondary granules with release of lysozyme (Gallin et al., 1980) and cationic proteins (Camussi et al., 1980), both of which can cause decreased neutrophil surface charge and can facilitate neutrophil adherence and aggregation. Various chemoattractants (e.g., PMA and N-formylated tripeptides), by altering intracellular cyclic nucleotide concentrations, cause selective secondary granule exocytosis (Gallin et al., 1975). Not all chemoattractants that cause neutrophil aggregation also cause degranulation (Craddock et al., 1980; O'Flaherty et al., 1978; Kaplan, 1982), suggesting that surface charge alone does not control cell–cell adhesion. The requirements of calcium, an intact neutrophil cytoskeleton, and degranulation for neutrophil adherence were demonstrated by inhibiting neutrophil adherence with low concentrations of calcium and lanthanum (O'Flaherty et al., 1978), cholchicine or vinblastine (Schneier et al., 1977), steroids, and glycolytic metabolic inhibitors (MacGregor et al., 1974).

Once stimulated by the chemoattractant, neutrophils have increased cellular adherence and show chemoattractant-dose-dependent cellular locomotion (Zigmond, 1978). The increased adherence may reflect surface-charge neutralization (Gallin, 1980a) or changes in the availability of chemoattractant receptors (Gallin et al., 1979). Increased availability of receptors may be a result of increased receptor numbers on the membrane surface, the reorganization of preexisting receptors, or an improved efficiency in communication between receptor and neutrophil cytoskeleton.

Neutrophil activation, after exposure to a chemoattractant, results from several events, including increased cytoplasmic ionized calcium, which triggers cellular events leading to granule secretion, increased metabolism, cytoskeletal changes, and cell movement (Romeo et al., 1975; Smolen et al., 1981; Snyderman and Goetzel, 1981). Increased intracellular calcium is the result of an influx from the extracellular environment and release from intracellular membrane-enclosed compartments (Pozzan et al., 1983). The increased calcium causes activation of phospholipases and increases intracellular cyclic nucleotides. Linkage of gelsolin to actin, resulting in the dissolution of actin-binding protein-bound actin, is also calcium dependent (Stendahl and Stossel, 1980). Polymerization of the actin lattice will result in the movement of neutrophil structures from regions of high calcium concentration to regions of lower calcium concentration.

Chemotaxis is dependent on transmethylation reactions mediated by S-adenosylmethionine (Schiffmann et al., 1979; Pike et al., 1978). This was demonstrated by treating cells with chemicals that indirectly inhibited S-adenosylmethionine-mediated methylation reactions. The concentration of membrane-bound methylated phospholipid is reduced in rabbit neutrophils after exposure to chemoattractants.

Chemoattractant-receptor-mediated enzyme activation causes membrane phospholipid cleavage, which leads to the production of arachadonic acid metabolites. This occurs by degradation of phosphatidylcholine via activation of phospholipase A_2 and results in the release of arachidonic acid (Hirata and Axelrod, 1980). Free arachidonic acid in leukocytes is converted to thromboxanes and prostaglandins (especially PGE_2) by cyclooxygenase and to hydroxyeicosatetraenoic acids (HETE) by lipoxygenase (Snyderman and Goetzel, 1981).

Lipooxygenase products may be involved in several neutrophil functions. Inhibition of lipooxygenation suppresses neutrophil migration, hexose monophosphate transport, aggregation, and degranulation (Bass et al., 1980; Naccache et al., 1981; Goetzel et al., 1980). The exact mechanism of inhibition is unclear, but some HETEs may be incorporated into membrane phospholipids (altering membrane properties) or may alter intracellular proteins and other polar constituents that are vital to cell function (Goldman and Goetzel, 1981).

Some chemoattractants also cause increased intraneutrophil concentrations of both cAMP and cGMP (Smolen et al., 1980; Simchowitz et al., 1980). The increased cAMP activates calcium-dependent protein kinase, which controls phosphorylation of critical proteins in neutrophil function (Snyderman and Goetzel, 1981). Additional chemoattractant-receptor-mediated changes include increased intracellular hydrogen ion concentration (Serhan et al., 1980; Bareis et al., 1982) and sodium and potassium fluxes (Gallin and Rosenthal, 1974; Boucek and Snyderman, 1976; Naccache et al., 1977).

After stimulation the neutrophil shape becomes polarized with topographical changes of cellular organelles and cytoskeletal components. The centrosome of stimulated neutrophils contains the cytoskeletal organizing center, the Golgi apparatus, and most of the primary and secondary granules. With increased time after chemoattractant stimulation there is an increase in the number and length of microtubules and transient separation of centrioles. The separated centrioles are each surrounded by an aster of microtubules, which is considered to be a reflection of chemoattractant-induced neutrophil stimulation (centrosome splitting) (Schliwa et al., 1982). Microtubules extend to, but do not penetrate, the microfilament-rich uropod and lamellipodium. Most of the intermediate filaments are found in the uropod (Snyderman and Goetzel, 1981). Microfilaments form a zone subjacent to the plasma membrane which excludes all other cell organelles and exists as electron-dense polymerized areas at sites of cell attachment (Gallin, 1980b). Thick filaments (10 nm) occupy the centrosome and core of the pseudopodia (Blose and Chacko, 1976). The nucleus moves to the rear of the neutrophil and is separated from the lamellipodial leading edge by most of the granules and the Golgi apparatus (Malech et al., 1977; Gallin et al., 1980). The cell membrane of the uropod contains almost all of the coated pits and vesicles in the polarized cell, as compared to a diffuse distribution found in the unstimulated neutrophil (Pfeiffer et al., 1980; Snyderman and Goetzel, 1981). Before the neutrophil can change the direction of the migration reorientation of the nucleus, centrioles and cytoskeletal elements must occur (Malech et al., 1977). Cytoskeletal changes are responsible for organelle rearrangement. Neutrophils are extremely sensitive to chemoattractant dose changes and can detect a 1% gradient difference between different regions of the cell surface (Zigmond, 1977; Zigmond, 1974).

Chemoattractants induce an array of other neutrophil responses, such as aggregation, enhanced oxidative metabolism, and increased expression of complement receptors (O'Flaherty et al., 1977; Anwar and Kay, 1977). These events do not seem to be involved in the initiation of chemotaxis, but may modulate the chemotactic response. Newly generated active oxygen radicals modify neutrophil function by the generation of chemotactic and chemokinetic factors from cellular and extracellular lipids. Late events induced by chemoattractants result in more efficient phagocytosis and microbicidal activity after the neutrophil has already been activated (Snyderman and Goetzl, 1981).

Defects of several events in neutrophil chemotaxis have been observed in naturally occurring diseases (Gallin, 1980c). Altered adherence is seen with diabetes mellitus; abnormal deformability is seen in neonates and in the Chediak–Higashi syndrome (e.g., Aleutian mink disease); abnormal random migration is seen in toxic neutrophils, actin dysfunction syndromes, thermal injury, and Kartagener's syndrome; abnormal directed migration is seen with hypogammaglobulinemia, α-mannosidase deficiency, and systemic lupus erythematosis.

Chemotactic rate (chemotactic index) and response to various chemoattractants varies between species (Smith et al., 1985; Chenoweth et al., 1980). Using migration under agarose as a measure of chemotactic index, pig neutrophils were shown to have a lower index than human neutrophils. Furthermore, pig neutrophils do not respond to some purified bacterial chemotactic factors (Chenoweth et al., 1980). The morphologic similarity between neutrophils from various species (Table I) would suggest chemotactic responsiveness could be attributable to membrane receptor or biochemical differences.

An experimental model for studying neutrophil chemoattractant-receptor concentration and response is the horse neutrophil. Horse neutrophils have a low responsiveness to the potent chemoattractant N-formylated methionyl-leucyl-phenylalanine (Camp and Leid, 1982). In neutrophil migration studies this peptide is frequently used to induce directed neutrophil migration. Equine neutrophils have high-affinity receptors for the N-formylated peptides (Snyderman and Pike, 1980) but the number of receptors is substantially reduced when compared to guinea pig, rabbit, or human neutrophils. Although the N-formylated peptides are not potent initiators of chemotaxis in horse neutrophils, they do induce degranulation and stimulate the production of superoxide anion. The mechanism for this type of response by equine neutrophils is not known, but there is a dose-dependent effect seen with these tripeptide chemoattractants (Zinkl and Brown, 1982).

V. Phagocytosis and Degranulation

Phagocytosis and degranulation are two interrelated processes which require intact neutrophilic leukocyte membranes (see Section II,C) and cytoskeletal elements (microtubules and microfilaments). Both processes can be inhibited by cold temperatures, vincristine, vinblastine, and cholchicine (Rungger-Brandle and Gabbiani, 1983), all of which act by altering microtubule function. Cell membrane stimulation by a phagocytizable particle causes cytoskeletal changes similar to those seen with chemotaxis (see Section IV) and also many changes in neutrophil metabolism (see Section III and Fig. 5). If the particle is opsonized by antibody, Fc receptors on the neutrophil membrane facilitate ingestion. Neutrophil pseudopodia are able to "wrap around" the particle by the coordinated action of microfilament polymerization, cell membrane fluidity, and Fc receptors.

Membrane components and functions differ in the region of pseudopodia formation (as occurs with phagocytosis) and lamellipodia formation (as occurs with chemotaxis). Membranes near pseudopodia formation accumulate ligand–receptor complexes (Albertini *et al.*, 1977; Berlin and Oliver, 1978) and are enriched in "coated" membranes (Pfeiffer *et al.*, 1980). Endocytotic function is restricted to this region, and there is exclusion of Fc receptors (Walker *et al.*, 1980). The uropodia of a neutrophil undergoing chemotaxis has receptor-mediated endocytosis, pinocytosis, and concentration of coated pits and vesicles (Davis *et al.*, 1982). The lamellipod membrane excludes coated pits and lacks pinocytotic activity but has preferential binding of immunoglobulin aggregates (Fc receptors) (Davis *et al.*, 1982).

Opsonization of a particle facilitates phagocytosis, but is not required. Opsonins such as antibody and certain complement fragments increase the rate of phagocytosis by several-fold (Bertram *et al.*, 1982). The rate of phagocytosis is also different between species of domestic animals. Using *in vitro* conditions, bovine blood neutrophils ingest opsonized *Staphylococcus aureus* more rapidly than equine blood neutrophils (T. A. Bertram, F. L. Coignoul, and J. A. Roth, 1985, unpublished data).

The earliest events of degranulation are associated with changes in granule morphology (Coignoul *et al.*, 1984b). These changes may be analogous to the morphological changes seen in mast cells during degranulation. Degranulation, like phagocytosis, depends on an intact cytoskeletal system and is closely linked to chemotaxis (see Section IV), ingestion, and neutrophil metabolism (see Section III and Fig. 5).

Secretion of granule proteins (controlled by microfilaments) such as

TABLE III

MORPHOMETRIC ANALYSIS OF EXUDATE NEUTROPHILS FROM HORSE AND PIG[a]

Species	Number of animals	Granule area (μm^2)	Neutrophil area (μm^2)	Nucleus area (μm^2)	Granule volume[b]
Equine	2	2.10 ± 0.2	32.24 ± 1.8	3.13 ± 0.2	6.5
Porcine	3	3.96 ± 0.3	37.86 ± 1.7	5.28 ± 0.4	10.5

[a]Horse neutrophils were collected from the uterus and pig neutrophils were collected from the lung. Exudates in both animals were produced using Gram-negative bacteria (*Hemophilus* sp.). The exudate was fixed in 2.5% glutaraldehyde in cacodylate buffer. The analysis was conducted as previously described by Bertram and Coignoul (1982).
[b]Percentage of neutrophil volume.

elastase and collagenase helps loosen interstitial ground substance which facilitates neutrophil migration. Granule enzymes may be autocrine-like in controlling neutrophil function by destroying hyaluronic acid which has been demonstrated to influence neutrophil adhesion and directed migration (Hakansson *et al.*, 1980). Granule exocytosis also results in the release of mediators thereby influencing the inflammatory response by inactivating and generating chemoattractants (Wright and Gallin, 1975; Bronza and Ward, 1977) (see Section VIII).

Secreted neutrophil enzymes could come from the cell cytoplasm, cell membrane, or primary and secondary granules. Results in Table III demonstrate that in pigs and horses some of these enzymes likely come from cytoplasmic granules. Equine neutrophils present in exudates have a 50% reduction in granule volume when compared with circulating blood neutrophils. The granule volume of pig neutrophils in exudates is approximately 30% less than the granule volume of blood neutrophils. These results demonstrate that the extent of neutrophil degranulation is species and/or location dependent. The relative contribution of these granule enzymes to the total amount of neutrophil enzymes released has not been established.

If neutrophil exocytosis is limited there is an increase in cell adhesiveness and in the number of chemoattractant receptors (Gallin *et al.*, 1978). If there is extensive granule release, neutrophils become less responsive to chemoattractant stimuli, are hyperadhesive, and have a change in cell surface charge (Gallin, 1980a; Gallin *et al.*, 1978). These changes may facilitate the localization of neutrophils in an inflammatory site.

Microtubule and microfilament polymerization are required to move granules from the centrosome to the phagosome membrane for intracellular release or to the plasma membrane for extracellular release. The onset of degranulation brings about the release of granule enzymes and initiates neutrophil oxidative metabolism (Fig. 5). Enzyme release leads to microbe killing, tissue damage (see Section III), and modulation of various inflammatory and immunologic processes (see Section VIII).

Differential degranulation of specific granules occurs *in vitro* when neutrophils are treated with PMA. This process may be related to cyclic nucleotide fluxes which control degranulation. Recently, differential inhibition of degranulation has been demonstrated (T. A. Bertram, P. Canning, and J. A. Roth, 1985, unpublished data). This was demonstrated using a nucleotide or nucleotide-like compound isolated from *Brucella abortus* (Canning *et al.*, 1985) which was capable of suppressing azurophil granule, but not specific granule release from bovine neutrophils stimulated with opsonized zymosan.

VI. Granulocytopoiesis

Granulocytes and macrophages differentiate from a common stem cell which is controlled by hematopoietic hormones called colony-stimulating factors (CSF) (Burgess *et al.*, 1977; Stanley and Heard, 1977; Golde and Cline, 1974). Leukocytes that produce CSF include mononuclear phagocytes (alveolar, peritoneal, and hepatic macrophages) and stimulated T lymphocytes of the helper series (Golde and Cline, 1972; Moore *et al.*, 1974; Saxon *et al.*, 1978). These cells are capable of responding to antigenic stimulation and thus provide possible mechanism for accelerated granulocytopoiesis during inflammation.

Factors released from mature neutrophils and macrophages can inhibit granulocytopoiesis. Mature neutrophils release a "chalone" (Paukovits, 1971) that is likely to be a direct inhibitor of neutrophil maturation (Herman *et al.*, 1978). An indirect system may exist whereby neutrophil development is controlled by macrophage secretion products which may promote (CSF) or inhibit (prostaglandins) granulocytopoiesis (Broxmeyer *et al.*, 1977). Release of these products may be modulated by the mature neutrophil (Kurland *et al.*, 1978). Macrophage release of CSF is reduced in the presence of extracts from mature neutrophils.

The bone marrow microenvironment is critical for normal granulocytopoiesis and stem cell differentiation. This was demonstrated by placing bone marrow stroma into laboratory animals and evaluating stem cell implantation patterns; erythroid colonies developed in the spleen, whereas granulocytic colonies were found in the bone marrow (Wolf, 1974). Appropriate microenvironmental conditions depend on the presence of phagocytic cells (mononuclear and epithelioid) and fat-laden giant cells in the spleen and bone marrow. *In vitro* stem cell proliferation and differentiation depend on the presence of and contact with these phagocytic cells (Cline *et al.*, 1977; Dexter and Moore, 1977). For appropriate granulocytopoiesis there must also be interaction (factor release or cell contact) between T lymphocytes, mononuclear phagocytes, polymorphonuclear phagocytes (neutrophils), and stromal cells of the bone marrow. Myeloid series diseases could result from an abnormality in any of these areas, including the bone marrow microenvironment. Hematopoietic stem cells and their microenvironmental requirements have been discussed extensively in various monographs (Golde and Cline, 1974; Robinson and Mangalik, 1975).

Neutrophil maturation consists of a mitotic phase of approximately 7.5 days and a nonmitotic (metamyelocyte) phase of 6.5 days (Baintain *et al.*, 1971). Histochemical and ultrastructural studies in various species have demonstrated many similarities in the process of neutrophil maturation (Baintain and Farquhar, 1966, 1968a,b; Ackerman, 1968; Nafsted and Nafsted, 1968; Campbell, 1968). Neutrophil function also develops in an ordered sequence. Using leukemic cells as a functional probe of neutrophil differentiation, the following sequence has been demonstrated for neutrophil functional maturation (Glasser, 1983): phagocytosis → microbial killing → random locomotion → chemotaxis. Receptors for Fc (Glasser, 1983) and C3 (Lotem and Sachs, 1977), which are important for phagocytosis, also develop in early stages of cell ontogeny. Newer methods of *in vitro* stem cell culture will provide more information on the interactions and control of granulocytopoiesis and how this process relates to cell membrane receptors.

VII. Neutrophils of the Circulating Blood (Neutrophil Heterogeneity)

Different populations of neutrophilic leukocytes exist in exudates and peripheral blood of man and animals. Based on differences in function and receptor population, at least two populations of neutrophils have been identified (Klempner and Gallin, 1978; Messner and Jelinek, 1970; Harvath and Leonard, 1982). Methods in these studies were based on the ability of neutrophils to form rosettes with IgG-coated human RBCs. Rosetting neutrophils were more adherent, were able to phagocytize more *Staphylococcus aureus,* and were more responsive to chemoattractants than were nonrosetting neutrophils. Phagocytosis of latex beads was not significantly different between the two neutrophil populations. A higher percentage of exudate neutrophils rosette IgG-coated erythrocytes than peripheral blood neutrophils (Klempner and Gallin, 1978).

When blood neutrophils are isolated and separated with a fluorescence-activated cell sorter, approximately 20% fail to respond to chemotactic stimuli (Seligmann *et al.,* 1981), some fail to ingest opsonized particles, and some do not mediate *in vitro* antibody-dependent cell-mediated cytotoxicity (Zighelboim *et al.,* 1976). This suggests circulating blood neutrophils are morphologically and functionally heterogeneous.

Impaired neutrophil function observed in some diseases may reflect the "normal" function of different populations of neutrophils rather than an induced change in the neutrophil itself. Humans receiving hemodialysis for renal failure have a neutropenia following treatment. A majority of the remaining neutrophils will not rosette IgG-coated erythrocytes (Klempner *et al.,* 1980). Impaired neutrophil function has been observed during acute Gram-negative infections (Baisero, 1973; Link *et al.,* 1979; Althaus *et al.,* 1980), and intravenous administration of endotoxin is associated with a reduced number of rosetting neutrophils in the circulating blood (Gallin *et al.,* 1980).

Bactericidal activity has been correlated with the ability of neutrophils to rosette IgG-coated RBCs. Nonrosetting cells have reduced bactericidal and chemotactic (directed migration) activity, but normal chemokinesis (random migration) and normal ingestion of nonopsonized latex particles. Lactoferrin and proteolytic enzyme concentrations were also different between the two populations of neutrophils (Broxmeyer *et al.,* 1980). Complement receptors for C4a, C3b, C3d, and C3bi were present in all groups (Whited *et al.,* 1981).

VIII. Neutrophil Function in Inflammatory and Immunologic Processes

The neutrophilic leukocyte's role in inflammation is more than simply margination, chemotaxis, degranulation, and phagocytosis. Neutrophils are involved in or control the release of vasoactive amines, the deposition of platelets, the production of leukotrienes, and vascular permeability. Even though the neutrophil is highly differentiated with limited metabolic and adaptive capabilities, there is reciprocal interaction with other cellular and humoral factors. This interaction allows modulation of the neutrophil's highly toxic and potentially lethal armamentarium.

Neutrophils are directly involved in some vascular changes of immune-complex diseases. Immune complexes attach to rabbit heterophils, inducing release of platelet activating factor (PAF) (Vinella et al., 1983; Lynch et al., 1979). This factor induces the release of vasoactive amines, leading to an increase in vascular permeability (Vinella et al., 1983), and may promote neutrophil chemotaxis (Ingraham et al., 1983). Increased vascular permeability may be needed for immune-complex deposition in extravascular tissues, which is a critical step in the development of localized tissue damage (Cochrane, 1971). Any potential vasoactive effects would be exacerbated by the release of neutrophil cationic proteins (also induced by immune complexes), which would act on basophils, leading to release of more PAF (Benveniste et al., 1977). In vivo work has demonstrated that platelets are selectively deposited in acutely inflamed tissues during neutrophil migration through vessel walls (Issekutz et al., 1983). This effect may be mediated through neutrophil endoperoxides and thromboxanes, which are potent platelet aggregators (Weissman et al., 1978).

Platelets can also influence neutrophil function. Activated platelets amplify granulocyte adherence to nylon fibers (Rasp and Repine, 1981), platelet factor IV can increase the activity of granulocyte proteases (Lanky and Wohl, 1981), and platelet release of serotonin promotes increased neutrophil cytotoxicity and adherence to endothelial cells. These in vitro data have been supported by work in rabbits, where platelet deposition and platelet–neutrophil aggregation occur in acutely inflamed areas of skin (Issekutz et al., 1983). The interaction of varying numbers of platelets and neutrophils may modify early inflammatory lesions.

Humoral factors generated in the inflammatory and immune response may also influence neutrophil function. Guinea pig neutrophils are aggregated by lymphokines, which also aggregate macrophages (Badenoch-Jones, 1982). Using Sephadex beads as a marker, leukotriene C_4 (LTC$_4$), leukotriene D_4 (LTD$_4$), and leukocyte chemotactic factor leukotriene B_4 (LTB$_4$) enhanced neutrophil adherence (Goetzl et al., 1983). LTC$_4$ and LTD$_4$, which are not chemotactic, were as active as the potent chemoattractant LTB$_4$. These findings suggest that the vasoactive leukotrienes, which have a significant role in inflammation, may also modify neutrophil function during the inflammatory process.

Antibodies may promote or inhibit neutrophil function. Bovine neutrophils have greatly reduced chemiluminescence if antibody is absent from cytotoxicity assays. This was shown not to be a direct relationship to the antibody concentration free in the media, since both the number and density of immunoglobulins attached to the target cell controlled chemiluminescence by the neutrophil (Weber and Peterhaus, 1983). Some myeloma antibodies (IgA) inhibit neutrophil chemotaxis (Van-Epps and Williams, 1976; Christophers and Schroder, 1983). The polymeric form of myeloma IgA restricts the access of chemoattractants to receptors on the cell membrane. Aggregated IgA may also inhibit neutrophil chemotaxis and chemokinesis (Kemp et al., 1980).

The potential influence of IgA on steric hindrance of receptors is demonstrated by the complementary role of immunoglobulin and complement receptors on the neutrophil membrane. The presence of these two receptors is not functionally redundant, because IgG–Fc receptors control internalization of the cell membranes, whereas C3b receptors facilitate recognition and adhesion by the neutrophil (Hakansson and Venge, 1982; Scribner and Fahrney, 1976; Mantovani, 1975). By blocking one of these receptors, neutrophil function can be altered. Complement receptors are more sensitive than antibody receptors to neutrophil oxygen radicals and proteases, which are released during phagocytosis and chemotaxis (Hakansson and Venge, 1982). This differential sensitivity may allow neutrophils to autoregulate their own function through degranulation and enzyme release.

The ability of neutrophils to mediate *in vitro* cytotoxicity of mammalian cells has been clearly demonstrated (Coignoul et al., 1984a,b; Weiss et al., 1981; Weiss and LoBuglio, 1980; Clark and Szot, 1981). Using *in vitro* methods, T and B lymphocytes were labeled with immune complexes and exposed to neutrophils. The results indicated that neutrophils can mediate lymphoid cell cytotoxicity and can alter lymphoid cell responses to mitogens (in the absence of cytotoxicity). Neutrophils have also been demonstrated to potentiate mevalonic acid-stimulated B lymphocyte replication in the absence of either lysosomal enzymes or active oxygen radicals (Yachnin and Richman, 1982). These results support the concept that activated neutrophils may influence (both suppress and help) various immunologic functions.

The influence of neutrophil toxic products on vascular endothelium, released as a result of neutrophil aggregation is usually considered a mechanism that leads to vascular damage. Occasionally, however, tissue damage is not seen with neutrophil aggregation (Shew and Hensen, 1982). A potential explanation was demonstrated using *in vitro* techniques; neutrophil aggregation was shown to not always depend on or precede degranulation (Korchak *et al.*, 1983), indicating that toxic enzymes and oxygen radicals necessary for tissue damage may not always be released. *In vitro* studies have also demonstrated that activated neutrophils disrupt endothelial monolayers by oxygen-radical-independent mechanisms requiring neutrophil–endothelial contact (Harlan *et al.*, 1985). These observations indicate that neutrophil activation does not always lead to degranulation.

Neutrophils may have a role in regulating local blood vascular responses during inflammation. Leukocyte cathepsin B cleaves angiotensinogen to its active components in the absence of renin and angiotensin-converting enzyme (Wintroub *et al.*, 1982). Angiotensin is one of the most potent vasoactive substances readily available in the circulating blood. This neutrophil-generated angiotensin may potentiate the hyperemia and increased vascular permeability seen during inflammation by increasing the blood pressure in areas of inflammation.

IX. Summary

Differences in neutrophil morphology between various species of domestic animals are evident when morphometric techniques are used. Morphometric analysis can be coupled with functional assays of degranulation to demonstrate changes in granule volume after neutrophil activation (Bertram and Jensen, 1984). Morphometric and functional analysis of the neutrophil can also be used to evaluate the response of neutrophils to infectious agents (Coignoul *et al.*, 1984a). Comparison of these assays between animal species may provide insight into the susceptibility of animals to various microbial pathogens.

The enzyme content of neutrophil granules has been extensively studied, but the process of enzyme release from granules is poorly understood. Granule contents are assumed to be released in an "all or none" fashion. The presence of unique forms of granules (granules with a flocculent matrix) seen in degranulating neutrophils suggests that partial granule-content release as well as total granule-content release may be controlled by similar processes. If a selective process of granule enzyme release occurs, a more refined control of degranulation may exist than has been previously believed.

Functions of neutrophilic leukocytes include phagocytosis, killing, and digestion of microbes which invade the host. The neutrophil is also able to increase vascular permeability, help or suppress some T and B lymphocyte responses, and modify some phases of the inflammatory process. Research into the role of neutrophils in killing tumor cells has demonstrated the potential beneficial effects of neutrophil-mediated tissue-damaging mechanisms.

REFERENCES

Ackerman, G. A. (1968). *Lab. Invest.* **19**, 290–302.
Agner, K. (1972). "Structure and Function of Oxidation-Reduction Enzymes" (A. Akeson and H. Ehrenburg, eds.), Vol. 18, pp. 329–335. Pergamon, Oxford.
Albertini, D. F., Berlin, R. D., and Oliver, J. M. (1977). *J. Cell Sci.* **26**, 57–75.
Allen, R. C., Stjernholm, R. L., and Steele, R. H. (1972). *Biochem. Biophys. Res. Commun.* **47**, 679–684.
Althaus, D., Keller, H. U., Hess, M. W., and Cottier, H. (1980). *Int. Arch. Allergy Appl. Immunol.* **61**, 321–328.
Ambruso, O. R., and Johnston, R. B., Jr. (1981). *J. Clin. Invest.* **67**, 352–360.
Amherdt, M., Baggiolini, M., Perrelet, A., and Orci, L. (1978). *Lab. Invest.* **39**, 398–404.
Anderson, B. R., Brendzel, A. M., and Lint, T. F. (1977). *Infect. Immun.* **17**, 62–66.
Anwar, A. R. E., and Kay, A. B. (1977). *Nature (London)* **269**, 522–525.
Arnold, R. R., Cole, M. F., and McGhee, J. R. (1977). *Science* **197**, 263–265.
Babior, B. M. (1978). *N. Engl. J. Med.* **298**, 659–668, 721–725.
Bachner, R. L., and Johnston, R. B., Jr. (1971). *Br. J. Haematol.* **20**, 277–285.
Badenoch-Jones, P. (1982). *J. Immunol.* **47**, 169–174.
Baggiolini, M. (1972). *Enzyme* **13**, 132–160.
Baggiolini, M. (1980). *In* "The Handbook of Inflammation" (G. Weissmann, ed.), Vol. 2, pp. 163–187. Elsevier, Amsterdam.
Baggiolini, M., DeDuve, C., Masson, P. L., and Heremans, J. F. (1970a). *J. Exp. Med.* **131**, 559–570.
Baggiolini, M., Hirsch, J. G., and DeDuve, C. (1970b). *J. Cell Biol.* **45**, 586–597.
Baggiolini, M., Bretz, U., and Gusus, B. (1974). *Schweiz. Med. Wochenschr.* **104**, 129–132.
Baggiolini, M., Amherdt, M., and Orci, L. (1976). *Experientia* **32**, 1400–1401.
Baggiolini, M., Bretz, U., and Dewald, B. (1978). *In* "Neutral Proteases of Human Polymorphonuclear Leukocytes" (K. Haverman and A. Janoff, eds.), pp. 3–17. Urban & Schwarzenberg, Baltimore.
Baggiolini, M., Horisberger, U., Gennaro, R., and Dewald, B. (1985). *Lab. Invest.* **52**, 151–158.
Baintain, D. F. (1977). *In* "The Granulocyte: Function and Clinical Utilization," pp. 1–27. Liss, New York.
Baintain, D. F., and Farquhar, M. G. (1966). *J. Cell Biol.* **28**, 277–301.
Baintain, D. F., and Farquhar, M. G. (1968a). *J. Cell Biol.* **39**, 286–298.
Baintain, D. F., and Farquhar, M. G. (1968b). *J. Cell Biol.* **39**, 299–317.
Baintain, D. F., Ullyot, J. L., and Farquhar, M. G. (1971). *J. Exp. Med.* **134**, 907–934.
Baisero, M. H. (1973). *Schweiz. Med. Wochenschr.* **103**, 1599–1605.
Bareis, D. L., Hirata, F., Schiffmann, E., and Axelrod, J. (1982). *J. Cell Biol.* **93**, 690–697.
Barrett, A. J. (1974). "Proteinase Inhibitors" (H. Fritz, H. Tschesone, L. J. Greene, and E. E. Truskhe, eds.), pp. 574–580. Springer-Verlag, Berlin and New York.

Bass, D. A., O'Flaherty, J. T., Szejda, P., DeChatelet, L. R., and McCall, C. E. (1980). *Proc. Natl. Acad. Sci. U.S.A.* **77,** 5125–5137.
Beard, M., and Novikoff, A. B. (1968). *J. Hystochem. Cytochem.* **16,** 512.
Beatty, P., Ochs, H., Harlan, J., Price, T., Rosan, H., Taylor, R., Hansen, J., and Klebanoff, S. (1984). *Lancet* **1,** 535–542.
Benveniste, J., LeCovedic, J. P., Polonsky, J., and Tence, M. (1977). *Nature (London)* **269,** 170–171.
Berlin, R. D., and Oliver, J. M. (1978). *J. Cell Biol.* **77,** 789–804.
Bertram, T. A., and Coignoul, F. L. (1982). *Vet. Pathol.* **19,** 534–543.
Bertram, T. A., and Jensen, A. E. (1984). *Am. J. Vet. Res.* **45,** 1099–1104.
Bertram, T. A. Coignoul, F. L., and Jensen, A. E. (1982). *Infect. Immun.* **37,** 1241–1247.
Blose, S. H., and Chacko, S. (1976). *J. Cell Biol.* **70,** 459–466.
Boucek, M. M., and Snyderman, R. (1976). *Science* **193,** 905–907.
Boxer, L. A., Watamabe, A. M., and Rister, M. (1976). *N. Engl. J. Med.* **295,** 1041–1045.
Boxer, L. A., Allen, J. M., Watamabe, A. M., Besch, H. R., and Baehner, R. L. (1978). *Blood* **51,** 1045–1050.
Boxer, L. A., Haak, R. A., Yang, H. H., Wolach, J. B., Butterick, C., and Boehner, R. L. (1982). *Clin. Res.* **30,** 517A (Abstr.).
Bretz, U. (1978). *Experientia* **34,** 934–938.
Bretz, U., and Baggiolini, M. (1973). *J. Cell Biol.* **59,** 696–707.
Bretz, U., and Baggiolini, M. (1974). *J. Cell Biol.* **63,** 251–269.
Briggs, R. T., Drath, D. B., Karnovsky, M. L., and Karnovsky, M. J. (1975). *J. Cell Biol.* **67,** 566–586.
Bronza, J. P., and Ward, P. A. (1977). *Fed. Proc., Fed. Am. Soc. Exp. Biol.* **36,** 1020.
Broxmeyer, H. F., Moore, M. A. S., and Ralph, P. (1977). *Exp. Haematol.* **5,** 87–102.
Broxmeyer, H. E., Ralph, P., Bognacki, J., Kincade, P. W., and Desousa, M. (1980). *J. Immunol.* **125,** 903–909.
Brune, K., and Spitznagel, J. K. (1973). *J. Infect. Dis.* **127,** 84–94.
Brune, K., Leffell, M. S., and Spitznagel, J. K. (1972). *Infect. Immun.* **5,** 283–287.
Bullen, J. J., Rogers, H. J., and Leigh, L. (1972). *Br. Med. J.* **1,** 69–75.
Burgess, A. W., Camkaris, J., and Metcalf, D. (1977). *J. Biol. Chem.* **252,** 1998–2003.
Camp, C. J., and Leid, R. W. (1982). *Am. J. Vet. Res.* **43,** 397–401.
Campbell, F. (1968), *J. Morphol.* **123,** 405–415.
Camussi, G., Tetta, C., Bussolino, F., Cappio, F. C., Coda, R., Masera, G., and Segolini, G. (1980). *Appl. Immunol.* **62,** 1–15.
Canning, P. C., Roth, J. A., Tabatabai, L. B., and Deyoe, B. L. (1985). *J. Infect. Dis.* **152.**
Chang, J., Freer, R., Stella, R., and Greenbaum, L. M. (1972). *Biochem. Pharmacol.* **21,** 3095–3106.
Chenoweth, D. E., Lane, T. A., Rowe, J. G., and Hugli, T. E. (1980). *Clin. Immunol. Immunopathol.* **15,** 525–535.
Cheson, B. D., Christensen, R. L., Sperling, R., Kohler, B. E., and Babior, B. M. (1976). *J. Clin. Invest.* **58,** 789–796.
Chibber, R., and Castle, A. G. (1983). *Comp. Biochem. Physiol.* **75B,** 335–340.
Christophers, E., and Schroder, J. M. (1983). *Immunobiology* **164,** 127–135.
Clark, R. A., and Szot, S. (1981). *J. Immunol.* **126,** 1295–1301.
Cline, M. (1973). *Clin. Res.* **21,** 595.
Cline, M. J., Le Feure, C., and Golde, D. W. (1977). *J. Cell. Physiol.* **90,** 105–116.
Cochrane, C. G. (1971). *J. Exp. Med.* **134,** 75s–89s.

Coignoul, F. L., Bertram, T. A., and Cheville, N. F. (1984a). *Am. J. Vet. Res.* **45**, 1972–1975.
Coignoul, F. L., Bertram, T. A., Roth, J., and Cheville, N. F. (1984b). *Am. J. Vet. Res.* **45**, 898–902.
Craddock, P. R., White, J. G., Weisdorf, D. J., and Hammerschmidt, D. E. (1980). *Inflammation* **4**, 381–395.
Davis, B. H., Walker, R. J., Pearson, C. B., Becker, E. L., and Oliver, J. M. (1982). *Am. J. Pathol.* **108**, 206–216.
DeDuve, C., and Wattiqux, R. (1966). *Annu. Rev. Physiol.* **28**, 435–492.
DePierre, J. W., and Karnovsky, M. L. (1974a). *J. Biol. Chem.* **249**, 7111–7120.
DePierre, J. W., and Karnovsky, M. L. (1974b). *J. Biol. Chem.* **249**, 7121–7129.
Dewald, B., Baggiolini, M., Curnutte, J. T., and Babior, B. M. (1979). *J. Blin. Invest.* **63**, 21–29.
Dexter, T. M., and Moore, M. A. S. (1977). *Nature (London)* **269**, 412–413.
Drazin, R. E., and Lehrer, R. I. (1977). *Infect. Immun.* **17**, 382–388.
Efrati, C., Sacks, T., Ne'eman, N., Lahov, M., and Ginsburg, I. (1976). *Inflammation* **1**, 371–407.
Elsbach, P. (1980). *Rev. Infect. Dis.* **2**, 106–128.
Fantane, J. C., and Ward, P. A. (1982). *Am. J. Pathol.* **107**, 397–418.
Fee, J. A., and Valentine, J. S. (1977). "Superoxide and Superoxide Dismutases" (A. M. Michelson, J. M. McCord, and I. Fridovich, eds.), pp. 19–60. Academic Press, New York.
Freese, E., Sheu, C. W., and Galiers, E. (1973). *Nature (London)* **241**, 321–325.
Gabig, T. G., and Babior, B. M. (1981). *Annu. Rev. Med.* **32**, 313–326.
Gallin, J. I. (1980a). *J. Clin. Invest.* **65**, 298–306.
Gallin, J. I. (1980b). *In* "The Handbook of Inflammation" (G. Weissman, ed.), Vol. 2, pp. 299–335. Elsevier, Amsterdam.
Gallin, J. I. (1980c). *Ann. Intern Med.* **2**, 520–538.
Gallin, J. I., and Rosenthal, A. S. (1974). *J. Cell Biol.* **63**, 594–609.
Gallin, J. I., Durocher, J. R., and Kaplan, A. P. (1975). *J. Clin. Invest.* **55**, 967–974.
Gallin, J. I., Wright, D. G., and Schiffmann, E. (1978). *J. Clin. Invest.* **62**, 1364–1374.
Gallin, J. I., Gallin, E. K., and Schiffmann, E. (1979). *In* "Advances in Inflammation Research" (G. Weissmann, ed.), Vol. 1, pp. 123–138. Raven, New York.
Gallin, J. I., Wright, D. G., Malech, H. L., Davis, J. M., Klempner, M. S., and Kirkpatrick, C. H. (1980). *Ann. Intern. Med.* **92**, 520–538.
Gennaro, R., Odzani, L., and Romeo, D. (1983a). *Infect. Immun.* **40**, 684–690.
Gennaro, R., Dewald, B., Horisberger, U., Gubler, H. U., and Baggiolini, M. (1983b). *J. Cell Biol.* **96**, 1651–1661.
Ginsburg, I., and Lahav, M. (1983). *Eur. J. Microbiol.* **2**, 186–191.
Glasser, L., *(1983)*. *Am. J. Clin. Pathol.* **79**, 45–51.
Goetzl, E. J., Waller, P. F., and Sun, F. F. (1980). *J. Immunol.* **124**, 926–933.
Goetzl, E. J., Brindley, L. L., and Goldman, D. W. (1983). *J. Immunol.* **50**, 35–41.
Golde, D. W., and Cline, M. J. (1972). *J. Clin. Invest.* **51**, 2981–2983.
Golde, D. W., and Cline, M. J. (1974). *N. Engl. J. Med.* **291**, 1388–1395.
Goldman, D. W., and Goetzl, E. J. (1981). *Fed. Proc., Fed. Am. Exp. Biol.* **40**, 1004.
Goldstein, I. M. (1976). *Prog. Allergy* **20**, 301–340.
Goldstein, I. M., and Weissman, G. (1974). *J. Immunol.* **113**, 1583–1588.
Goldstein, I. M., Cerqueira, M., Lind, S., and Kaplan, M. B. (1977). *J. Clin. Invest.* **59**, 249–254.
Graham, R. C., and Karnovsky, M. J. (1966). *J. Histochem. Cytochem.* **14**, 291–302.

Green, I., Kirkpatrick, C. H., and Dale, D. C. (1971). *Proc. Soc. Exp. Biol. Med.* **137,** 1311–1317.
Greenbaum, L. M. (1972). *Am. J. Pathol.* **68,** 613–623.
Haber, F., and Weiss, J. (1934). *Proc. R. Soc. London Ser. A* **147,** 332–351.
Hakansson, L., and Venge, P. (1982). *Immunology* **47,** 687–694.
Hakansson, L., Hallgren, R., and Venge, P. (1980). *J. Clin. Invest.* **66,** 298–305.
Hanker, J. S., and Giammara, B. L. (1983). *Science* **220,** 415–417.
Hardin, J. H., Spicer, S. S., Greene, W. B., and Horn, R. G. (1968). *J. Histochem. Cytochem.* **16,** 510.
Harlan, J., De Chatelet, L. R., Iverson, D. B., and McCall, C. E. (1977). *Infect. Immun.* **15,** 436–443.
Harlan, J., Schwartz, B. R., Reidy, M. A., Schwartz, S. M., Ochs, H. D., and Harker, L. A. (1985). *Lab. Invest.* **52,** 141–150.
Harrison, J. E., and Schultz, J. (1976). *J. Biol. Chem.* **251,** 1371–1374.
Harvath, L., and Leonard, E. J. (1982). *Infect. Immun.* **36,** 443–449.
Healy, P. J. (1982). *Res. Vet. Sci.* **33,** 275–279.
Held, H. M., and Hurst, J. K. (1978). *Biochem. Biophys. Res. Commun.* **81,** 878–885.
Henson, P. M., and Shew, J. O. (1982). *Am. J. Pathol.* **108,** 17–23.
Herman, S. P., Golde, D. W., and Cline, M. J. (1978). *Blood* **51,** 207–219.
Hirata, F., and Axelrod, J. (1980). *Sci.* **209,** 1082–1085.
Hoffstein, S., and Weissman, G. (1975). *Arthritis Rheum.* **18,** 153–165.
Hoover, R. L., Briggs, R. T., and Karnovsky, M. J. (1978). *Cell* **14,** 423–428.
Horn, R. G., and Spicer, S. S. (1964). *Lab. Invest.* **13,** 1–15.
Horn, R. G., and Spicer, S. S. (1965). *Am. J. Pathol.* **46,** 197–213.
Ingraham, L. M., Chenetic, P. E., Boxer, L. A., and Baehner, R. L. (1983). *Fed. Proc., Fed. Am. Soc. Exp. Biol.* **42,** 385 (Abstr. No. 542).
Issekutz, A. C., Ripley, M., and Jackson, J. R. (1983). *Lab. Invest.* **49,** 716–724.
Jacques, Y. V., and Bainton, D. F. (1978). *Lab. Invest.* **39,** 179–185.
Jain, N. C. (1967). *Folia Haematol.* **88,** 297–304.
Jain, N. C. (1968). *Acta Haematol.* **39,** 51–59.
Jain, N. C. (1969). *Acta Haematol.* **41,** 249–253.
Jain, N. C. (1970a). *Blut* **22,** 133–143.
Jain, N. C. (1970b). *Folia Haematol.* **94,** 49–63.
Jensen, M. S., and Baintain, D. F. (1973). *J. Cell Biol.* **56,** 379–388.
Kakinuma, K. (1970). *J. Biochem.* **68,** 177–185.
Kaplan, H. B. (1982). *Biochim. Biophys. Acta* **721,** 55–63.
Karnovsky, M. L. (1968). *Semin. Hematol.* **5,** 156–165.
Kemp, A. S., Cripps, A. W., and Brown, S. (1980). *Clin. Exp. Immunol.* **40,** 388–395.
Kim, H., Pangalis, G. A., Payne, B. C., Kadin, M. E., and Rappaport, H. (1982). *Am. J. Pathol.* **106,** 204–223.
Klebanoff, S. J. (1975a). *In* "The Phagocytic Cell In Host Resistance" (J. A. Bellanti and D. H. Dayton, eds.), pp. 45–56. Raven, New York.
Klebanoff, S. J. (1975b). *Semin. Hematol.* **12,** 117–142.
Klebanoff, S. J., and Clark, R. A. (1978). *In* "The Neutrophil: Function and Clinical Disorders," pp. 5–51, 409–489, 217–218. North-Holland Publ., Amsterdam.
Klebanoff, S. J., Durack, D. T., and Rosen, H. (1977). *Infect. Immun.* **17,** 167–173.
Klempner, M. S., and Gallin, J. I. (1978). *Blood* **51,** 659–669.
Klempner, M. S., Gallin, J. I., Balow, J. E., and Van Kammen, D. P. (1980). *Blood* **55,** 777–783.
Korchak, H. M., and Weismann, G. (1978). *Proc. Natl. Acad. Sci. U.S.A.* **75,** 3818–3822.

Korchak, H. M., Roos, D., Giedd, K. N., Wynkoop, E. M., Vienne, K., Rutherford, L. E., Buyon, J. P., Rich, A. M., and Weissmann, G. (1983). *Proc. Natl. Acad. Sci. U.S.A.* **80**, 4968–4972.
Kurland, J. I., Bockman, R. S., Broxmeyer, H. E., and Moore, M. A. S. (1978). *Science* **199**, 552–555.
Lanky, S. A., and Wohl, H. (1981). *J. Clin. Invest.* **67**, 817–826.
Latimer, K. S., and Prasse, K. W. (1982). *Am. J. Vet. Res.* **43**, 525–527.
Lehrer, R. I. (1972). *J. Clin. Invest.* **51**, 2566–2572.
Lehrer, R. I., Ladra, K. M., and Hake, R. B. (1975). *Infect. Immun.* **11**, 1226–1234.
Link, A. S., Jr., Bass, D. A., and McCall, C. E. (1979). *J. Infect. Dis.* **140**, 517–526.
Lotem, J., and Sachs, L. (1977). *Proc. Natl. Acad. Sci. U.S.A.* **74**, 5554–5558.
Lynch, J. M., Lotner, G. Z., Betz, S. J., and Henson, P. M. (1979). *J. Immunol.* **123**, 1219–1226.
McCall, C. E., Katayama, I., Cotran, R. S., and Finland, M. (1969). *J. Exp. Med.* **129**, 267–293.
MacGregor, B. R. (1980). *In* "The Handbook of Inflammation." (G. Weissmann, ed.), Vol. 2, pp. 267–298. Elsevier, Amsterdam.
MacGregor, R. R. (1976). *Clin. Res.* **24**, 348.
MacGregor, R. R., Spangnulo, P. J., and Lentnek, A. L. (1974). *N. Engl. J. Med.* **291**, 642–646.
Malech, H. L., Root, R. K., and Gallin, J. I. (1977). *J. Cell Biol.* **75**, 666–693.
Mandell, G. L. (1970). *Proc. Soc. Exp. Biol. Med.* **134**, 447–449.
Mantovani, B. (1975). *J. Immunol.* **115**, 15–17.
Messner, R. P., and Jelinek, J. (1970). *J. Clin. Invest.* **49**, 2165–2171.
Moore, M. A. S., Spitzer, G., Metcalf, D., and Pennington, O. G. (1974). *Br. J. Haematol.* **27**, 47–55.
Naccache, P., Freer, R. J., Showell, H. J., Becker, E. L., and Sha'afi, R. I. (1977). *J. Cell Biol.* **73**, 428–444.
Naccache, P. H., Borgent, P., Goetzel, E. J., and Sha'afi, R. I. (1981). *J. Clin. Invest.* **67**, 1584–1587.
Nafstad, H. J., and Nafstad, I. (1968). *Pathol. Vet.* **5**, 451–470.
Nakamura, S., Yoshinaga, M., and Hayashi, H. (1976). *J. Immunol.* **117**, 1–6.
Odeberg, H., and Olsson, I. (1975). *J. Clin. Invest.* **56**, 1118–1124.
Odeberg, H., and Olsson, I. (1976). *Infect. Immun.* **14**, 1269–1275.
O'Donnell, R. T., and Anderson, B. R. (1982). *Infect. Immun.* **38**, 351–359.
O'Flaherty, J. T., Craddock, P. R., and Jacob, H. S. (1977). *Blood* **48**, 987–993.
O'Flaherty, J. T., Showell, H. J., Becker, E. L., and Ward, P. A. (1978). *Am. J. Pathol.* **92**, 155–166.
Ohlsson, K., Olsson, I., and Spitznagel, J. K. (1977). *Hoppe-Seylers Z. Physiol. Chem.* **358**, 361–366.
Oseas, R. S., Yang, H. H., Baehner, R. L., and Boxer, L. A. (1981). *Blood* **57**, 939–945.
Parmely, R. T., Takagi, M., Barton, J. C., Boxer, L., and Austin, R. L. (1982). *Am. J. Pathol.* **109**, 343–358.
Paukovits, W. R. (1971). *Cell Tissue Kinet.* **4**, 539–547.
Penniall, R., and Spitznagel, J. K. (1975). *Proc. Natl. Acad. Sci. U.S.A.* **72**, 5012–5015.
Pfeiffer, J. R., Oliver, J. M., and Berlin, R. D. (1980). *Nature (London)* **286**, 727–730.
Piatt, J. F., and O'Brien, P. J. (1979). *Eur. J. Biochem.* **93**, 323–332.
Pike, M. C., Kredich, N. M., and Snyderman, R. (1978). *Proc. Natl. Acad. Sci. U.S.A.* **75**, 3928–3941.

Plow, E. F., and Edington, T. S. (1975). *J. Clin. Invest.* **56**, 30–38.
Pozzan, T., Lew, D. P., Wollheim, C. B., and Tsien, R. Y. (1983). *Science* **221**, 1413–1415.
Pryzwansky, K. B., Martin, L. E., and Spitznagel, J. K. (1978). *J. Reticuloendothel. Soc.* **24**, 295–310.
Rasp, F. L., and Repine, J. E. (1981). *J. Lab. Clin. Med.* **97**, 812–819.
Rausch, P. G., and Canonico, P. G. (1975). *Infect. Immun.* **12**, 687–693.
Rausch, P. G., and Moore, T. G. (1975). *Blood* **46**, 913–919.
Rausch, P. G., Canonico, P. G., and Chapple, F. E., III (1974). *Fed. Proc., Fed. Am. Soc. Exp. Biol.* **33**, 257.
Reijngoud, D. J., and Tager, J. M. (1977). *Biochim. Biophys. Acta* **472**, 419–449.
Repine, J. E., Eaton, J. W., Anders, M. W., Hoidal, J. R., and Fox, R. B. (1979). *J. Clin. Invest.* **64**, 1642–1651.
Rest, R. F., Cooney, M. H., and Spitznagel, J. K. (1978a). *Infect. Immun.* **19**, 131–137.
Rest, R. F., Cooney, M. H., and Spitznagel, J. K. (1978b). *Biochem. J.* **174**, 53–59.
Robinson, W. A., and Mangalik, A. (1975). *Semin. Hematol.* **12**, 7–25.
Romeo, D., Zabucchi, G., Miani, N., and Rossi, F. (1975). *Nature (London)* **253**, 542–544.
Root, R. K., and Cohen, M. S. (1981). *Rev. Infect. Dis.* **3**, 565–598.
Root, R. K., and Metcalf, J. A. (1977). *J. Clin. Invest.* **60**, 1266–1279.
Rosen, H., and Klebanoff, S. J. (1977). *J. Biol. Chem.* **252**, 4803–4810.
Rosen, H., and Klebanoff, S. J. (1979). *J. Clin. Invest.* **64**, 1725–1729.
Roth, J. A., and Kaeberle, M. L. (1981). *Vet. Immunol. Immunopathol.* **2**, 157–174, 1981.
Rungger-Brändle, E., and Gabbiani, G. (1983). *Am. J. Pathol.* **110**, 361–391.
Sagone, A. L., Jr., King, G. W., and Metz, E. N. (1976). *J. Clin. Invest.* **57**, 1352–1358.
Saxon, A., Stevens, R. H., and Golde, D. W. (1978). *Ann. Intern. Med.* **88**, 323–326.
Sbarra, A. J., and Karnovsky, M. L. (1969). *J. Biol. Chem.* **234**, 1355–1362.
Schiffmann, E., O'Dea, R. F., Chiang, P. K., Verkatasubramanian, K., Corcoran, B., Hirata, F., and Axelrod, J. (1979). In "Modulation of Protein Function" (D. E. Atkinson and F. C. Fox, eds.). Academic Press, New York.
Schliwa, M., Pryzwansky, K., and Eutenever, U. (1982). *Cell* **31**, 705–717.
Schneier, J., Gall, J. A., Carpe, A. I., and Boggs, D. R. (1977). *Scand. J. Haematol.* **19**, 435–442.
Scribner, D. J., and Fahrney, D. (1976). *J. Immunol.* **116**, 892–897.
Seligmann, B., Chesed, T. M., and Gallin, J. I. (1981). *J. Clin. Invest.* **68**, 1125–1131.
Serhan, C. N., Korchak, H. M., and Weissmann, G. (1980). *J. Immunol.* **125**, 2020–2024.
Shew, J. O., and Hensen, P. M. (1982). *Am. J. Pathol.* **108**, 17–23.
Simchowitz, L., Fischbein, L. C., Spilberg, I., and Atkinson, J. P. (1980). *J. Immunol.* **124**, 1482–1491.
Smith, G. S., Lunsden, J. E., and Wilcock, B. P. (1985). *Can. J. Comp. Med.* **49**, 43–49.
Smolen, J. E., and Weissman, G. (1978). *Biochim. Biophys. Acta* **512**, 525–538.
Smolen, J. E., Korchak, H. M., and Weissmann, G. (1980). *J. Clin. Invest.* **65**, 1077–1085.
Smolen, J. E., Korchak, H. M., and Weissmann, G. (1981). *Biochim. Biophys. Acta* **677**, 512–521.
Snyderman, R., and Goetzl, E. (1981). *Science* **213**, 830–837.
Snyderman, R., and Pike, M. C. (1980). *Science* **209**, 493–495.
Sonoda, M., and Koboyashi, K. (1966). *Jpn. J. Vet. Res.* **14**, 71–77.
Sonoda, M., and Kobayashi, K. (1970a). *Jpn. J. Vet. Res.* **18**, 63–65.
Sonoda, M., and Kobayashi, K. (1970b). *Jpn. J. Vet. Res.* **18**, 37–41.
Spagnuolo, P. J., Ellner, J. J., Hassid, J. J., and Dunn, M. J. (1980). *J. Clin. Invest.* **66**, 406–412.

Spicer, S. S., and Hardin, J. H. (1969). *Lab. Invest.* **20**, 488–497.
Spitznagel, J. K. (1977). In "The Granulocyte: Function and Utilization" (T. J. Greenwalt and G. A. Jamieson, eds.), pp. 103–131. Liss, New York.
Spitznagel, J. K., Dalldorf, F. G., Lefell, M. S., Folds, J. D., Welsh, I. R. H., Cooney, M. H., and Martin, L. E. (1974). *Lab. Invest.* **30**, 774–785.
Stanley, E. R., and Heard, P. M. (1977). *J. Biol. Chem.* **252**, 4305–4312.
Stendahl, O. I., and Stossel, T. P. (1980). *Biochem. Biophys. Res. Commun.* **92**, 675–680.
Tauber, A. I., and Babior, B. M. (1977). *J. Clin. Invest.* **60**, 374–379.
Tynelius-Bratthall, G., and Lindhe, J. (1974). *Arch. Oral Biol.* **19**, 97–101.
Valone, F. H., and Goetzl, E. J. (1983). *Am. J. Pathol.* **113**, 85–94.
Van Epps, D. E., and Williams, R. C. (1976). *J. Exp. Med.* **144**, 1227–1242.
Venge, P., and Olsson, I. (1975). *J. Immunol.* **115**, 1505–1508.
Vincent, P. C., Chanana, A. D., Cronkite, E. P., and Joel, D. D. (1974). *Blood* **43**, 371–377.
Vinella, G., Lopes-Vinella, M. F., Shuler, C., Sherwood, T., Espinosa, G. A., Winocour, P., and Colwell, J. A. (1983). *J. Immunol.* **50**, 43–51.
Vischer, T. L., Bretz, U., and Baggiolini, M. (1976). *J. Exp. Med.* **144**, 863–872.
Voetman, A. A., Loos, J. A., and Roos, D. (1980). *Blood* **55**, 741–747.
Walker, R. J., Berlin, R. D., Pfeiffer, J. R., and Oliver, J. M. (1980). *J. Cell Biol.* **86**, 199–211.
Ward, P. A., and Hill, J. H. (1970). *J. Immunol.* **104**, 535–543.
Ward, P. A., and Zvaifler, A. J. (1970). *J. Clin. Invest.* **50**, 606–616.
Wasserman, H. H., and Murray, R. W. (1979). "Singlet Oxygen." Academic Press, New York.
Weber, L., and Peterhaus, E. (1983). *Immunobiology* **164**, 333–342.
Weinstein, J., and Bielski, B. H. J. (1979). *J. Am. Chem. Soc.* **101**, 58–62.
Weiss, J., Beckerdite-Quagliata, S., and Elsbach, P. (1980). *J. Clin. Invest.* **65**, 619–628.
Weiss, J., and Elsbach, P. (1977). *Biochim. Biophys. Acta* **466**, 23–33.
Weiss, S. J., and LoBuglio, A. F. (1980). *Blood* **55**, 1020–1024.
Weiss, J., Franson, R. C., Beckerdite, S., Schmeidler, K., and Elsbach, P. (1975). *J. Clin. Invest.* **55**, 33–42.
Weiss, J., Elsbach, P., Olsson, I., and Odeberg, H. (1978a). *J. Biol. Chem.* **253**, 2664–2672.
Weiss, S. J., Rustagi, P. K., and LoBuglio, A. F. (1978b). *J. Exp. Med.* **147**, 316–324.
Weiss, S. J., Young, J., LoBuglio, A. F., Slivka, A., and Nimeh, N. F. (1981). *J. Clin. Invest.* **68**, 714–721.
Weiss, S. J., Lampert, M. B., and Test, S. T. (1983). *Science* **222**, 625–628.
Weissman, G., Smolen, J. E., and Hoffstein, S. (1978). *J. Invest. Dermatol.* **71**, 95–99.
Welsh, I. R. H., and Spitznagel, J. K. (1971). *Infect. Immun.* **4**, 97–102.
Wetzel, B. K., Horn, R. G., and Spicer, S. S. (1963). *J. Histochem. Cytochem.* **11**, 812–814.
Wetzel, B. K., Horn, R. G., and Spicer, S. S. (1967a). *Lab. Invest.* **16**, 349–382.
Wetzel, B. K., Spicer, S. S., and Horn, R. G. (1967b). *J. Histochem. Cytochem.* **15**, 311–334.
Whited, S. C., Santaella, M., Frank, M. M., Gaither, T., and Gallin, J. I. (1981). *Inflammation* **5**, 103–114.
Wintroub, B. U., Kaempfer, C. E., and Klickstein, L. B. (1982). *Fed. Proc., Fed. Am. Soc. Exp. Biol.* **41**, 734 (Abstr. No. 2707).
Wolf, N. S. (1974). *Cell Tissue Kinet.* **7**, 89–98.
Woodin, A. M., and Wieneke, A. A. (1970a). *Biochim. Biophys. Acta* **233**, 702–715.
Woodin, A. M., and Wieneke, A. A. (1970b). *J. Gen. Physiol.* **56**, 16–32.

Wright, D. G., and Gallin, J. I. (1975). *Inflammation* **1**, 23–39.
Yachnin, S., and Richman, D. P. (1982). *Cell. Immunol.* **72**, 248–262.
Yamada, Y., and Sonoda, M. (1970). *Jpn. J. Vet. Res.* **18**, 83–89.
Zeya, H. I., and Spitznagel, J. K. (1966). *Science* **154**, 1049–1051.
Zeya, H. I., and Spitznagel, J. K. (1971). *Lab. Invest.* **24**, 237–245.
Zighelboim, J., Gale, R. P., and Kedar, E. (1976). *Transplantation* **21**, 524–526.
Zigmond, S. H. (1974). *Nature (London)* **249**, 250–252.
Zigmond, S. H. (1977). *J. Cell Biol.* **75**, 606–616.
Zigmond, S. H. (1978). *J. Cell Biol.* **77**, 269–287.
Zinkl, J. G., and Brown, P. D. (1982). *Am. J. Vet. Res.* **43**, 613–616.
Zucker-Franklin, D. (1968). *Semin. Hematol.* **5**, 109–133.

Pathobiology of Animal Platelets

KENNETH M. MEYERS

Department of Veterinary and Comparative Anatomy, Pharmacology, and Physiology, Washington State University, Pullman, Washington

I.	Introduction	131
II.	Acquisition	132
III.	Ultrastructure	134
IV.	Basic Platelet Response	138
	A. Dense Granule Pathway	140
	B. Arachidonic Acid Pathway	144
	C. Platelet-Activating Factor	148
	D. Additional Agonists	150
	E. Summary	150
V.	Modulators	151
	A. PGI_2 and cAMP	151
	B. Epinephrine	152
	C. Epinephrine as a Gain Controller	154
VI.	Agglutinating Agents	155
	A. von Willebrand Factor	155
	B. Endotoxin	155
VII.	Platelet Membrane Glycoproteins	156
VIII.	Tumor Cells	157
IX.	Thrombocytopenia	159
	References	159

I. Introduction

Platelets, the smallest formed element in blood, participate in the stopping of hemorrhage. This is accomplished by platelets secreting or forming vasoconstrictive substances and by platelets adhering to the subendothelium and then aggregating to prevent mechanically the loss of blood by forming a platelet plug. Platelets have a demanding role. They provide adequate protection against hemorrhage in a system in which blood is flowing at a high velocity. At the same time, inappropriate intravascular responses leading to intravascular platelet aggregation (thrombosis) do not occur.

This review is concerned with the pathobiology of animal platelets.

II. Acquisition

Acquisition of a blood sample for platelet studies requires special precautions. Platelets are stimulus–response cells and the venipuncture must be done cleanly to avoid the generation of compounds that may affect platelet yield and function. The withdrawal must be controlled, not so rapid as to activate mechanically the platelets but fast enough to ensure adequate mixture of the anticoagulant. Care must be taken to ensure that the interior of the vessel is not traumatized; this could produce prostaglandins which inhibit platelet function. Furthermore, the animal should not be unduly stressed during the withdrawal; this could also affect platelet function.

Animal platelets are routinely obtained using either chemical or physical restraint and an anticoagulant. Common procedures for obtaining a blood sample are presented in Table I. The method of restraint and the anticoagulant used vary with the species. Citrate, used at a concentration of $0.11\ M$ (one part citrate per nine parts blood), is the most frequently used anticoagulant. In some animals, such as the rat, this citrate concentration depresses platelet aggregation responses (Dwyer and Meyers, 1985a; Furlow and Bass, 1976). In the dog, Clemmons and Meyers (1984) report that it is difficult to routinely obtain platelets in adequate numbers that function in a predictable manner. To overcome these problems, heparin has been used successfully in the rat (Dwyer and Meyers, 1985a; Furlow and Bass, 1976) and a higher citrate concentration has been suggested for the dog (Clemmons and Meyers, 1984).

The choice of restraint is dictated by the nature of the species. Where possible, physical restraint is used. This is not without problems, and it is difficult to obtain blood from pigs without restraint stress. Most cats, some dogs, rats, mink, and monkeys require chemical restraint. A variety of anesthetics have been used. We have used ketamine HCl to anesthetize mink (Meyers *et al.*, 1978), methoxyflurane to anesthetize rats (Dwyer and Meyers, 1985a), and thiamylal Na to anesthetize dogs (Meyers *et al.*, 1983a) and cats (Meyers *et al.*, 1981), even though platelet responses are known to be inhibited by barbiturates (MacKenzie *et al.*, 1972). Platelets obtained from dogs lightly anesthetized

TABLE I

SUMMARY OF ACQUISITION OF PRP FROM ANIMALS

Animals	Method of restraint			Anticoagulant		Centrifugation[a]	Site[b]
	Physical	Chemical		Citrate	Heparin		
Companion animals							
Cat		Thiamyl Na		0.11 M		High/low-3	J
Dog	×	Thiamyl Na		0.11 or 0.18 M		High	J
Horse	×			0.11 M		Low-1	J
Food-producing animals							
Cow	×			0.11 M		High/low-2	J
Pig	×			0.11 M		High/low-3	IVC
Sheep	×			0.11 M		High/low-2	J
Laboratory animals							
Gerbil							H
Guinea pig							H
Monkey		Phencyclidine HCl					
Mouse	×						
Rabbit				0.11 M			CEA
Rat		Methoxyflurane			5 or 50 U/ml		H
Mink		Ketamine HCl		0.11 M			H

[a] High gravitational force, 1200 g × 2.5 min; low gravitational force, 1 = 150 g × 15 min; 2 = 250 g × 30 min; 3 = 750 g × 30 min.
[b] J, jugular vein; IVC, inferior vena cava; H, heart; CEA, central ear artery.

with thiamylal Na did not respond differently to ADP (2.5–10 μM) than did those from the same dogs when they were not anesthetized. Platelet counts in the lightly barbiturate-anesthetized dogs were reduced, presumably as a result of splenic sequestering. Recently methoxyflurane has been used to anesthetize rats for platelet studies and was found to provide platelet yields comparable to other anesthetics (Dwyer and Meyers, 1985a), and in addition, platelet function was not depressed or exaggerated. Phencyclidine has been used to anesthetize monkeys (Addonizio et al., 1979).

III. Ultrastructure

The mean volume of platelets from most species ranges from 4.1 fl in the goat to 15 fl in the cat (Meyers et al., 1982a; Clemmons et al., 1983) (Table II). Platelet counts vary from slightly less than 200,000/μl in the horse to over 2,000,000/μl in rats (Table II). The nonstimulated, or resting, platelets are diskoid shaped, and when sectioned perpendicularly to the equatorial plane they are elliptical (Fig. 1). There is a circumferential band of microtubules, which in bovine platelets

TABLE II

CHARACTERISTICS OF ANIMAL PLATELETS

Animals	Count (platelets/μl) × 10^{-5}		Size (fl)	Protein content (mg/10^{11} platelets)
	Whole blood	PRP		
Companion animals				
Cat	1.89		12.0	185
Dog	2.74		7.5	153
Horse	1.07		5.1	99
Food-producing animals				
Cow	3.17		5.0	102
Pig	6.34		6.9	177
Sheep	4.07		4.4	
Laboratory animals				
Gerbil				
Guinea pig			4.5	
Mouse			3.3	
Rabbit		4.73	3.3	127
Rat			4.7	
Mink		3.65	8.0	184

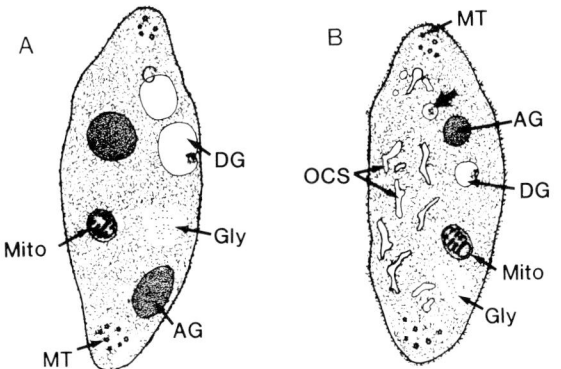

FIG. 1. Representation of (A) bovine and (B) feline platelets. Mito, Mitochondria; Gly, glycogen; MT, microtubules; AG, α-granule; DG, dense granule; OCS, open or surface-connected canalicular system.

number 19 (Meyers et al., 1982c). Mitochondria are present in numbers less than one per platelet section. They are usually small and are either round or oval.

There are two prominent types of granules: dense granules and α-granules. The dense granules contain adenine nucleotides (predominantly ATP and ADP), amines [primarily 5-hydroxytryptamine (5-HT) or serotonin], and bivalent cations (Mg^{2+} and Ca^{2+}). If the platelet 5-HT content is high, such as in bovine platelets (Meyers et al., 1982c), then the granules have a core that is intensely electron dense. The core is usually eccentrically positioned on or against the granule membrane. Surrounding the core is an extremely electron-lucent area. Occasionally, sections through the granule are obtained in which the core is not included; in this case only the electron-lucent area is seen. On the other hand, sections may include only the area of the granule in which the core is located. Here, the core will predominate and the translucent area will be minor. Occasionally, two dense cores can be seen. There are species variations in the appearance and number of dense granules. Species that have a high serotonin concentration will have numerous dense granules and the core will be very dense (Meyers et al., 1982c). In species that have less serotonin, the dense granules are less prominent.

The other granule type that is readily identifiable is the α-granule. This granule is more numerous than the dense granule and is typically homogeneous with a moderately electron-dense matrix. It is not unusual, at least in bovine platelets, to observe oval and drumstick-like granules with heterogeneous straining densities. α-Granules in animal platelets have not been studied extensively and little is known about their composition. In man, α-granules contain proteins that presumably function in coagulation, inflammation, and the healing of wounds (Kaplan, 1981). Some of these granule proteins, those with antiheparin activity, are unique to the platelet. Antiheparin activity has been found in monkey, horse, pig, cow, sheep, rabbit, and rat platelets in addition to human platelets (Fabrizi et al., 1981). Thomas et al. (1970) reported that the heparin-neutralizing activity of cat and pig platelets was greater than that of human platelets, but that of rabbit and guinea pig platelets was less. Antiheparin proteins from rabbit (Ginsberg et al., 1979), pig (Rucinski et al., 1983), and cattle (Claglowski et al., 1981) platelets have been purified. Two heparin-binding proteins that are secreted from pig platelets have been identified by Rucinski et al. (1983): platelet factor 4 and porcine basic protein. When comparing the similar human proteins to the porcine proteins, some common antigenic determinants were identified. However, the commercially available antibodies to human platelet factor 4 will not cross-react with platelets from other species, including porcine platelets. Since these antiheparin proteins are unique, it was anticipated that the circulating levels of these proteins would increase during platelet activation and therefore be diagnostic for participation of platelets in the pathophysiology of vascular lesions (Zahavi and Kakkar, 1980). Unfortunately, this potential has not been realized (Files et al., 1981).

The less prominent types of granules in human platelets that have been identified include peroxisomes and lysomes (Bentfeld-Barker and Bainton, 1982). Granule-like structures with unusual characteristics have been identified in cattle platelets (Meyers et al., 1982c). Occasionally, large granules that have a structure resembling microtubules are seen adjacent to the granule membrane. There is another membrane-bound structure that is similar in size to the dense granule and has a loose, disorganized matrix. It is present in the platelets of normal cattle and those of cattle with the Chediak–Higashi syndrome that are virtually devoid of platelet dense granules (Meyers et al., 1982c; Prieur et al., 1976). It is not known whether these structures are normal variants of α- or dense granules or whether they are a different granule.

Two types of smooth membrane systems are present in platelets of most species: the dense tubular system (DTS) and the open or surface-connected canalicular system (SCCS). The dense tubular system is less readily identified in resting platelets than in stimulated platelets. It has been suggested that in human platelets the DTS is involved with Ca fluxes (White, 1972). Structures resembling the SCCS in human platelets are seen in platelets from most species. In human platelets the SCCS is in continuity with the cell membrane via pits that can be seen in freeze-fractured replicas (White, 1973). The extent of the SCCS can be seen in platelets incubated with cationized ferritin and peroxidase (Zucker-Franklin, 1981). The SCCS was not observed in thin sections of resting bovine platelets (Meyers *et al.*, 1982c). Recently, pits were not seen in replicas of freeze-fractured platelets (Zucker-Franklin *et al.*, 1985). Cationized ferritin, ruthenium red, and peroxidase were localized on the outer plasma membrane and were not interiorized, demonstrating that the SCCS is not present in resting bovine platelets (Zucker-Franklin *et al.*, 1985). Species differences in the SCCS may account for the variations observed in the way bovine platelets adhere to glass. When human, cat, and mink platelets are placed on glass slides, the granules are located in the center of the platelet and are surrounded by a skirt of cytoplasm. In contrast, bovine platelets have a stellar-like appearance, with one or two long pseudopods and several smaller pseudopods protruding from the central granule core.

When stimulated, the response of bovine platelets, which lack the SCCS, is different from those that have the SCCS. If the platelets are prevented from aggregating and are treated with low agonist concentration, the platelets lose their diskoid shape and acquire an oval shape with an irregular, convoluted surface (Meyers *et al.*, 1982c). Associated with the convolutions are granules that protrude from the platelet. The microtubules are organized, but follow a tortuous route within the cell. In contrast to human platelets (White, 1971), granule centralization is only rarely observed in bovine platelets. With increasing concentrations, the change in the shape of bovine platelets becomes more pronounced as the centrifugal movement of platelet granules becomes more prominent. Pseudopods are present at this time. Organized groups of microtubules are seen only in the pseudopods. With increasing agonist concentration, the number of platelet granules decreases. When maximal release is induced, approximately 90% of the α-granules disappear. While not proven, the impression is that the granules are being secreted and that the granule membrane is fusing with the plasma membrane. Furthermore, it appears the granules may be releasing their constituents into channels formed earlier in the secretory event by the fusion of other granule membranes and the plasma membrane.

When these platelets are stirred in the presence of fibrinogen and calcium, platelet aggregation is observed. When the ultrastructure of bovine platelets is studied during the aggregation response, a progressive change in platelet structure is observed (Meyers *et al.*, 1982c).

During the initial phase, the platelets acquire an irregular shape and platelet-to-platelet contact may occur. This is followed by platelets aggregating in a mass. Each platelet is a separate entity and extracellular space is readily observed. It is likely that these platelets could separate and aggregation could be reversed. However, in the latter stages of the aggregation response, irreverisble platelet aggregates appear. There are two types. In one type, the core of the aggregate is composed of degranulated platelets, boundaries are difficult or impossible to see, and the platelets appear fused. The more peripheral platelets are usually intact and contain granules. In the second type of aggregate, the platelets in the center are in close cell-to-cell contact, but they contain granules, and the individual platelets are easily recognized. The periphery of the aggregate is composed mostly of degranulated platelets with pseudopods that extend into the center of the aggregate.

IV. Basic Platelet Response

Platelets from all mammalian species studied to date respond to a variety of stimuli by first changing shape and then aggregating (Fig. 2). The aggregation response depends upon the type of inducer, or agonist, the strength of the agonist, and the origin of the platelets. The initial aggregation response is reversible; the platelets aggregate and then dissociate. With increasing concentration of an appropriate agonist, irreverisble aggregation is observed and platelets will not dissociate. As the aggregation response proceeds from reversible to irreversible, the aggregation curve may either appear monophasic throughout or it may have a biphasic appearance.

The species variation is, for the most part, quantitative and not qualitative, since the *sequence* of a change in platelet shape, reversible aggregation, and irreversible aggregation does not change. However, *progression* along this sequence does change. For example, an agonist in one species may produce only a change in platelet shape, while in another species, platelets may change shape and aggregate but the aggregation is reversible. In still another species, the agonist may induce irreversible aggregation.

There are several types of agonists of animal platelets (Holmsen, 1982). Agonists can be low-molecular-weight substances such as 5-HT, ADP, thromboxane A_2, prostaglandin endoperoxides (PGG_2 and PGH_2), and platelet activating factor (PAF). These compounds are formed by the platelet. Other physiological agonists include proteolytic

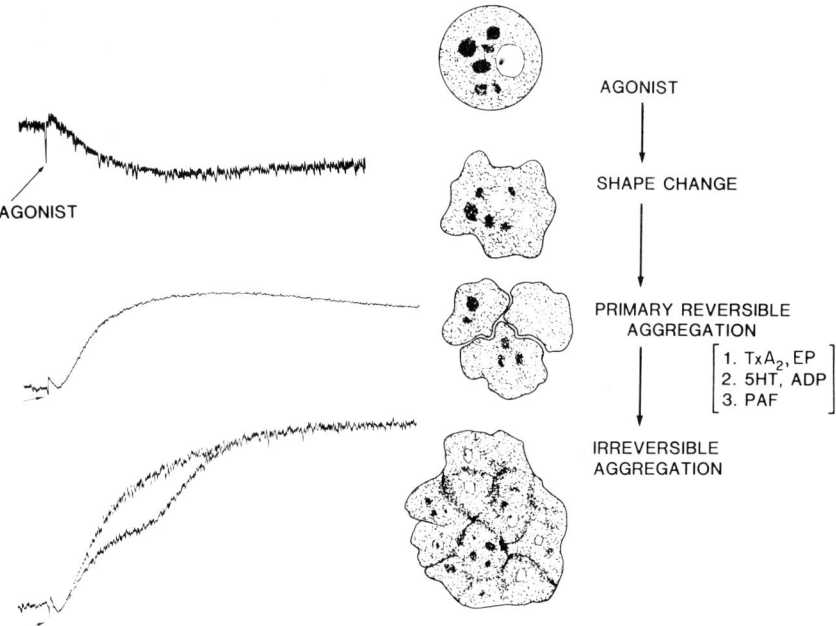

FIG. 2. The sequence of platelet responses to increasing agonist concentration. Aggregation tracings are at the left and platelet ultrastructure in the middle. The initial response is a change in shape, with the platelets acquiring an irregular appearance; this is shown by a decrease in the aggregation tracing as the amount of light transmitted through the aggregation cuvette decreases. The next event is platelet-to-platelet contact, which is indicated by an increase in the aggregation tracing as the amount of light transmitted through the aggregation cuvette is increased. This initial aggregation can reverse. With increasing agonist concentration, a biphasic irreversible or monophasic irreversible aggregation is seen. The formation of agonists from arachidonic acid (TxA_2, EP), the secretion of dense granule agonists (5-HT, ADP), and possibly the formation of PAF by platelets is thought to be responsible for the biphasic response and to contribute to irreversible aggregation.

enzymes such as thrombin and particulate matter such as collagen fibrils. Other compounds will cause platelet agglutination, including antiplatelet antibody, aggregated immune complexes, zymosan, ristocetin plus factor VIII, and snake venom extract plus factor VIII. Furthermore, other substances may not act as agonists, but instead may change the sensitivity of the platelet to an agonist. These are termed "modifiers" and include epinephrine (Scrutton and Wallis, 1981; Meyers et al., 1983a), prostaglandin I_2 (Weiss and Turitto, 1979), or prostacyclin, and, in human platelets, vasopressin (Haslam and Rossen, 1972).

Agonists may induce the formation of prostaglandins (PG) G_2 and H_2 and thromboxane (Tx) A_2 from arachidonic acid (AA), the formation of platelet activating factor, and the secretion of granule constituents by platelets. This may occur during aggregation. The formation or secretion of additional agonists by the platelet in response to an agonist can be considered a positive feedback process that ensures the platelet reaction will go to completion. The liberation and metabolism of arachidonic acid is termed the "arachidonic acid pathway." The dense granule pathway refers to the secretion of 5-HT and ADP into the suspension medium, while the formation of PAF is termed the "PAF pathway." Platelets from the species studied appear to have each of the three feedback pathways, but the participation of each pathway in platelet aggregation varies as species lines are crossed. The importance of each pathway depends upon the amount of agonist present and the sensitivity of the platelet to the agonist.

A. Dense Granule Pathway

Dense granules contain adenine nucleotides, ATP and ADP, an amine, 5-HT, and bivalent cations Ca^{2+} and/or Mg^{2+} (Table III). Within the granule these constituents are thought to form a high-molecular-weight complex, thereby allowing the nucleotides and amines to be stored in large amounts without imposing an osmotic force (Pletscher et al., 1971). Agonists stored in platelet-dense granules, ADP and 5-HT, are important for normal platelet function. This is shown by studies that employ animals whose platelets are deficient in adenine nucleotides and 5-HT and studies that describe the action of these compounds on platelets. Platelets that lack or are deficient in dense granule constituents are termed "storage-pool deficient" (SPD). SPD platelets have been described in mink (Meyers et al., 1978), cattle (Bell et al., 1976; Meyers et al., 1979d, 1983b), cats (Meyers et al., 1981), mice (Holland, 1976), and most humans with the Chediak–Higashi syndrome (CHS) (Bell et al., 1976; Boxer et al., 1977; Parmley et al., 1979), mice that have pigmentary abnormalities (Novak et al., 1981, 1984), and fawn-hooded rats (Tschopp and Zucker, 1972). Associated with the storage-pool deficiency is a bleeding tendency; the time of bleeding is prolonged, and collagen-induced platelet aggregation is impaired. The CHS platelets are characterized by reduced ATP, ADP, and Mg content and a virtual absence of 5-HT. Protein and acid hydrolase contents, on the other hand, are normal.

Most of the dense granule constituents are located in other compartments within the platelet. To determine if the granule pool is deficient,

TABLE III

SUMMARY OF DENSE GRANULE CONSTITUENTS AND RESPONSE TO ADP AND 5-HT

Animals	Content								Response			
	5-HT dense granule[a]	Total[b]	Ca^{2+} dense granule	Mg^{2+} dense granule	ATP dense granule	ADP dense granule	Total		ADP aggr.[c]	Biphasic aggr.[c]	5-HT aggr.[c]	Biphasic aggr.[d]
Companion animals												
Cat	0.9	3.5	2.7	3.2	2.1	0.9	3.5		++	+	++	+
Dog	0.6	1.8	2.0	3.7	1.8	0.7	2.5		++	+/−	+/++	+/−
Horse	0.6	1.5	3.0	1.4	0.5	0.5	1.2		++	+/−	+	−
Food-producing animals												
Cow	2.3	10.0	3.5	1.5	1.0	0.8	3.3		++	−	−	
Pig	1.2	5.7	4.8	9.4	3.3	2.0	9.8		++	−		
Sheep									++	−	−	
Laboratory animals												
Gerbil									++			
Guinea pig									++	+	−	
Mouse									++			
Rabbit	4.0	23.9	2.4	3.5	4.1	0.7	4.2		++	−	+	−
Rat									++	+/−	−	
Mink	1.5	5.5	3.7	4.2	3.3	1.7	6.2		++	−		

[a] Amount (μmol/10^{11} platelets) secreted assuming all 5-HT is located within the dense granule and corrected for 100% 5-HT release.
[b] Total values (μM) refer to the maximal amount of ADP or 5-HT that can be released from platelets in PRP and were calculated from the platelet count (10^8 platelets/ml PRP) and maximal secretable ADP or 5-HT per 10^8 platelets.
[c] Response presented as +, reversible; ++, irreversible; +/++, inconsistent response of reversible–irreversible aggregation. −, no response; +/−, inconsistent response.
[d] +, Presence of biphasic aggregation; −, absence of biphasic aggregation; +/−, inconsistent response.

platelets can be treated with an agonist, such as thrombin, that will induce maximal granule secretion without causing platelet lysis. Then the amount of secreted material released into the extracellular fluid is determined. To distinguish between the metabolic nucleotide pool and the dense granule nucleotide pool, the platelets are incubated with [^{14}C]adenine (Meyers *et al.*, 1979c; Holmsen and Weiss, 1972). The radiolabeled adenine is taken up by the platelet and is converted into [^{14}C]ATP, [^{14}C]ADP, and [^{14}C]AMP. For short periods of time the labeled nucleotides remain within the metabolic pool and do not exchange with the storage pool (Reimers *et al.*, 1975, 1977). When platelets are treated with thrombin to induce maximal granule secretion, nucleotides released into the suspension medium have a low specific radioactivity, indicating that they originated from the granule pool.

The importance of dense granule agonists to normal platelet function depends upon the amount of the agonist formed and the sensitivity of the platelet. While other nucleotides can be stored in dense granules, the adenine nucleotides ATP and ADP are present in the largest amounts (Da Prada *et al.*, 1981). The total granule adenine nucleotide pool and the ATP/ADP ratio vary between species (Meyers *et al.*, 1982a). The amount of secretable ATP and ADP of platelets from rabbits, pigs, and humans exceeds 4 μmol/10^{11} platelets, but in platelets from dogs, cats, and mink it is >1 but <4 μmol/10^{11} platelets. The secretable fraction of adenine nucleotides of cattle and horse platelets is less than 1 μmol/10^{11} platelets. The ATP/ADP ratio of the secretable fraction varies from 5.8 in rabbit platelets to 0.4 in human platelets. Except for human and rabbit platelets, the ATP/ADP in the secretable pool from the other species studied varies from 1 to 2.8. The plasma ADP concentration due to platelet secretion is in close agreement as species lines are crossed, even though there is considerable variation in the platelet granule content of ADP (Table III). When platelet counts in platelet-rich plasma (PRP) and the maximal amount of ADP that can be secreted by platelets are considered, the maximal plasma concentration that can be achieved for ADP is between 1.2 and 10 μM for the eight species mentioned above.

Platelets from some species are affected by ATP and AMP as well as ADP. Platelets from humans (Mustard and Packham, 1971) and pigs and rabbits (Packham *et al.*, 1969) are inhibited by AMP, while rat platelets (Haskel *et al.*, 1980) are not affected. ATP induces aggregation of guinea pig (Lefort and Vargaftig, 1978) and rat (Haskel *et al.*, 1980; Ts'so, 1976) platelets, presumably by being converted into ADP. Conversely, ATP inhibits human and rabbit platelet aggregation.

ADP appears to be the universal platelet agonist (Table III). The action of ADP has been studied on platelets from 14 species and has been found to induce aggregation in each case. Maximal aggregation occurred between 1.5 and 14 μM and, except in pigs and rabbits, it was irreversible (Packham *et al.*, 1969; Thomas *et al.*, 1970). Whether a biphasic aggregation curve is observed or not depends upon the species. ADP has not been reported to induce a biphasic aggregation response of platelets from mice (Rosenblum *et al.*, 1983), cattle (personal observation), monkeys (Addonizio *et al.*, 1979), or pigs and rabbits (Packham *et al.*, 1969; Thomas *et al.*, 1970). Occasionally, biphasic aggregation is seen in platelets from humans (Thomas *et al.*, 1970), dogs (Clemmons and Meyers, 1984), and horses (Meyers *et al.*, 1979a), while guinea pig (Lefort and Vargaftig, 1978; Thomas *et al.*, 1970) and cat (Tschopp, 1970; Thomas *et al.*, 1970; Meyers *et al.*, 1981) platelets routinely generate biphasic aggregation. In addition to being a platelet agonist, ADP induces a refractory state if incubated with unstirred platelets. This has been shown for human (O'Brian, 1966), rabbit (Packham *et al.*, 1969), rat (Simard-Duquesne, 1973), pig (Born and Cross, 1963), and cattle (Okada *et al.*, 1978) platelets. In summary, ADP is an important agonist since platelets from all species studied to date contain and secrete ADP and aggregate to ADP.

Serotonin is found in platelets in amounts ranging from 0.3 to 4.0 μmol/10^{11} platelets (Meyers *et al.*, 1982a). Based on the platelet count and the amount of 5-HT that can be secreted maximally, plasma concentrations of between 0.9 and 24 μM can be obtained, depending upon the species (Table III). Rabbits can obtain a plasma 5-HT concentration of 24 μM; this is followed by cattle at 10 μM. The concentration of 5-HT in the plasma of other species studied was pig (5.7 μM), mink (5.5 μM), cat (3.5 μM), dog (1.8 μM), horse (1.5 μM), and human (0.9 μM). Serotonin is not the only amine found in animal platelets. Platelets from rabbits (DaPrada *et al.*, 1967) and pigs (Lorenz *et al.*, 1971; Ugurbil *et al.*, 1984) contain histamine, but it does not appear to complex with nucleotides such as 5-HT within the dense granule.

Serotonin is not a potent agonist of platelets from most species, and the action of serotonin does not appear to be correlated to the amount of 5-HT within the platelet (Table III). Platelets from some dogs (Clemmons and Meyers, 1984) (those that irreversibly aggregate to arachidonic acid) and cats (Meyers *et al.*, 1978, 1981) exhibit biphasic, irreversible aggregation, and this response is coupled to the secretory response and the formation of TxB_2. In dogs, the aggregation response waxes and wanes as the concentration increases from 1 μM to 1 mM. Human platelets, rabbit platelets (Drummond, 1976; Baumgartner,

1969), and some dog platelets (Clemmons and Meyers, 1984) (those that aggregate reversibly to AA) exhibit only a slight reversible aggregation response. Platelets from cattle (personal observation), sheep (R. Clemmons, personal communication), rats (Drummond, 1976), guinea pigs (Drummond, 1976), and mink (Meyers et al., 1978) do not aggregate to 5-HT. Serotonin potentiates the action of other agonists in all species studied except the guinea pig (Drummond, 1976; Dodds, 1978). The response of the platelets seemed to be correlated to 5-HT binding sites (Leysen et al., 1983a,b). The specific binding of 5-HT to membranes from feline platelets could be demonstrated but not to membranes from human, cattle, horses, pigs, or sheep platelets. In summary, it appears that 5-HT is not a major agonist in all species but may have an important function in potentiating the action of other agonists. Red meat-eating carnivores studied to date have a well-developed 5-HT pathway that reaches peak importance in the cat, where these platelets contain significant amounts of 5-HT, and 5-HT can induce AA metabolism and dense granule secretion.

B. Arachidonic Acid Pathway

Arachidonic acid is released from the 2 position of phosphatidylinositol and phosphatidylcholine (Rittenhouse-Simmons and Deykin, 1981) (Fig. 3). This is mediated, in part, by a phospholipase (PL) A_2 (Broekman et al., 1981). In addition, agonists can also activate PLC, leading to the production of 1,2-diacylglycerol (DG) (Bell and Majerus, 1980; Rittenhouse-Simmons, 1980; Prescott and Majerus,

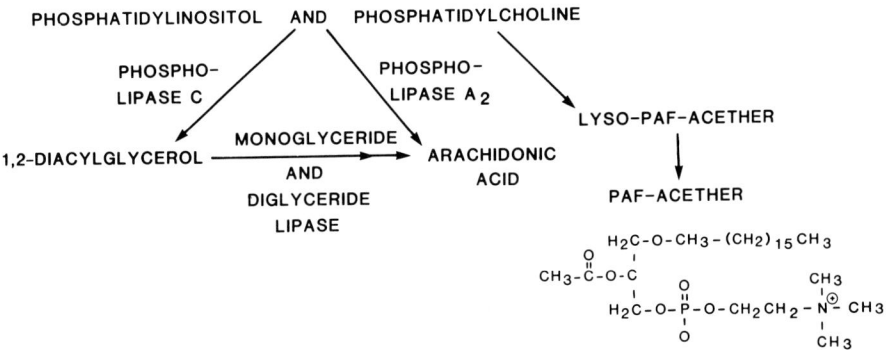

Fig. 3. Liberation of arachidonic acid from phospholipids and the formation and structure of PAF-acether.

1983). Arachidonic acid can then be liberated from 1,2-DG by the action of diglyceride and monoglyceride lipase. In human (Siess and Lapetina, 1983), cattle (Hakata et al., 1982), and horse (Siess and Lapetina, 1983; Billah, 1980) platelets, PLC is soluble and Ca dependent. In the horse, PLC is activated early, leading to the formation of diacylglyceride (Lapetina and Cuatrecasas, 1979a) which, in the presence of ATP and DG kinase, is converted to phosphatidic acid (PA) (Lapetina et al., 1981). Acting as an ionophore, PA could cause PLA_2 activation and the liberation of AA. In support of this, the formation of PA has been shown to precede AA release (Lapetina and Cuatrecasas, 1979b; Lapetina, 1982). This process may not occur in human platelets, since the release of AA occurs before PA formation (Neufeld and Majerus, 1983), or in canine platelets (Sutherland and Amin, 1982), since PLA_2 activity cannot be demonstrated. Like equine platelets, rat platelets (Sutherland and Amin, 1982) have PLA_2, PLC, and DG lipase activity, but the temporal relationships between AA release and PA metabolism have not been described.

The released AA can be metabolized by cyclooxygenase and by lipoxygenase (Fig. 4). The primary product of lipoxygenase is 12-HPETE, which is then converted to 12-HETE (Hamberg and Samuelsson, 1974a,b). When the concentration of 12-HPETE is elevated, there is nonenzymatic conversion of 12-HPETE to THETE. While the stabile 12-HETE does not appear to affect platelet function, the labile 12-HPETE could modify platelet function by stimulating guanylate cyclase (Vanderhoek et al., 1982) and inhibiting the enzymes responsible for thromboxane production (Hammarstrom and Falardeau, 1977; Siegel et al., 1979).

Prostaglandins G_2 and PGH_2 are the AA-derived products of cyclooxygenase; they are unstable, and TxA_2 and 12-hydroxy-5,8,10-heptadecatrienoic acid (HHT) and malondialdehyde (MDA) are formed rapidly. Thromboxane A_2 has a short half-life, converting quickly to TxB_2. Minor amounts of PGD_2, PGE_2 and PGF_2 are formed. This general scheme, evolved from studies on human platelets, has been followed in studies of AA metabolism in animal platelets (Rosenblum et al., 1983; Van Rollings et al., 1980; Lapetina and Cuatrecasas, 1979b; Lapetina et al., 1978). Unusual products derived from AA were not observed. However, there are species differences in the amounts of TxB_2 and MDA that are formed when platelets are treated with thrombin or AA (Table IV). Platelets from humans, dogs, mice, rats, and rabbits form more TxB_2 than do equine platelets, which, in turn, form more than mink, pig, and cattle platelets (Meyers et al., 1980). Arachidonic acid metabolism appears to be important for normal feline

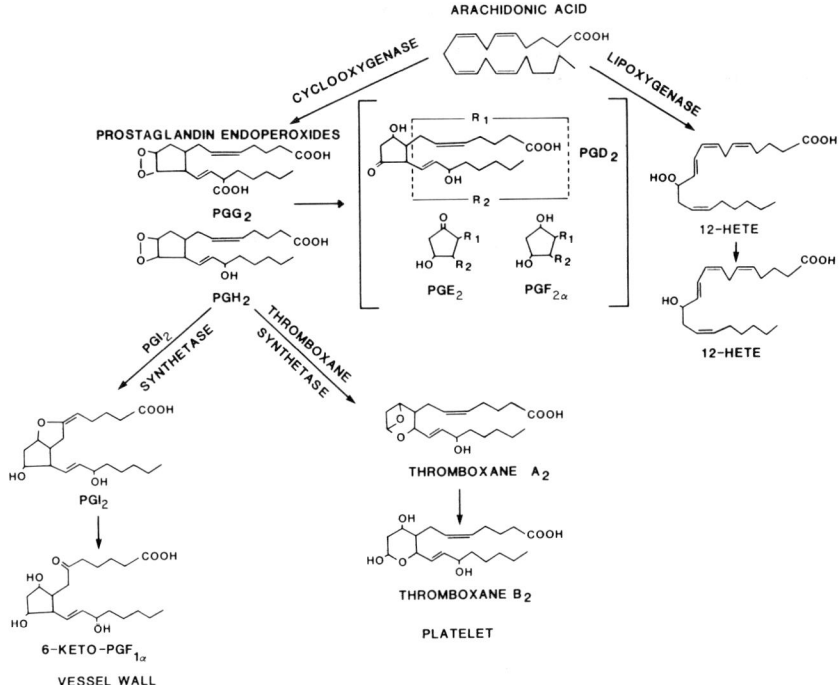

FIG. 4. Metabolism of arachidonic acid by platelets and blood vessels.

platelet aggregation, but large individual variations in the amount of TxB_2 formed have been reported (Meyers et al., 1980). Arachidonic acid is an essential fatty acid for the cat (Rivers et al., 1975), and platelet response can be modified by changing the diet (MacDonald et al., 1984), but whether the variation in TxB_2 in the general cat population is a reflection of diet or AA assimilation is not clear.

The prostaglandin endoperoxides and TxA_2 are platelet agonists that can act, as was shown in rabbit (Harfenist et al., 1982), cat, (Meyers et al., 1979c), and human (Charo et al., 1977) platelets, independently of secreted dense granule agonists. With the exception of canine platelets, AA-induced aggregation is related to the amount of TxB_2 formed (Meyers et al., 1980) (Table IV). Human, rat (Nishizawa et al., 1983; Furlow and Bass, 1976; Gordon et al., 1983), and rabbit (Cattaneo et al., 1980; Naito et al., 1983; Smith and Jubiz, 1981) platelets, which form relatively large amounts of TxB_2, irreversibly aggregate to arachidonic acid, as do platelets from cats (Meyers et al., 1979c, 1981), mice (Rosenblum et al., 1983), gerbils (Agwu et al., 1983),

TABLE IV

FORMATION OF TxB$_2$ AND RESPONSE TO AA

Animals	Amount of TxB$_2$ formed (nmol/10^{11} platelets)	Change of shape	Response to AA		Inhibition with increasing concentration
			Aggregation		
			Reversible	Irreversible	
Companion animals					
Cat				×	
Dog	>50	×	×	×	×
Horse	~50		×	×	
Food-producing animals					
Cow	<50	×			
Pig	<50	×			
Sheep		×			
Laboratory animals					
Gerbil					
Guinea pig				×	
Mouse				×	
Rabbit				×	×
Rat				×	×
Mink	<50	×			

and guinea pigs (LeFort and Vargaftig, 1978). Equine platelets commonly give a reversible aggregation response (Meyers *et al.*, 1979a,b), but irreversible aggregation has been observed (R. Clemmons, personal communication). Arachidonic acid induced only a change in the shape of mink and bovine platelets (Meyers *et al.*, 1980). Porcine platelets exhibited a slight, almost negligible (Meyers *et al.*, 1980) aggregation response.

Canine platelets have been reported both to respond and not respond to AA (Harris *et al.*, 1981; Clemmons and Meyers, 1984). Platelets from thiamylal sodium-anesthetized dogs or unanesthetized dogs that have been conditioned to sampling where sodium citrate (0.18 M) has been used as the anticoagulant exhibit two types of responses when Ca has been added back to the platelet-rich plasma. First, platelets from some dogs either did not aggregate to arachidonic acid or, as was most common, exhibited only reversible aggregation. Second, platelets from other dogs exhibited monophasic, irreversible aggregation and then (depending upon the dog) remained irreversible, became biphasic, or reversed as the concentration increased to 1 mM. The response exhibited by a given dog was constant and did not vary when tested repeatedly. The waxing and waning of aggregation with increasing AA concentration is not unique to the dog and has been reported with rabbit (Cattaneo et al., 1980) and rat (Vargaftig, 1978) platelets (Table IV). In the latter, a pronounced biphasic aggregation response is seen when heparin is used as the anticoagulant (Dwyer and Meyers, 1985a). Minor platelet inhibition has also been seen in human platelets at high AA concentrations (Linder et al., 1979).

Within a species there are breed (Clemmons and Meyers, 1984) and strain (Dwyer and Meyers, 1985b) differences. Certain breeds of dogs have a high incidence of individuals whose platelets exhibit one type of response (Clemmons and Meyers, 1984). Within the Scottish terrier and English setter breeds, there is a high number of dogs whose platelets aggregate irreversibly to AA. On the other hand, a high percentage of greyhounds do not or only reversibly aggregate to AA. In mongrels about 50% of the dogs irreversibly aggregate to AA, while in beagles the incidence is 33%.

Platelets from different strains of rats can respond quite differently. In a study by Dwyer and Meyers (1985a), the responses of Sprague–Dawley, Lewis, Holtzman, and NBR rats were compared. There were differences in the sensitivity to AA with the rank order of NBR > Holtzman > Sprague–Dawley = Lewis.

The species differences in the AA pathway may have pharmacological significance. For those species in which the AA pathway is well developed, such as dogs and cats, treatment with agents that modify this pathway, such as nonsteroidal antiinflammatory agents (DeClerck and David, 1981) or certain penicillin derivatives (Johnson et al., 1978), may result in inadequate platelet responses. On the other hand, this may not be a problem for those species in which this pathway is less important.

C. Platelet-Activating Factor

A factor was found to be released from circulating antigen-stimulated, IgE-sensitized basophils that induced the aggregation of rabbit platelets and the release of vasoactive amines (Benveniste et al., 1972). This factor was termed platelet-activating factor (Benveniste et al., 1972). The structure of PAF from rabbit basophils and porcine leukocytes has been identified as 1-O-alkyl-2-acetylglyceryl-3-phosphorylcholine (AGEPC or PAF-acether) (Demopoulos et al., 1979; Benveniste et al., 1979). In addition to the formation of PAF by basophils,

PAF has been shown to be released from platelets (Chignard et al., 1979a), macrophages (Mencia-Huerta and Benveniste, 1979), monocytes (Lynch et al., 1979), and polymorphonuclear neutrophils (Lotner et al., 1980). PAF appears to be formed, at least in part, by a deacylation–reacylation pathway (Snyder et al., 1983). Upon stimulation of the cell, a phospholipase A_2 reaction results in the deacylation of phosphatidylcholine analogs and the formation of lyso-PAF-acether. A second acetylating reaction involving an acetyltransferase catalyzes the formation of PAF-acether. The acetyltransferase appears to be a regulated enzyme, becoming activated and inactivated as a consequence of phosphorylation and dephosphorylation (Lenihan and Lee, 1984). PAF is rapidly inactivated and is degraded by both plasma and platelets (Alam et al., 1983a).

PAF is an important mediator of inflammations and allergic hyperreactions. When administered *in vivo* it induces a systemic hypotension (Halonen et al., 1981), acute respiratory distress (Halonen et al., 1981), neutropenia (McManus et al., 1980), and thrombocytopenia (McManus et al., 1980). The systemic hypotension is due to vasodilation of peripheral arterial blood vessels and to be effective requires the presence of endothelium (Kasuya et al., 1984). The respiratory distress is due, in part, to PAF-induced bronchoconstriction (Vargaftig et al., 1980). PAF also induces degranulation of neutrophils and is chemotactic (Shaw et al., 1981). It also increases vascular permeability (Wedmore and Williams, 1981).

There are marked species differences in the response of platelets to PAF. Platelets from some species (guinea pig, rabbit, horses, and cattle) are very sensitive to PAF and will exhibit maximal aggregation responses at PAF concentrations of less than 40 nM (Cargill et al., 1983; Liggit et al., 1984). Maximal aggregation of guinea pig platelets has been reported at concentrations as low as 0.4 nM (Cargill et al., 1983). Human platelets are less sensitive to PAF and require a PAF concentration of 30–400 nM to achieve maximal aggregation (Cargill et al., 1983). The large range in the dose required to achieve aggregation is a reflection of the large individual variation within a species. Platelets from rats and mice do not aggregate to PAF (Namm et al., 1982). Similar differences between human and rabbit platelets have been reported.

The action of PAF on rabbit platelets has been studied extensively. PAF is formed by rabbit platelets upon stimulation with thrombin and collagen (Chignard et al., 1980) or the calcium ionophore A23187 (Chignard et al., 1980; Alam et al., 1983b) but not with ADP or AA (Chignard et al., 1980). PAF induces granule secretion (Namm et al.,

1982; Henson, 1976) and aggregation (Bussolino and Camussi, 1980; Cazenave et al., 1979). Aggregation is not dependent upon ADP release or AA formation (Cazenave et al., 1979). PAF acts synergistically with ADP and epinephrine (Vargaftig et al., 1982). The mechanism(s) by which PAF activates platelets has not been fully described. PAF did not alter basal levels of cAMP but did antagonize PGE_1-induced increase in cAMP (Haslam and Vanderivel, 1982). PAF also induces the formation of TxB_2 (Vargaftig et al., 1982), increases the uptake of Ca^{2+} (Lee et al., 1981), and causes a rapid loss of phosphatidylinositol 4,5-biphosphate (PIP_2) (Billah and Lapetina, 1982). The loss of PIP_2 from the plasma membrane has been suggested by Billah and Lapetina (1982) to trigger the phosphatidylinositol cycle. This would subsequently lead to the activation of phospholipase C and the formation of PA, which has been suggested to serve as an intracellular Ca^{2+} ionophore (Lapetina, 1982).

There are conflicting views of the role PAF may play in platelet aggregation. Undoubtedly PAF plays an important role in platelet responses that are PAF sensitive (rabbit and guinea pig) and is not important in those species that do not respond to PAF (rat and mouse). It may have only a minor role in the activation of human platelets by thrombin (Kloprogge et al., 1983). The marked variation in the response of platelets to PAF suggests that PAF is not a general platelet agonist, like ADP, but that PAF is one of the platelet-derived agonists formed during activation. Like TxA_2 and 5-HT, the importance of PAF in the basic platelet response depends upon the species.

D. Additional Agonists

Platelets from some species also respond to some low-molecular-weight compounds, the physiological significance of which is not clear. Canine platelets aggregate and secrete in response to acetylcholine (Chuang et al., 1974). These responses are mediated by muscarinic receptors. Vasopressin includes aggregation of human platelets and induces canine platelets to change shape, but will not induce any part of the basic platelet response of porcine or rabbit platelets (Haslam and Rossen, 1972).

E. Summary

Animal platelets respond to thrombin and collagen in a sequential manner, from the platelet changing shape to irreversible aggregation. As part of the process, the platelet may secrete or form substances that act to drive the platelet response to completion. There are three such platelet-derived positive feedback pathways: the dense granule pathway, the arachidonic acid pathway, and the platelet-activating pathways. As species lines are crossed, there are marked differences in the importance of these pathways. In some species (rodents, man, and red meat-eating carnivores) the arachidonic acid pathway is well developed and important for normal platelet responses. In large domestic animals and mink, a white meat-eating carnivore, this pathway may be very rudimentary. ADP released during secretion appears to be a universal agonist, with platelets from different species releasing equivalent amounts and being equally sensitive to ADP. The other dense granule agonist, 5-HT, may have a potentiating role but appears to act as an agonist only in canine and, especially, feline platelets. The PAF pathway is a recently described pathway. Based only on sensitivity, this pathway may prove to be well developed in the rabbit and the larger domestic animals.

V. Modulators

A. PGI_2 AND cAMP

The sensitivity of platelets can be changed by modifiers formed outside the platelet. Prostacyclin, or PGI_2, is an example of an inhibitory modulator. PGI_2 is formed by the endothelium, which metabolizes the endoperoxides formed from AA to PGI_2 rather than TxA_2 (Weksler et al., 1977). Other inhibitory PGs are PGE_1, PGE_2, and PGD_2. However, they are either not formed by the endothelium or by platelets or they are formed in small amounts (Rosenblum et al., 1983; Van Rollings et al., 1980; Lapetina et al., 1978). PGI_2 is the most potent inhibitory PG reported to date and may be a universal modifier (Whittle et al., 1978; McFarlane et al., 1974). Platelets from every species studied to date are inhibited by PGI_2 (Whittle et al., 1978). There is very little species variation in the dose required for platelet inhibition: 0.5–3.7 ng/ml of PGI_2 inhibits platelet function (Whittle et al., 1978).

There is profound inhibition of platelet function by PGI_2, including the expression of fibroinogen receptors (Kinlough-Rathbone et al., 1975), the release of AA (Dembinska-Kieo et al., 1979; Lapetina et al., 1977), and the secretion of granule constituents (Bussolino and Camussi, 1980). These effects are associated with an increase in cAMP within the platelet (McDonald and Stuart, 1973; Best et al., 1977; Gorman et al., 1977; Tateson et al., 1977). The increase of cAMP within the plastelet, whether the result of activation of adenyl cyclase or the inhibition of phosphodiesterase, leads to platelet inhibition. As would be expected, the inhibition of platelet function is associated with the activation of β-catecholamine receptors (Yu and Latour, 1977) when platelets have these receptors following treatment with adenosine and its analogs (Haslam and Rossen, 1975) and with inhibitors of phosphodiesterase, such as papaverine, pyrimidopyrimidines, and methylxanthines (Tang and Frojmovic, 1980).

B. Epinephrine

Platelets from some species respond to epinephrine. An unusual aggregation response is elicited by epinephrine in human platelets (Mills and Roberts, 1967). A primary aggregation wave is followed by a biphasic response. The aggregation response is unique since it occurs in the absence of a platelet shape change. At low concentrations of epinephrine that do not induce aggregation of human platelets, epinephrine potentiates the aggregation induced by agonists. Potentiation without shape change or aggregation is also seen in platelets from rabbits (Hallam *et al.*, 1981, 1982; Grant and Scrutton, 1980), rats (personal observation), mice (Rosenblum *et al.*, 1983), dogs (Meyers *et al.*, 1983a; Clemmons and Meyers, 1984; Chignard and Vargaftig, 1978; Johnson *et al.*, 1980), and cats (Tschopp, 1970). Platelets from some dogs (Clemmons and Meyers, 1984) and cats (MacDonald *et al.*, 1984) have been reported to aggregate in response to epinephrine. In both species this aggregation is unique since it is delayed in onset and resembles collagen-induced aggregation. In dogs this epinephrine response is seen only in individuals whose platelets irreversibly aggregate to AA, and it can be prevented by treating platelets with cyclooxygenase inhibitors (personal observation). Platelets from cattle and sheep (personal observations), pigs (Drummond, 1976), horses (Meyers *et al.*, 1979a), and guinea pigs (Glusa and Markwardt, 1983) do not aggregate to epinephrine, nor does it potentiate the response to other agonists.

The potentiating effect of epinephrine on canine platelets has been studied by Meyers *et al.* (1983a). Epinephrine did not induce a change in any part of the basic platelet that could be detected in the aggregometer, such as a change in platelet shape or aggregation, indicating that unless the platelet is exposed to an agonist, the effect of epinephrine is without functional consequence. However, when confronted with an agonist of the epinephrine-treated platelet, the response to the agonist is augmented. This potentiation has been observed with all agonists tested, including ADP, 5-HT, collagen, thrombin, and PAF. The potentiation is marked, and an irreversible aggregation response to collagen of epinephrine-treated platelets is observed, while the same platelets that were not treated with epinephrine would only change shape. Similarly, platelets that otherwise would not irreversibly aggregate to AA do so in the presence of epinephrine. An *in vivo* role for epinephrine is suggested by the finding that the potentiation observed *in vitro* occurs at epinephrine concentrations that are potentially physiological. Furthermore, aggregation to arachidonic acid of platelets obtained from dogs before and following iv epinephrine administration is potentiated following epinephrine treatment.

The potentiating action of epinephrine on canine platelets appears to be mediated through α receptors. The α receptor antagonists prevent the action of epinephrine, and α receptor agonists such as clonidine and norepinephrine mimic the action of epinephrine. Platelets are considerably less sensitive to norepinephrine than they are to epinephrine. This suggests that under physiological conditions epinephrine may be the only catecholamine that modifies platelet responses.

α receptors are divided into two types: α_1 and α_2. When originally described in the peripheral nervous system, α_1 receptors were postsynaptic, while α_2 receptors were presynaptic and modulated the release of norepinephrine. When characterized in platelets from other species, the platelet α receptor appears to be similar to the α_2 receptor (Grant and Scrutton, 1979, 1980; Glusa and Markwardt, 1983). Recently, Kerry *et al.* (1984) determined the density of α_2 adrenoreceptors on platelets from several species and found the following order: human = rabbit > rat >> guinea pig.

Canine platelets, as well as platelets from other species, have β receptors (Yu and Latour, 1977; Kerry and Scrutton, 1983). When characterized, they have been identified as β_2 adrenoreceptors. The rank order of the density of β_2 adrenoreceptors on platelets from different species was rat > rabbit >> guinea pig (Kerry and Scrutton, 1983). Activation of the β receptors leads to inhibition of platelet function, presumably because cAMP is elevated. The net potentiation observed in canine platelets is probably due to a greater number of α receptors than β receptors. The presence of two types of receptors for epinephrine that elicit two different types of platelet responses provides the potential for potentiation, inhibition, or some temporal sequence of potentiation and inhibition. Whether or not this does occur remains to be seen.

The mechanism that mediates epinephrine-induced potentiation of canine platelets is not known. As is the case for other receptors, it is possible that there is a second messenger. Epinephrine is known to inhibit adenyl cyclase (Jacobs, 1983). This inhibition would result in a reduction in cAMP, which, in turn, could result in an increased sensitivity of the platelet. However, Haslam *et al.* (1978) showed that platelet responses do not require a reduction in cAMP. The adenyl cyclase inhibition could also be a coupled event that would prevent any elevation of cAMP and the subsequent inhibition, thereby ensuring potentiation. Since epinephrine potentiates the response to all agonists, its action could be focused on a common pathway. Many agonists activate the AA pathway and epinephrine potentiates AA-induced aggregation; however, epinephrine-induced potentiation can still be observed when AA metabolism by cyclooxygenase is prevented (Meyers *et al.*, 1983a). The potentiating action of epinephrine to all agonists may be focused on the final common pathway for all agonists, Ca^{2+}. This is supported by the observation that epinephrine markedly potentiates the action of A23187, the calcium ionophore (Meyers *et al.*, 1983a). Here, epinephrine is able to induce irreversible aggregation in platelets that without epinephrine would only change shape when treated with A23187. If it is assumed that A23187 allows Ca^{2+} to move according to its electrochemical gradient, then epinephrine may act to induce a change in the sensitivty of the platelet to Ca^{2+} or cause an affinity change which allows more Ca^{2+} to become translocated from internal stores.

C. Epinephrine as a Gain Controller

Hemostasis is a highly controlled process in which there is an instant response to hemorrhage. Inappropriate activation that could lead to intravascular thrombosis and reduced blood flow posterior to the thrombus should be prevented. Some animals, such as carnivores and small herbivores, place stress on this system since in the wild they are frequently confronted with traumatic situations. In these species, it may be advantageous to augment the hemostatic competence of the animal at times of potential trauma and then reduce it when the stress has dissipated. In some species, epinephrine may modulate platelet function, by serving as a gain controller of platelet function, to change the relationship between the actuating signal and the response. In these species, when adrenal medullary secretion of epinephrine is low, the sensitivity of the platelet to agonists is low. Exposure of an animal to a fight-or-flight situation often results in activation of the sympathoadrenal system and an accompanying increase in epinephrine secretion. Epinephrine markedly increases the sensitivty of the platelet to all agonists without causing the platelet to change shape or aggregate. Therefore, the platelet circulates in the normal manner until it is exposed to an agonist such as collagen, thrombin, or one of the platelet-derived agonists, at which time the response would be augmented. With the passing of the stress, plasma epinephrine levels would decrease and platelet reactivity would return to the resting level. The specificity of the α receptor response to epinephrine ensures that norepinephrine will have little effect.

VI. Agglutinating Agents

A. von Willebrand Factor

There are compounds that induce clumping of platelets that have been treated with fixative or depleted of energy. This type of platelet clumping is termed "agglutination." In the presence of von Willebrand factor (vWF), the antibiotic ristocetin (Meyers *et al.*, 1978) and bovine coagulation factor VIII (Donati *et al.*, 1973) induce clumping of human platelets in plasma. The requirement of vWF factor has led to the use of ristocetin-induced agglutination in the diagnosis of human vWF (Hoyer, 1981). Normal canine platelets are not agglutinated by ristocetin in plasma but when they are suspended in a balanced salt solution ristocetin-induced agglutination can occur (Johnson *et al.*, 1978). A nonimmunological method of assaying human plasma vWF using *Bothrops jararaca* venom has been termed the "venom coagglutination assay" (Read *et al.*, 1978). This test uses formaldehyde-fixed platelets that have been lyophilized. These platelets retain their ability to interact with vWF. In the assay, prepared platelets are incubated with venom coagglutinin (VC) and the test plasma. The rate and extent of platelet agglutination are dependent upon the vWF concentration of test plasma. Recently, R. M. Clemmons (personal communication) has been able to fix canine platelets with paraformaldehyde and have them retain their ability to agglutinate in the presence of vWF and VC. This suggests that a test could be developed to nonimmunologically determine vWF.

B. Endotoxin

Endotoxin can induce close platelet-to-platelet contact. Rabbit platelets are sensitive to endotoxin, and platelet clumping accompanied by release of granule constituents is observed (Morrison *et al.*, 1978). Endotoxin induces canine platelet agglutination, as evidenced by the presence of close platelet-to-platelet contact of energy-depleted platelets (Meyers et al., 1982b). In addition, this was not modified by conditions that affect platelet aggregation, such as PGI, adenosine, indomethacin, CP/CPK, methylsergide, and local anesthetics (Fletscher and Ramwell, 1980). Endotoxin did not induce repeatable agglutination of equine or bovine platelets (Meyers et al., 1982b).

VII. Platelet Membrane Glycoproteins

An appreciation of the surface protein composition has functional as well as pathological significance. Physiological responses such as adherence and aggregation are initiated by agonists interacting with platelet plasma membrane receptors. In addition to the receptor sites, platelet plasma membranes have numerous uptake sites for low-molecular-weight compounds such as serotonin (Murray et al., 1983).

Phillips and Agin (1977) were able to identify seven glycoproteins (GP), using a reduced/nonreduced gel system, which they numbered I–VII. Using two-dimensional gel systems and under reduced conditions, up to 28 or 32 different glycoproteins have been identified (Sixma and Schiphorst, 1980; McGregor et al., 1980). Glycoprotein I is a complex of at least two distinct glycoproteins, GPIa and GPIb (Clemetson et al., 1977). These are associated with two other proteins: GPIc, which does not stain with periodic acid–Schiff reagent and is probably not a glycoprotein, and glycocalicin (Okumura and Jamieson, 1976). The GPIb is absent in Bernard–Soulier platelets, which lack the receptor for the factor VIIIc–vWF complex (Nurden and Caen, 1978). There appears to be a close structural relationship to a GPII (GPIIb) and a GPIII (GPIIIa). The two proteins are antigenically different and structurally distinct but may exist in a complex on the platelet surface (McEver et al., 1982; Leung et al., 1981). They are thought to be important for normal platelet-to-platelet interactions. Glanzmann's thrombasthenia is an inherited bleeding disorder in which platelet adhesion is reduced (Caen et al., 1966). Agonist-induced platelet aggregation is defective, but agonist-induced platelet secretion is normal. Platelets from thrombasthenic patients are deficient in or lack GPIIb and GPIIIa (McGregor et al., 1981). A role for GPV in the interaction of thrombin with platelets has been suggested, and it has been shown that thrombin splits off a 64-kDa fragment from GPV (Berndt and Phillips, 1981). A thrombasthenic thrombopathy in otterhounds was described by Raymond and Dodds (1979); it is characterized by a prolonged bleeding time, variable thrombocytopenia, impaired clot restriction and glass bead retention, abnormal platelet factor 3 production, and defective platelet aggregation to ADP, collagen, and thrombin. Platelets from these dogs were larger than normal. The glycoprotein profile indicated an elevation of GPI, a variable expression of GPII, and a reduction in GPIII.

von Willebrand's disease is an autosomal condition that has been described in dogs (Dodds, 1975), humans (Hoyer, 1981), and pigs (Hogan et al., 1941). It is characterized by prolonged bleeding times, reduced factor VIII, and defective platelet adhesion, but normal aggregation responses to collagen (Larrieu et al., 1968). The factor VIII molecule is considered to be a complex of two proteins (Gralnick et al., 1977): coagulation factor VIII (VIII:C) and vWF. Factor VIII:C is a regulator of the intrinsic coagulation cascade that may participate with factor IX, Ca^{2+}, and phospholipids to activate factor X. Several functional deficiencies, including increased bleeding time, are present in von Willebrand's disease that cannot be attributed to VIII:C deficiency. The factor in plasma or cryoprecipitate that corrects these defects is vWF (Brinkhous et al., 1981). von Willebrand's factor appears to be the only plasma protein that mediates the adhesion and spreading of platelets to the subendothelium following vascular injury (Sakariassen et al., 1979). It is thought to be synthesized by the endothelium (Jaffe et al., 1973) and the megakaryocyte (Nachman et al., 1977). von Willebrand's Factor formed by the endothelium is probably the source of plasma vWF and subendothelium vWF. The vWF found stored within platelets is probably derived from the megakaryocyte.

Activated platelets contain specific receptors which bind the vWF, whether it be plasma derived or secreted by the platelet. The receptor for VIII:C–vWF is presumed to be glycoprotein Ib in human platelets (Nurden and Caen, 1978). The finding that GPIb is the receptor for VIII:C–vWF is derived in part from studies on human patients with Bernard–Soulier (BS) syndrome. These patients have an increased bleeding time and a deficiency in platelet GPIb (Nurden and Caen, 1978). These BS syndrome patients have normal levels of VIII:C–vWF, but their platelets do not agglutinate to ristocetin (Nurden and Caen, 1979). Bleeding problems with abnormalities in platelets adhering to the subendothelium can be caused by either a deficiency of vWF, as in von Willebrand's disease, or inappropriate binding, as in the Bernard–Soulier syndrome.

VIII. Tumor Cells

Some transformed cells may induce aggregation of platelets *in vitro*. The response depends upon the type of tumor cell and the species origin of the platelets. For example, Ehrlich ascites tumor cells induce

TABLE V

Causes and Treatment of Thrombocytopenia Published from 1978 to 1984

Species	Etiology	Treatment	Reference
Canine	Immune[a]	Prednisone	Ward (1980)
	Immune[a]	Prednisone	Clark et al. (1980)
	Immune	Vincristine	Green et al. (1982)
	Drug—aurothioglucose?	Stop treatment	Fadok and Janney (1982);
	Drug—dapsone; DIC		Lee et al. (1979)
	Drug—phenylbutazone	Stop treatment	Schalm (1979)
	Drug—estrogen; immune[a]	Splenectomy	Davis (1984)
	Modified live vaccines[b]	Levamisole	Pineau et al. (1980)
	Infectious canine hepatitis		Wigton (1978)
	Lymphohematopoietic neoplasms[c]		Madewell et al. (1980)
	Metastic tumors of bone marrow or spleen		O'Donnel et al. (1981)
Equine	Lymphosarcoma		Reef et al. (1984)
	Immune (n = 2)[a]	Dexamethasone	Larson, et al. (1983)
	DIC		Morris and Beech (1983)
	Myelonocytic myeloproliferative disease		Brumbaugh et al. (1982)
Feline	Drug—propyluracil; consumption		Peterson et al. (1984)
	Unknown	Supportive	Harvey and Gaskins (1980)
	FIP–DIC		Weiss et al. (1980)
Ferrets	Estrogen-induced marrow suppression		Bernard et al. (1983)

[a]Suspected but not proven.
[b]Reduces platelet counts one-third to one-half.
[c]In more than 50% of the cases.

the aggregation of human platelets but not platelets from sheep or rabbits (Evans and Crowie, 1983).

Excessive bleeding can occur in human neoplastic disease and is commonly associated with a thrombocytopenia. The thrombocytopenia is usually due to impaired production, but it can also be accompanied by increased utilization. O'Donnel et al. (1981) studied platelet and fibrinogen kinetics in 53 dogs with naturally occurring tumors that were not treated, and only 6 dogs had platelet counts outside the normal range. These dogs had metastatic tumors involving the spleen or bone marrow, sites of platelet destruction and production. That platelets are being affected by neoplasias is shown by the finding that platelet survival was decreased in 40% of the dogs with localized tumors and in 80% of the dogs with metastasis. In a follow-up study, the shortened platelet survival could be improved with treatments that alter platelet arachidonic acid or cAMP systems (Slichter et al., 1982).

IX. Thrombocytopenia

Thrombocytopenia has been reported in a variety of different species. A thrombocytopenia occurs when the platelet count falls below 90,000 or 100,000 platelets per microliter. There is risk of bleeding with platelet counts below 50,000 per microliter. The thrombocytopenia can be due to inadequate production and is associated with inadequate megakaryocyte numbers or inappropriate platelet consumption, which is associated with normal megakaryocytes in the bone marrow and a shortened platelet survival. There are several causes of thrombocytopenia, including disseminated intravascular coagulation, systemic lupus erythrematosus, sepsis, drug action or reaction, and an autoimmune state. Autoimmune thrombocytopenia has been recently discussed by Dodds (1983). A summary of information on thrombocytopenia published from 1980 to 1984 is presented in Table V.

References

Addonizio, V. P., Edmunds, L. H., and Coleman, R. W. (1979). *J. Lab. Clin. Med.* **91,** 989–997.
Agwu, D. E., Holub, B. J., Johnson, I. B., and Crane, S. (1983). *Can. J. Comp. Med.* **47,** 203–206.
Alam, I., Smith, J. B., and Silver, M. J. (1983a). *Lipids* **18,** 534–538.
Alam, I., Smith, J. B., and Silver, M. J. (1983b). *Thromb. Res.* **30,** 71–79.
Baumgartner, H. R. (1969). *J. Physiol. (London)* **201,** 409–423.
Bell, R. L., and Majerus, P. W. (1980). *J. Biol. Chem.* **255,** 1790–1792.
Bell, T. C., Meyers, K. M., Prieur, D. J., Fauci, A. S., Wolff, S. M., and Padgett, G. A. (1976). *Blood* **48,** 175–184.
Benard, S. L., Leathers, C. W., Brobst, D. F., and Gorham, J. R. (1983). *Am. J. Vet. Res.* **44,** 657–661.
Bentfeld-Barker, M. E., and Bainton, D. F. (1982). *Blood* **59,** 472–581.
Benveniste, J., Henson, P. M., and Cochrane, C. G. (1972). *J. Exp. Med.* **136,** 1356–1377.
Benveniste, J., Tence, M., Varenne, P., Bidault, J., Boullet, C., and Polansky, J. (1979). *C.R. Acad. Sci. Paris* **289,** 1017–1040.
Berndt, Mc., and Phillips, D. R. (1981). *J. Biol. Chem.* **256,** 59–61.
Best, L. C., Martin, T. J., Russel, R. G. G., and Preston, F. E. (1977). *Nature (London)* **267,** 850–852.
Billah, M. M. (1980). *J. Biol. Chem.* **255,** 10227–10231.
Billah, M. M., and Lapetina, E. G. (1982). *J. Biol. Chem.* **257,** 12705–12708.
Born, G. V. R., and Cross, M. J. (1963). *J. Physiol. (London)* **168,** 178–195.

Boxer, G. J., Holmsen, H., Robrin, L., Bang, N. U., Boxer, L. A., and Baehner, R. L. (1977). *Br. J. Haematol.* **35**, 521–533.
Brinkhous, K. M., Read, M. S., Reddick, R. L., and Griggs, T. R. (1981). *Ann. N.Y. Acad. Sci.* **370**, 191–204.
Broekman, M. J., Ward, J. W., and Marcus, A. J. (1981). *J. Biol. Chem.* **256**, 8271–8274.
Brumbaugh, G. W., Sitzel, K. A., Zinkl, J. G., and Feldman, B. F. (1982). *J. Am. Vet. Med. Assoc.* **180**, 313–316.
Bussolino, F., and Camussi, G. (1980). *Prostaglandins* **20**, 781–791.
Caen, J. P., Castaldi, P. A., Leclerc, J. C., Inceman, S., Larrieu, M. J., Probst, M., and Benard, J. (1966). *Am. J. Med.* **41**, 4–26.
Cargill, D. I., Cohen, D. S., Van Valen, R. G., Kimek, J. J., and Levine, R. P. (1983). *Thromb. Haemostasis* **49**, 294–307.
Cattaneo, M., Kinlough-Rathbone, R. L., Perry, D. W., Chahil, A., Vickers, J. D., Lam, S. C. T., Packham, M. A., and Mustard, J. F. (1980). *Blood* **60**, 1179–1187.
Cazenave, J.-P., Benveniste, J., and Mustard, J. F. (1979). *Lab. Invest.* **41**, 275–285.
Charo, I. F., Feinman, R. D., Detwiler, T. C., Smith, J. B., Ingerman, C. M., and Silver, M. J. (1977). *Nature (London)* **269**, 66–69.
Chignard, M., and Vargaftig, B. B. (1978). *Biochem. Biophys. Res. Commun.* **85**, 1631–1639.
Chignard, M., LeCouldic, J. P., Tence, M., Vargaftig, B. B., and Benveniste, J. (1979). *Nature (London)* **279**, 799–800.
Chignard, M., LeCouldic, J. P., Vargaftig, B. B. and Benveniste, J. (1980). *Br. J. Haematol.* **46**, 455–464.
Chuang, H. Y. K., Shermer, R. W., and Mason, R. G. (1974). *Res. Commun. Chem. Pathol. Pharmacol.* **7**, 333–346.
Ciaglowski, R. E., Snow, J. W., and Walz, D. A. (1981). *Ann. N.Y. Acad. Sci.* **370**, 668–697.
Clark, H. C., Childress, R. D., and Coleman, N. C. (1980). *Vet. Med. Small Anim. Clin.* 427–430.
Clemetson, K. J., Pfueller, S. L., Loscher, E. F., and Jenkins, C. S. P. (1977). *Biochim. Biophys. Acta* **464**, 493–508.
Clemmons, R. M., and Meyers, K. M. (1984). *Am. J. Vet. Res.* **45**, 137–144.
Clemmons, R. M., Bliss, E. L., Dorsey-Lee, M. R., Seachord, C. L., and Meyers, K. M. (1983). *Thromb. Haemostasis* **50**, 838–843.
DaPrada, M., Pletscher, A., Tranzer, J. P., and Knuchel, H. (1967). *Nature (London)* **216**, 1315–1316.
DaPrada, M., Richards, J. G., and Kettler, K. (1981). *In* "Platelets in Biology and Pathology 2" (J. L. Gordon, ed.), pp. 107–145. North-Holland Publ., Amsterdam.
Davis, W. M. (1984). *J. Am. Vet. Med. Assoc.* **185**, 976–977.
DeClerck, F., and David, J. L. (1981). *J. Cardiovasc. Pharmacol.* **3**, 1388–1412.
Dembinska-Kieo, A., Rucker, W., and Schonhofer, P. S. (1979). *Atheroslerosis* **33**, 217–226.
Demopoulos, C. A., Pinckard, R. N., and Hanahan, D. J. (1979). *J. Biol. Chem.* **254**, 9355–9358.
Dodds, W. J. (1975). *Blood* **45**, 221–230.
Dodds, W. J. (1978). *In* "Plastelets: A Multidisciplinary Apprach" (G. DeGaetano and S. Garattini, eds.), pp. 45–49. Raven, New York.
Dodds, W. J. (1983). *Adv. Vet. Sci. Comp. Med.* pp. 163–195.
Donati, M. B., DeGaetano, G., and Vermylen, J. (1973). *Thromb. Res.* **2**, 97–104.

Drummond, A. H. (1976). In "Platelets in Biology and Patholgoy I" (J. L. Gordon, ed.), pp. 203–239. North-Holland Publ., Amsterdam.
Dwyer, S. D., and Meyers, K. M. (1985a). Thromb. Res., in press.
Dwyer, S. D., and Meyers, K. M. (1985b). Thromb. Res., in press.
Evens, P. M., and Crowie, F. P. (1983). Cell Biol. Int. Rep. **7,** 771–778.
Fabrizi, P., Barbarulli, G., Castellani, M., and Tarli, P. (1981). Thromb. Res. **21,** 165–168.
Fadok, V. A., and Janney, E. H. (1982). J. Am. Vet. Med. Assoc. **181,** 261–262.
Files, J. C., Malpass, T. W., Yee, E. K., Ritchie, J. C., and Harker, L. A. (1981). Blood **58,** 607–619.
Fletscher, J. R., and Ramwell, P. W. (1980). Circ. Shock **7,** 299–308.
Furlow, T. W., and Bass, N. H. (1976). Neurology **26,** 297–304.
Ginsberg, M. H., Hoskins, R., Segirst, P., and Painter, R. (1979). J. Biol. Chem. **254,** 12365–12371.
Glusa, E., and Markwardt, F. (1983). Haemostasis **13,** 96–101.
Gordon, P. B., Browning, J. D., and O'Dell, B. L. (1983). J. Nutr. **113,** 766–772.
Gorman, R. R., Bunting, S., and Miller, O. V. (1977). Prostaglandins **13,** 377–388.
Gralnick, H. R., Collier, B. S., Shulman, N. R., Anderson, J. C., and Hilgartner, M. (1977). Ann. Intern. Med. **86,** 598–616.
Grant, J. A., and Scrutton, M. C. (1979). Nature (London) **277,** 659–661.
Grant, J. A., and Scrutton, M. C. (1980). Br. J. Pharmacol. **71,** 121–134.
Green, C. G., Scoggins, J., Thomas, J. E., and Barsanti, J. A. (1982). J. Vet. Med. Assoc. **180,** 140–143.
Hakata, H., Kambayashi, J. I., and Kosaki, G. (1982). J. Biochem. **92,** 929–935.
Hallam, T. J., Scrutton, M. C., and Wallis, R. B. (1981). Thromb. Res. **20,** 413–424.
Hallam, T. J., Scrutton, M. C., and Wallis, R. B. (1982). Thromb. Res. **27,** 435–445.
Halonen, M., Palmer, J. D., Lohman, I. C., McManus, L. M., and Packard, R. N. (1981). Am. Rev. Respir. Dis. **124,** 416–421.
Hamberg, M., and Samuelsson, B. (1974a). Biochem. Biophys. Res. Commun. **61,** 942–949.
Hamberg, M., and Samuelsson, B. (1974b). Proc. Natl. Acad. Sci. U.S.A. **71,** 3400–3404.
Hammarstrom, S., and Falardeau, P. (1977). Proc. Natl. Acad. Sci. U.S.A. **74,** 3691–3695.
Harfenist, E. J., Guccione, M. A., Packham, M. A., Kinlough-Rathbone, R. L., and Mustard, J. F. (1982). Blood **59,** 956–962.
Harris, R. H., Nichols, R., Schmeling, J. W., and Ramwell, R. W. (1981). Thromb. Res. **23,** 521–532.
Harvey, J. W., and Gaskin, J. M. (1980). Fel. Pract. **10,** 25–31.
Haskel, E. J., Agarwal, K. C., and Parks, R. E. (1980). Thromb. Haemostasis **42,** 1580–1588.
Haslam, R. J., and Rossen, G. M. (1972). Am. J. Physiol. **223,** 958–967.
Haslam, R. J., and Rossen, G. M. (1975). Mol. Pharmacol. **11,** 528–544.
Haslam, R. J., and Vanderivel, M. (1982). J. Biol. Chem. **257,** 6879–6885.
Haslam, R. J., Davidson, M. M. L., and Desjardins, J. V. (1978). Biochem. J. **176,** 83–95.
Henson, P. M. (1976). J. Exp. Med. **143,** 937–951.
Hogan, A. G., Muhren, M. E., and Bogart, R. (1941). Proc. Soc. Exp. Biol. **48,** 217–219.
Holland, J. M. (1976). Proc. Soc. Exp. Biol. Med. **151,** 32–39.
Holmsen, H. (1982). In "Hemostasis and Thrombosis" (R. W. Coleman, J. Hirsh, V. J. Marden, and E. W. Salzman, eds.), pp. 390–403. Lippincott, Philadelphia.

Holmsen, H., and Weiss, H. J. (1972). *Blood* **39**, 197–209.
Hoyer, L. W. (1981). *Blood* **58**, 1–13.
Jakobs, K. H. (1983). *Eur. J. Biochem.* **132**, 125–130.
Jaffe, E. A., Hoyer, L. W., and Nachman, R. L. (1973). *J. Clin. Invest.* **52**, 2757–2764.
Johnson, G. J., Rao, G. H. R., and White, J. G. (1978). *Am. J. Pathol.* **91**, 85–106.
Johnson, G. S., Benson, R. E., and Dodds, W. J. (1979). *Thromb. Res.* **15**, 835–846.
Johnson, G. J., Rao, G. H., Leis, L. A., and White, J. G. (1980). *Blood* **55**, 722–729.
Kaplan, K. L. (1981). *In* "Platelets in Biology and Pathology 2" (J. L. Gordon, ed.), pp. 77–89. Elsevier, Amsterdam.
Kasuya, Y., Masuda, Y., and Shigenober, K. (1984). *J. Pharmacobio Dyn.* **7**, 138–142.
Kerry, R., and Scrutton, M. C. (1983). *Br. J. Pharmacol.* **79**, 681–691.
Kerry, R., Scrutton, M. C., and Wallis, R. B. (1984). *Br. J. Pharmacol.* **81**, 91–102.
Kinlough-Rathbone, R. L., Chahil, A., Packham, M. A., Reimers, H. J., and Mustard, J. F. (1975). *Thromb. Res.* **7**, 435–449.
Kloprogge, E., DeHass, G. H., Gorter, G., and Akkerman, J. W. N. (1983). *Thromb. Res.* **30**, 107–112.
Lapetina, E. G. (1982). *Trends Pharmacol.* **3**, 115–118.
Lapetina, E. G., and Cuatrecasas, P. (1979a). *Biochim. Biophys. Acta* **573**, 394–402.
Lapetina, E. G., and Cuatrecasas, P. (1979b). *Proc. Natl. Acad. Sci. U.S.A.* **76**, 1212–125.
Lapetina, E. G., Schmitges, C. J., Chandrabose, K. A., and Cuatrecasas, P. (1977). *Biochem. Biophys. Res. Commun.* **76**, 828–835.
Lapetina, E. G., Chandrabose, K. A., and Cuatrecasas, P. (1978). *Proc. Natl. Acad. Sci. U.S.A.* **75**, 818–822.
Lapetina, E. G., Billah, M. M., and Cuatrecasas, P. (1981). *J. Biol. Chem.* **256**, 5037–5040.
Larrieu, M. J., Caen, J. P., Meyer, D. O., Vainer, H., Sultan, Y., and Bernard, S. (1968). *Am. J. Med.* **45**, 354–372.
Larson, V. L., Perryman, V., and Stevens, J. B. (1983). *J. Am. Vet. Med. Assoc.* **183**, 328–330.
Lee, G. E., McKeever, P. J., and Ruth, G. R. (1979). *J. Am. Vet. Med. Assoc.* **175**, 49–52.
Lee, T.-C., Malone, B., and Snyder, F. (1981). *Biochem. Biophys. Res. Commun.* **102**, 1262–1268.
Lefort, J., and Vargaftig, B. B. (1978). *Br. J. Pharmacol.* **63**, 35–42.
Lenihan, D. J., and Lee, T.-C. (1984). *Biochem. Biophys. Res. Commun.* **120**, 834–839.
Leung, L. L. K., Kinoshita, T., and Nachman, R. L. (1981). *J. Biol. Chem.* **256**, 1994–1997.
Leysen, J. E., Gommeren, W., and DeClerck, F. (1983a). *Arch. Int. Pharmacodyn. Ther.* **263**, 322–324.
Leysen, J. E., Gommeren, W., and DeClerck, F. (1983b). *Eur. J. Pharmacol.* **88**, 125–130.
Liggit, H. D., Leid, R. W., Huston, L. (1984). *Vet. Immunol. Immunopathol.* **7**, 81–87.
Linder, B. L., Chernoff, A., Kaplan, K. L., and Goodman, D. S. (1979). *Proc. Natl. Acad. Sci. U.S.A.* **76**, 4107–4111.
Lorenz, W., Barth, H., Kusche, J., Reimann, H. J., Schmal, A., Matejaka, E., Mathias, C., Hutzel, M., and Werle, E. (1971). *Eur. J. Pharmacol.* **14**, 155–175.
Lotner, G. Z., Lynch, J. M., Betz, S. J., and Henson, P. M. (1980). *J. Immunol.* **124**, 667–684.
Lynch, J. M., Lotner, G. Z., Betz, S. J., and Henson, P. M. (1979). *J. Immunol.* **123**, 1219–1226.
MacDonald, M. L., Rogers, Q. R., and Morris, J. G. (1984). *Comp. Biochem. Physiol.* **78**, 123–126.

McDonald, J. W. D., and Stuart, R. K. (1973). *J. Lab. Clin. Med.* **81,** 838–849.
McEver, R. P., Baenziger, J. V., and Majerus, P. W. (1982). *Blood* **59,** 80–85.
MacFarlane, D. E., Smith, J. B., Mills, D. C. B., and Silver, M. J. (1974). *Blood* **44,** 947.
McGregor, J. L., Clemetson, K. J., James, E., Loscher, E. F., and Dechavanne, M. (1980). *Biochim. Biophys. Acta* **599,** 473–483.
McGregor, J. L., Clemetson, K. J., James, E., Capitanio, A., Greenland, T., Loscher, E. F., and Dechavanne, M. (1981). *Eur. J. Biochem.* **116,** 379–388.
MacKenzie, F. N., Svensjo, E., and Arfors, K.-E. (1972). *Microvasc. Res.* **4,** 42–50.
McGowan, E. B., Ding, A.-H., and Detwiler, T. C. (1983). *J. Biol. Chem.* **258,** 11243–11248.
McManus, L. M., Hanahan, D. J., Demopoulos, C. A., and Pinckard, R. N. (1980). *J. Immunol.* **124,** 2919–2924.
Madewell, B. R., Feldman, B. F., and O'Neal, S. O. (1980). *Thromb. Haemostasis* **44,** 35–38.
Mencia-Huerta, J. M., and Benveniste, J. (1979). *Eur. J. Immunol.* **9,** 409–415.
Meyer, D., McKee, P. A., Hoyer, L. W., Zimmerman, T. S., and Gralnick, H. R. (1978). *Thromb. Haemostasis* **40,** 245–251.
Meyers, K. M., Holmsen, H., Seachord, C. L., Hopkins, G. E., and Gorham, J. (1978). *Am. J. Haematol.* **7,** 137–146.
Meyers, K. M., Lindner, C., and Grant, B. (1979a). *Am. J. Vet. Res.* **40,** 260–264.
Meyers, K. M., Lindner, C., Katz, J., and Grant, B. (1979b). *Am. J. Vet. Res.* **40,** 265–270.
Meyers, K. M., Seachord, C. L., Holmsen, H., Smith, B. J., and Prieur, D. J. (1979c). *Nature (London)* **282,** 331–333.
Meyers, K. M., Holmsen, H., Seachord, C. L., Hopkins, G. E., Borchard, R. E., and Padgett, G. A. (1979d). *Am. J. Physiol.* **237,** R239–R248.
Meyers, K. M., Seachord, C. L., Holmsen, H., Smith, J. B., and Prieur, D. J. (1979e). *Nature (London)* **282,** 331–333.
Meyers, K. M., Katz, J. B., Clemmons, R. M., Smith, J. B., and Holmsen, H. (1980). *Thromb. Res.* **20,** 13–24.
Meyers, K. M., Seachord, C. L., Holmsen, H., and Prieur, D. J. (1981). *Am. J. Haematol.* **11,** 241–253.
Meyers, K. M., Holmsen, H., and Seachord, C. L. (1982a). *Am. J. Physiol.* **243,** R454–461.
Meyers, K. M., Boehme, M., and Inbar, O. (1982b). *Am. J. Vet. Res.* **43,** 1721–1728.
Meyers, K. M., Hopkins, G., Holmsen, H., Benson, K., and Prieur, D. J. (1982c). *Am. J. Pathol.* **106,** 364–377.
Meyers, K. M., Huston, L. Y., and Clemmons, R. M. (1983a). *Am. J. Physiol.* **245,** R100–R109.
Meyers, K. M., Seachord, C. L., Benson, K., Fukami, M., and Holmsen, H. (1983b). *Am. J. Physiol.* **245,** H150–H158.
Mills, D. C. B., and Roberts, G. C. K. (1967). *J. Physiol. (London)* **193,** 443–453.
Morris, D. D., and Beech, J. (1983). *J. Am. Vet. Med. Assoc.* **183,** 1067–1072.
Morrison, D. C., Kline, L. F., and Oades, Z. G. (1978). *Infect. Immun.* **20,** 744–751.
Murray, T. F., DeBarrows, B. R., Prieur, D. J., and Meyers, K. M. (1983). *Neurochemistr.* **22,** 781–784.
Mustard, J. F., and Packham, M. (1971). *Pharmacol. Rev.* **22,** 97–187.
Nachman, R., Levine, R., and Jaffe, E. A. (1977). *J. Clin. Invest.* **60,** 914–921.
Naito, S., Komatsu, H., Ujiie, A., Hamano, S., Kubota, T., and Tsuboshima, M. (1983). *Eur. J. Pharmacol.* **91,** 41–48.
Namm, D. H., Tadepalli, A. S., and High, J. A. (1982). *Thromb. Res.* **25,** 341–350.
Neufeld, E. J., and Majerus, P. W. (1983). *J. Biol. Chem.* **258,** 2461–2467.

Nishizawa, E. E., Williams, D. J., and Connell, C. L. (1983). *Thromb. Res.* **30**, 289–296.
Novak, E. K., Hui, S. W., and Swank, R. T. (1981). *Blood* **57**, 38–43.
Novak, E. K., Hui, S. W., and Swank, R. T. (1984). *Blood* **63**, 536–544.
Nurden, A. T., and Caen, J. P. (1978). *Br. J. Haematol.* **38**, 155–158.
Nurden, A. T., and Caen, J. P. (1979). *Semin. Haematol.* **16**, 234–250.
O'Brian, J. R. (1966). *Nature (London)* **212**, 1057–1058.
O'Donnell, M. R., Slichter, S. J., Weiden, P. L., and Storb, R. (1981). *Cancer Res.* **41**, 1379–1383.
Okada, M., Okamoto, H., and Inada, Y. (1978). *FEBS Lett.* **89**, 227–229.
Okumura, T., and Jamieson, G. A. (1976). *J. Biol. Chem.* **251**, 5944–5949.
Packham, M. A., Ardlie, N. G., and Mustard, J. F. (1969). *Am. J. Physiol.* **217**, 1009–1017.
Parmley, R. T., Poon, M. C., Crist, W. M., and Malluh, A. (1979). *Am. J. Haematol.* **6**, 51–60.
Peterson, M. E., Hurvitz, A. I., Leib, M. S., Cavanagh, P. G., and Dutton, D. E. (1984). *J. Am. Vet. Med. Assoc.* **184**, 806–808.
Phillips, D. R., and Agin, P. P. (1977). *J. Biol. Chem.* **252**, 2121–2126.
Pineau, S., Belbeck, W., and Moore, S. (1980). *Can. Vet. J.* **21**, 82–84.
Pletscher, A., DaPrada, M., Berneis, K. H., and Tanzer, J. P. (1971). *Experientia* **27**, 993–1120.
Prescott, S. M., and Majerus, P. W. (1983). *J. Biol. Chem.* **258**, 764–769.
Prieur, D. J., Holland, J. M., Bell, T. C., and Young, D. M. (1976). *Lab. Invest.* **35**, 197–204.
Raymond, S. L., and Dodds, W. J. (1979). *J. Lab. Clin. Med.* **93**, 607–613.
Read, M. S., Shermer, R. W., and Brinkhous, K. M. (1978). *Proc. Natl. Acad. Sci. U.S.A.* **75**, 4514–4518.
Reef, V. B., Dyson, S. S., and Beech, J. (1984). *J. Am. Vet. Med. Assoc.* **184**, 313–317.
Reimers, H. J., Mustard, J. F., and Packham, M. A. (1975). *J. Cell Biol.* **67**, 61–67.
Reimers, H. J., Packham, M. A., and Mustard, J. F. (1977). *Blood* **49**, 89–100.
Rittenhouse-Simmons, S. (1980). *J. Biol. Chem.* **255**, 2259–2262.
Rittenhouse-Simmons, S., and Deykin, D. (1981). *In* "Platelets in Biology and Pathology 2" (J. L. Gordon, ed.), pp. 349–372. North-Holland Publ., Amsterdam.
Rivers, J. P., Sinclair, A. J., and Crawford, M. A. (1975). *Nature (London)* **258**, 171–173.
Rosenblum, W. I., Nelson, G. H., Cockrell, C. S., and Ellis, E. F. (1983). *Thromb. Res.* **30**, 347–355.
Rucinski, B., Poggi, A., James, P., Holt, J. C., and Niewiarkowski, S. (1983). *Blood* **61**, 1072–1080.
Sakariassen, K. S., Bolhuis, P. A., and Sixma, J. J. (1979). *Nature (London)* **279**, 636–638.
Schalm, O. W. (1979). *Canine Proc.* **6**, 47–50.
Scrutton, M. C., and Wallis, R. B. (1981). *In* "Platelets in Biology and Pathology-2" (S. L. Gordon, ed.), pp. 179–210. Elsevier, Amsterdam.
Shaw, J. O., Pinckard, R. N., Ferrigni, K. S., McManus, L. M., and Hanahan, D. J. (1981). *J. Immunol.* **127**, 1250–1255.
Siegal, M. I., McConnell, R. T., Abrahams, S. L., Ponter, N. A., and Cuatrecasas, P. (1979). *Biochem. Biophys. Res. Commun.* **89**, 1273–1270.
Siess, W., and Lapetina, E. G. (1983). *Biochem. Biophys. Res. Commun.* **752**, 329–338.
Simard-Duquesne, N. (1973). *Thromb. Diath. Haemorrh.* **29**, 445–449.
Sixma, J. J., and Schiphorst, M. E. (1980). *Biochim. Biophys. Acta* **603**, 70–83.

Slichter, S. J., Weiden, P. L., O'Donnell, M. R., and Storb, R. (1982). *Blood* **59**, 1252–1258.
Smith, J. B., and Jubiz, W. (1981). *Prostaglandins* **22**, 353–363.
Snyder, F., Lee, T.-C., Blank, M. L., Cabot, M. C., Malone, B., and Albert, D. H. (1983). *In* "Platelet-Activating Factor and Structural Related Ether-Lipids" (J. Benveniste and B. Arnoux, eds.), pp. 253–261. Elsevier, Amsterdam.
Sutherland, C. A., and Amin, D. (1982). *J. Biol. Chem.* **257**, 14006–14010.
Tang, S. S., and Frojmovic, M. M. (1980). *J. Lab. Clin. Med.* **95**, 241–257.
Tateson, J. E., Moncada, S., and Vane, J. R. (1977). *Prostaglandins* **13**, 389–397.
Thomas, D. P., Niewiarkowski, S., and Ream, V. J. (1970). *J. Lab. Clin. Med.* **75**, 607–617.
Ts'so, C. (1976). *Am. J. Pathol.* **85**, 581–592.
Tschopp, T. B. (1970). *Thromb. Diath. Haemorrh,* **23**, 601–620.
Tschopp, T. B., and Zucker, M. B. (1972). *Blood* **40**, 217–226.
Ugurbil, K., Fukami, M. H., and Holmsen, H. (1984). *Biochemistry* **23**, 416–428.
Van Rollings, M., Ho, S. H., Greenwald, J. G., Alexander, M., Dorman, N. J., Wong, L. K., and Horrocks, L. A. (1980). *Prostaglandins* **2**, 571–577.
Vanderhoek, J. Y., Bryant, R. W., and Bailey, J. M. (1982). *Biochem. Pharmacol.* **33**, 3464–3467.
Vargaftig, B. B. (1978). *J. Pharm. Pharmacol.* **30**, 101–104.
Vargaftig, B. B., Lefort, S., Chignard, M., and Benveniste, J. (1980). *Eur. J. Pharmacol.* **65**, 185–192.
Vargaftig, B. B., Foqgue, F., Benveniste, J., and Odiot, J. (1982). *Thromb. Res.* **28**, 557–573.
Ward, M. V. (1980). *Vet. Med. Small Anim. Clin.* **8**, 1263–1268.
Wedmore, C. V., and Williams, T. J. (1981). *Br. J. Pharmacol.* **74**, 916P.
Weiss, H. J., and Turitto, V. T. (1979). *Blood* **35**, 244–250.
Weiss, R. C., Dodds, W. J., and Scott, F. W. (1980). *Am. J. Vet. Res.* **41**, 663–671.
Weksler, B. B., Marcus, A. J., and Jaffe, E. A. (1977). *Proc. Natl. Acad. Sci. U.S.A.* **74**, 3922–3926.
White, J. G. (1971). *In* "The Circulating Platelet" (S. A. Johnson, ed.), pp. 45–121. Academic Press, New York.
White, J. G. (1972). *Am. J. Pathol.* **66**, 295–312.
White, J. G. (1973). *Am. J. Pathol.* **70**, 45–56.
Whittle, B. J. R., Moncada, S., and Vane, J. R. (1978). *Prostaglandins* **16**, 373–388.
Wigton, D. H. (1978). *Vet. Clin. Pathol.* **7**, 16–17.
Yu, S. K., and Latour, J. G. (1977). *Thromb. Haemostasis* **37**, 413–422.
Zahavi, J., and Kakkar, V. V. (1980). *Thromb. Haemostasis* **44**, 23–29.
Zucker-Franklin, D. (1981). *J. Cell Biol.* **91**, 706–715.
Zucker-Franklin, D., Benson, K. A., and Meyers, K. M. (1985). *Blood,* **65**, 241–244.

The Pathology of Prosimians, Especially Lemurs

K. BENIRSCHKE,[*,†] C. MILLER,[‡] R. IPPEN,[§] A. HELDSTAB[¶]

[*]*Zoological Society of San Diego, San Diego, California and* [†]*Departments of Pathology and Reproductive Medicine, University of California San Diego, La Jolla, California,* [‡]*School of Veterinary Medicine, University of California at Davis, Davis, California,* [§]*Akademie der Wissenschaften der DDR, Forschungsstelle für Wirbeltierforschung, Berlin, German Democratic Republic,* [¶]*Institute of Animal Pathology, University of Bern, Bern, Switzerland*

I.	Introduction	167
II.	Review of the Literature	168
III.	General Considerations	172
IV.	Perinatal Mortality	173
V.	Congenital Anomalies	180
VI.	Infections	184
VII.	Hemosiderosis; Hepatoma	187
VIII.	Hyperplasia of the Islets of Langerhans	195
IX.	Pectus Excavatum	196
X.	Miscellaneous Conditions	200
XI.	Conclusions	205
	References	206

I. Introduction

The prosimians comprise six families of animals with greatly variable characteristics, and consequently there is some disagreement regarding the wisdom of inclusion of various taxa. For instance, controversy exists as to the inclusion of the insectivore-like tupaias among the order primates and also of the families Lorisidae and Tarsiidae. Since only relatively few of these animals have been kept in captivity sufficiently long, little is known about their physical needs, diseases, behavior, and causes of death. The most experience has been with the lemurs, one of the three families of Malagasy primates. For this reason this article concentrates on the diseases and biological peculiarities of lemurs. The hope is that from such a study will come some insight as to how to deal with these animals better in captivity and how to more successfully prevent their diseases. The final goal is to aid in their ultimate survival in captive populations.

II. Review of the Literature

Only one report in the literature has comprehensively reviewed the causes of mortality in lemurs. Coulanges et al. (1979) summarized the deaths of 126 animals from the zoo in Tsimbazaza (Malagasy Republic) occurring between 1964 and 1969. Their findings can be summarized as follows.

Pulmonary diseases (congestion, pneumonia, pleurisy)	45
Peritonitis with appendicitis, necrotizing enteritis	17
Aortic aneurysm	15
Hepatic diseases (jaundice, cirrhosis, hepatitis)	8
Toxoplasmosis	6
Internal hemorrhage	3
Intestinal invagination	2
Septicemia, staphylococcal	2
Skin mycoses (organism not identified)	2
Tuberculosis (organism not identified)	3
Neoplasms	3
Other causes	25

These authors made the point that pulmonary disase is frequent at that zoo because of the sensitivity of lemurs to the cold climate at the zoo's altitude. Deaths due to pulmonary disease occurred primarily due to *Klebsiella pneumoniae* and *E. coli* organisms. Enterocolitis was also primarily the result of *Klebsiella* infection and has practically disappeared following the systematic addition of sulfonamides to the diet. The frequent aortic aneurysms were attributed to the presence of the nematode *Spirocerca lupi,* thought to be acquired from ingested insects. The nature of mycotic skin infections remains unknown but was readily controlled by the application of quaternary ammonia. A variety of intestinal microorganisms were identified, including *Salmonella* sp., but *Yersinia enterocolitica* and *Listeria* were absent. Experimentally, lemurs can contract infection with *Neisseria* and are susceptible to plague. Among parasitic infections, these authors listed *Plas-*

modium girardi, P. foleyi, and, experimentally, *P. falciparum* infection. Moreover, the animals were found to be very susceptible to *Toxoplasma gondii,* which causes rapid death. Toxoplasma was found to be the cause of death in seven *Lemur catta,* two *Varecia variegata,* and one *Propithecus verreauxi,* but the mode of acquisition of *Toxoplasma* is not described. *Cysticercus* caused the death of a black lemur and a "rich fauna" of nematodes was discovered, including *Dipetalonema petteri* and *Spirocerca lupi,* the cause of aneurysms. Lemurs are also said to be susceptible to schistosomiasis.

So far as susceptibility to virus infection is concerned, Coxsackie, herpes, and reoviruses are pathogenic but poliomyelitis virus does not affect the animals. Echo II and Mengo virus caused paralysis. Lemurs may also develop antibodies to influenza virus during epidemics.

Griner (1983) described the principal causes of death in 83 prosimians at the San Diego Zoo, 44 of which were lemurs. Perinatal mortality accounted for 47% of the deaths and was highest in tarsiers. Another important cause of death was stress and, in Sifakas, the lack of knowledge for their proper nutrition. Infections were uncommon and included two cases of salmonellosis, one of pulmonary cryptococcosis, and candidiasis of a neonate. Parasites were infrequently encountered but cardiovascular disease occurred in four animals: a black lemur with aortic atherosclerosis, aneurysm, biliary calculi, hepatoma, and cataracts; myocardial degeneration in a sifaka and a tree shrew; and arteriosclerosis in a galago. Pilobezoars, pneumonia, enteritis, arthritis, and nephritis were other scattered findings. Two hepatomas were found in lemurs without metastases, and a mammary adenocarcinoma of a tree shrew had metastasized.

Ruch (1959) mentioned three neoplasms in his review of primate pathology: an osteosarcoma of the hand in a ring-tailed lemur, myeloid metaplasia in a male "striped lemur," and a less convincing lymph node enlargement in a ringtailed lemur. He also reviewed renal atrophy or hypoplasia in a ringtail and cystic kidney in *Microcebus* and reviewed the infertility of captive male brown lemurs. It would appear to us, however, that the cellular testicular "atrophy" is more likely the result of the pronounced seasonality seen in lemurs. Malaria in brown lemurs and echinococcosis in a brown lemur and ringtails are the infectious diseases mentioned by Ruch.

Demineralization of bones with hyperphosphatemia and hypocalcemia was described in *L. catta* and *Varecia variegata variegata* by Tomson and Lotshaw (1978). The disease was rectified by dietary change and is most likely a form of rickets. This report and a few notes in other literature suggest not only that prosimians are susceptible to vitamin D deficiency but also that their dietary intake needs careful supervision.

An apparently hereditary anomaly of the chest, pectus excavatum, was described by us to occur in *V. v. variegata* (Benirschke, 1980). As in the human condition, it is interspersed with flat chest and represents the manifestation of an autosomal recessive trait confined to this species. Other skeletal anomalies with lethal outcome (scoliosis, kinked tail) were associated with growth retardation but not proven to be the result of genetic influences (Benirschke *et al.*, 1981). A pedigree of ruffed lemur at London Zoo produced four nude neonates, which are thought to be the result of inbreeding, presumably due to a recessive autosomal gene (Goodwin, 1980). The condition was likened to the human BIDS (brittle hair, intellectual impairment, decreased fertility, short stature) syndrome (Jackson *et al.*, 1974). Hairless mutants are well known in a variety of species (Swanson, 1980).

Trichobezoars apparently occur in lemurs more commonly than in other species. Janssen *et al.* (1979) found trichobezoars in two ruffed lemurs, and Keller *et al.* (1979) saw three trichobezoars in a ruffed lemur with obstruction. In all three cases the large hairball was removed from the stomachs by laparotomy without difficulty. It is believed that the condition results from the combination of two factors—a less than normal content of roughage in the lemur diet and hair grooming and chewing because of boredom. To prevent recurrences we now administer Petromalt, a mild intestinal lubricant, to our animals twice weekly.

An important observation of hepatoma in a black lemur was recorded by Brygoo *et al.* (1964). This adult female had been in captivity in a Madagascar zoo for 4 years when she died from hepatocellular cancer with widespread pulmonary metastases. There was massive hepatic and pulmonary siderosis, sparing the tumor, and marked liver cirrhosis. The authors suggested a nutritional etiology and reviewed the animal's food habits in the wild and in captivity. While at the zoo the staple diet was banana with other fruit added. Just precisely how the excess iron was acquired is not mentioned but will be discussed subsequently.

Adenocarcinoma of the breast in two female ringtailed lemurs was found by Wadsworth *et al.* (1980), who also reviewed other tumors in tree shrews, galagos, and various simians. It is of parenthetic interest that one of these animals also had a vulvar squamous papilloma and ankylosis of the lumbar spine.

A pheochromocytoma in a male ringtailed lemur of at least 22 years age was described by Reichard *et al.* (1981). The tumor was found in the adrenal and thymus glands. Other lesions found in this animal from the San Diego Zoo will be discussed later in this review.

Boraski (1981) reviewed the occurrence of renal disease in prosimians. The most prominent lesion, membranoproliferative glomerulonephritis, was most commonly found in galagos but a unified concept of the pathogenesis did not emerge.

A series of deaths from necrotizing enterocolitis occurred in the lemur colony of the Cologne Zoo (Anonymous, 1983). The deaths were associated with parakeratosis of mucous membranes and extensive *E. coli* growth. No specific cause was determined, other than suspected food contamination.

A variety of fungi, particularly *Candida albicans,* was cultured from the stool of numerous primates by Schneider *et al.* (1983). These included several lemurs, and it was suggested that the organisms were introduced from a hand-raised animal that had suffered a generalized mycosis in youth.

Poley (1969) described the death of a ringtailed lemur from staphylococcal infection thought to have been acquired by food ("milk rice").

The high frequency of perinatal deaths in lemurs (21%) was discussed by Benirschke *et al.* (1980), who commented on the relative infrequency of congenital anomalies in nonhuman primates when compared to man. An evaluation of the causes of perinatal deaths, it was proposed, demanded among other things greater knowledge of the degree of maturity in neonates. This led to an investigation of the birth weights and histologic criteria for term births (Benirschke and Miller, 1981). Renal cortical maturation was found to be a useful indicator of term pregnancy, as is the case in human neonates.

The composition of milk from three lemur species was determined by Buss *et al.* (1976), who found significant differences between various species' milk lactose and protein contents. The authors suggested that these findings may serve as indicators for different species in cases where species designation is still disputed. Ratomponirina *et al.* (1982) studied the spermatogenesis of some intra- and interspecific lemur hybrids. In some cases (*L. fulvus* × *L. macaco*) fertile hybrids occur, while in others (*L. f. collaris* × *L. macaco*) fertility is absent, probably due to abnormal meiosis resulting from chromosomal differences. These authors also reviewed briefly the extensive cytogenetic characterization of lemur species that has recently been undertaken.

Lemurs have a pronounced seasonal reproductive cycle whose understanding is necessary for the evaluation of pathologic material. The highly seasonal animals depend upon light cycles for normal reproduction. In the northern hemisphere copulation occurs around December and birth in April–May. The length of gestation and estrus vary considerably among species, as do the external genitalia. Thus, in winter testes enlarge and vaginae are closed in *V. v. variegata* (except at estrus), while they are open in *L. macaco,* etc. These aspects have been reviewed in numerous morphological, behavioral, and hormonal studies of captive colonies (Bogart *et al.,* 1977a,b; Shideler and Lindburg, 1982). Of particular interest are the marked seasonal testicular cycle and the extensive prostatic development that are well documented in the studies by Petter-Rousseaux (1964). Multiple births occur commonly in several lemur species but are most characteristic of ruffed lemurs. Hill (1973) reported its frequency as 63.8% in *V. v. variegata,* 16.4% in *L. catta,* 8.2% in *L. mongoz,* and only 2.9 and 2.4%, respectively, in *L. fulvus* and *L. macaco.* He regarded multiple births as a "primitive" character. On the basis of pedigree information, Pasztor and Van Horn (1976) concluded that the twinning in *L. catta* is genetically determined and is usually of the dizygotic type, a conclusion they also reached with respect to their galago colony. In ruffed lemurs multiple pregnancies appear to be polyzygotic, and transplacental hematopoietic chimerism has not been identified. Triplets and quadruplets are common in this species, and quintuplets have been reported.

Finally, it is of considerable interest to note that in several species of prosimians there exists extensive postnatal and even postpubertal oogenesis, contrasting these animals from other mammals. Butler (1969) described this phenomenon in galagos and reviewed the evidence published for *Loris, Nycticebus,* and *Perodicticus.* The same phenomenon has been seen in adult *Daubentonia* (Petter-Rousseaux and Boulière, 1965) and is found in several lemur species to be described here.

III. General Considerations

The article is based on the examination of all autopsy records in prosimians available to us from the institutions listed. In almost all cases all of the histologic slides were examined and special stains were performed, and at times additional studies were undertaken to clarify controversial diagnoses. In many cases we were the prosectors.

It is apparent from Table I that an overwhelming perinatal mortality is responsible for over one-half of the autopsies performed. Among the remaining adults a few principal causes for death exist which will be examined in greater detail. For convenience, then, this

TABLE I
DISTRIBUTION OF MORTALITIES OF PROSIMIANS

Species	Stillborn		Neonatal			Adult (1 yr+)			Total
	M	F	M	F		M	F	(?)	
Varecia v. variegata	5	7	15	18		3	5	(1)	54
Varecia variegata ruber	4	2	6	6			1		19
Lemur catta	3	3	8	12		3	3	(5)	37
Lemur macaco	1		3	1	(2)	3	11	(5)	26
Lemur fulvus		1				1	1	(1)	4
Lemur coronatus						1			1
Propithecus verreauxi coqueli				1		3	2		6
Indri indri						1			1
Nycticebus coucang						2	5		7
Loris tardigradus						3	1		4
Perodicticus potto potto						1	1		2
Galago alleni						1	1	(1)	3
Galago crassicaudatus						1	2		3
Subtotal	13	13	32	38	(2)	23	33	(13)	
Total	26		72			69			167

article is divided into sections of major contributors to prosimian disease and mortality.

IV. Perinatal Mortality

In a previous publication we examined the perinatal deaths of mammals at San Diego Zoo (Benirschke et al., 1980). The overall mortality in primates was 31% and that of lemurs was 21%, while a majority of tupaias and tarsiers experienced perinatal death. Although in these previous studies abortions and stillbirths outnumbered neonatal deaths, this is no longer the case in our updated experience (Table I), where as many animals were stillborn as died in the immediate neonatal period. For the purposes of enumeration, four animals, two of age 6 weeks, one each 3 and 5 months old, were counted as perinatal deaths. Of three red ruffed lemurs the first died from maternal neglect, the others from salmonellosis and generalized candidiasis, respectively. One 6-week-old ringtail had rupture of the liver from a fall and slight bronchopneumonia. All others died within 25 days, the vast majority within 3 days. All adults listed in Table I were at least 1 year of age; the oldest with known age, a black and white ruffed lemur, was 15 years old.

In order to ideally assess the maturity of neonates, one should know the precise dates of conception. While this is the case in some specific animals under intense study, frequently this information is not available. Thus, when stillborns or neonates come to autopsy, their birth weight and length have served as a general guide, particularly when animals appeared normal. In malformed animals or those seemingly too small for term birth, more objective data are desirable to adjudge whether growth retardation or prematurity accounts for the deviation in size. Benirschke and Miller (1981) examined this question and found that in lemurs, at least, the histologic appearance of the renal cortex serves as a good guide. In temporally mature neonates the glomerulopoiesis has ceased, as is the case in human neonates, and the outermost glomeruli have separated from the capsule. In growth-retarded mature animals the same is true, while premature infants have continued subcapsular formation of new glomeruli (Figs. 1 and 2). As is stated in that report, neonates of *Varecia variegata ruber* may have weights from 73 to 111 g, *V. v. variegatus* from 80 to 125 g, and *Lemur catta* from 50 to 70 g. The variation may well be responsible for some neonatal problems in the smaller neonates and results from uterine position in the often polytocous animal. Three neonatal singleton black lemurs in our series weighed 55, 70, and 75 g.

Other important biological features of neonatal prosimian species must be appreciated for an understanding of the pathologic features of prosimians. For instance, when searching for parathyroid glands, one may find them embedded in thyroid tissue (Fig. 3). Also, the lemuridae have a pronounced fetal zone of the adrenal cortex, not unlike that seen in most other primates studied (Benirschke *et al.*, 1956) but also seen in a few other species (Moser and Benirschke, 1962). This fetal zone, which in humans is known to secrete weak androgens before birth, is comprised of large eosinophilic cells and makes up 80% of the cortical width. It undergoes involution, at times massive hemorrhagic necrosis, soon after birth. In most lemurs observed in this series the involution of the fetal zone commenced on the first day of life, was nearly complete by 4 days, and in 3 weeks only fibrous tissue separated the much widened definitive cortex from the medulla (Figs. 4, 5, and 6). Thus, most stillborns had a wide zone, with three exceptions in mature stillborn black and white ruffed lemurs. One was a runt (45 g) with mature kidneys and multiple congenital anomalies. Its fetal zone as well as the interstitial tissue of the testes was completely involuted (Fig. 11). The other two were triplet stillborns: these two had similar

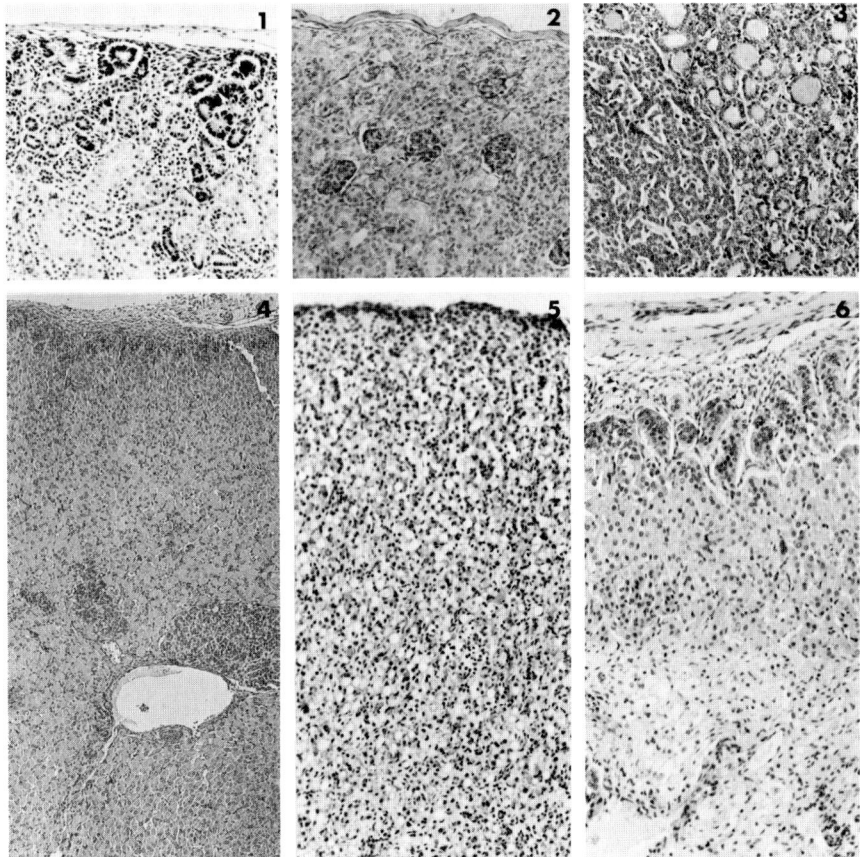

Fig. 1. Renal cortex of a *L. catta* abortus. Note the prominent glomerulopoiesis beneath the capsule (H & E, ×120). Autopsy No. 18888.

Fig. 2. Renal cortex of a *L. catta*, age 4 days. Glomerulopoiesis has ceased, and the glomeruli have moved away from the capsule (H & E, ×120). Autopsy No: 16747.

Fig. 3. Parathyroid (left) in the thyroid gland of a neonatal *V. v. variegata* (H & E, ×120). Autopsy No: 13035.

Fig. 4. Adrenal gland of a neonatal *V. v. variegata*. Note the narrow, dark, definitive cortex, the wide gray fetal zone, and the central vein with dark medullary cells adjacent (H & E, ×45). Autopsy No: 16189.

Fig. 5. Adrenal gland of a 4-day-old *L. catta*. The fetal zone is actively degenerating (H & E, ×120). Autopsy No: 16415.

Fig. 6. Adrenal gland of a 3.5-week-old *L. macaco*. The fetal zone below is completely involuted and replaced by fibrous tissue (H & E, ×120). Autopsy No: 16580.

severe congenital anomalies (one was partially eaten and histologically not available) and the other a normally structured littermate. Involution is thought to be under endocrine control, and one must therefore assume that the prenatal endocrine milieu for these two pregnancies was severely different. It might be added that the runt's cotriplets survived and appear normal. The testes of neonatal lemurs also have an unusual appearance. The sparse tubules seemingly disappear in a sea of hyperplastic Leydig cells that have a similar involutional fate, as does the fetal zone of the adrenal (Figs. 7, 8, 9, and 10). We have speculated that the steroid product of these interstitial cells is reflected by the urinary estrone output of the dam (Shideler et al., 1983). The ovaries of newborn prosimians are also remarkable in their size but not because of an obvious endocrine component (Figs. 12 and 13). Compared with simians, oogenesis is not complete at birth but continues well into the neonatal period (Butler, 1969; Petter-Rousseaux and Boulière, 1965). Consequently, Graafian follicles were never observed in the perinatal deaths of this study. The male accessory organs of lemurs are incomparably large and distended with secretions in neonatal lemurs, unlike most simians. As is true of most other neonates, there is squamous debris from aspirated vernix in the neonatal lemurs' lungs and the cerebellum has a peripheral outer granular layer that has completely disappeared by age 5 months (Fig. 14). A prominent pineal gland is also present in neonatal lemurs.

Perinatal mortality is conveniently subdivided into stillbirths and neonatal deaths, the latter being much more numerous in our study, which included 26 stillbirths and 72 neonatal deaths. Nine of 26 still-

FIG. 7. Testis of a *L. catta* abortus (H & E, ×120). Autopsy No. 18888.
FIG. 8. Testis of a *V. v. variegata* neonate (H & E, ×120). Autopsy No: 16189.
FIG. 9. Testis of a *L. catta* at age 2 days. The interstitial cells are beginning to involute (H & E, ×120). Autopsy No: 13801.
FIG. 10. Testis of a *L. catta* at age 4 days. The interstitial cells are nearly completely involuted (H & E, ×120). Autopsy No: 15464.
FIG. 11. Testis of a stillborn growth-retarded *V. v. variegata* with multiple anomalies. The interstitial cells are prematurely involuted (H & E, ×120). Autopsy No: 14061.
FIG. 12. Ovary of a neonatal *V. v. variegata* showing active oogenesis in the periphery (H & E, ×120). Autopsy No: 17723.
FIG. 13. Ovary of a 4-day-old *L. catta* with completed oogenesis (H & E, ×120). Autopsy No: 16747.
FIG. 14. Cerebellum of a neonatal *V. v. variegata* showing a prominent outer granular cell layer (H & E, ×188). Autopsy No: 13036.
FIG. 15. Papillary cardiac muscle of a 2-day-old *V. v. variegata* with growth retardation showing old central calcification. The animal died from bronchopneumonia (H & E, ×120). Autopsy No: 15209.

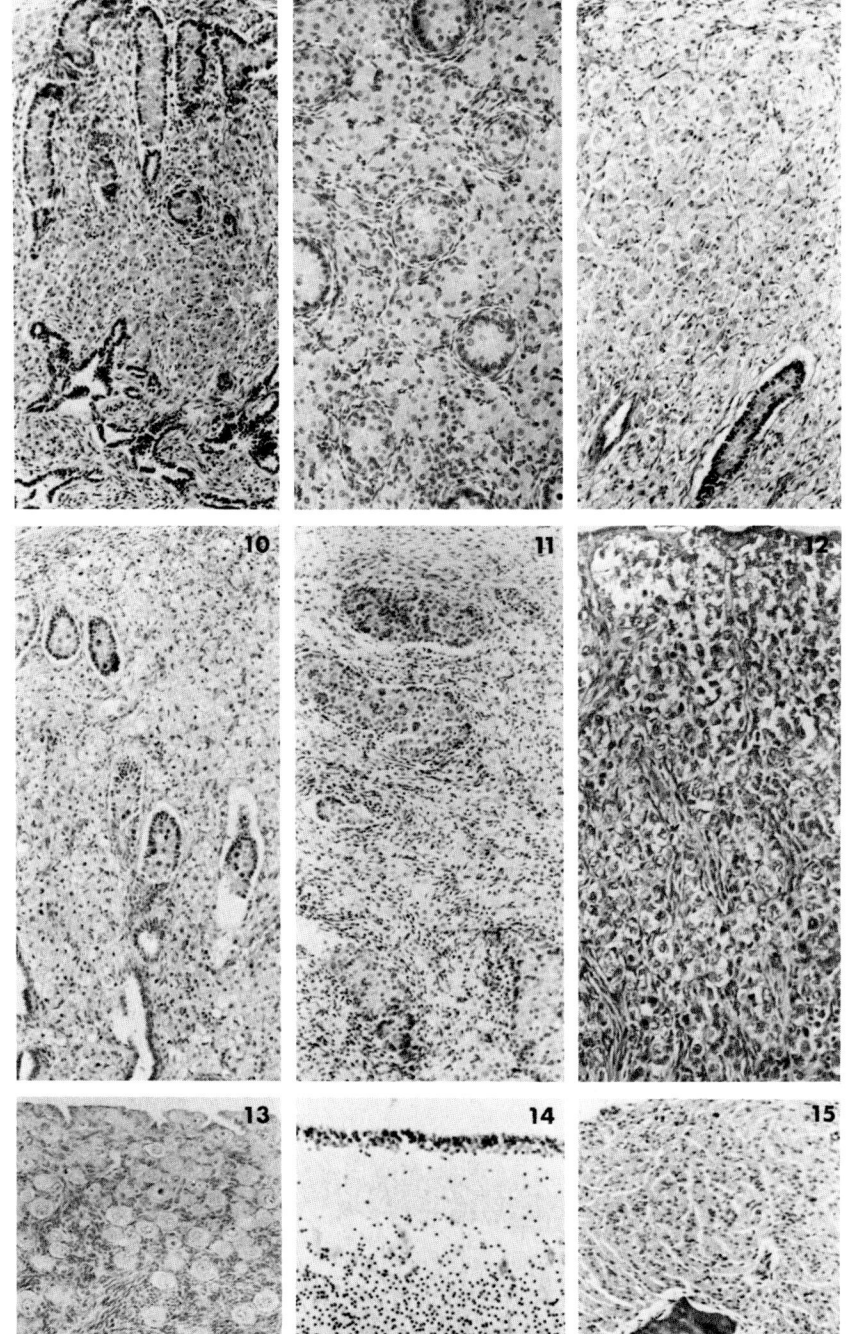

births may be classified as abortions. Two sets of twins of black and white ruffed lemurs (*Varecia variegata variegata, V. v. v.*) were macerated at birth and had histologically immature kidneys. The births of the first set (77 and 90 g) were accompanied by chorioamnionitis and, in the smaller, diaphragmatic hernia. The other twins were remarkable by their disparity, one weighing 90 g, the other representing a fetus papyraceus and weighing only 15 g. The cause of these abortions is unknown. Five of the other eight stillborn *V. v. v.* were malformed and growth retarded; one other with growth retardation was the twin to an anomalous fetus. One histologically mature stillborn (75 g) had abdominal eventration, presumably produced by maternal predation; the other (91 g) was one of normal surviving triplets. Of the six red ruffed lemurs (*Varecia variegata ruber, V. v. r.*) that were stillborn, two were littermates (79 and 111 g) of triplets and were predated at birth—the survivor died at 3 months from salmonellosis. One immature triplet stillborn (60 g) lost his littermates neonatally from neglect. One pair of large stillborns (115 and 130 g) were mature and their cause of death was not discerned. Finally, a 78-g female, mature stillborn was the smallest of quintuplets who, with a female neonatally dead littermate (90 g), had unexplained cataracts. The latter also had scoliosis; the three male littermates survived normally.

Five of the six stillborn ringtailed lemurs (*Lemur catta, L. c.*) were counted as abortuses. One weighed only 6.5 g, another macerated fetus weighed 40 g, the weight of one is unknown, and only in one set of macerated twins (36 and 54 g) with histologically immature kidneys were pathologic findings (placental infarcts) made.

The causes of death of the 72 neonatal deaths are more difficult to summarize. All of the 33 *V. v. v.* neonatal deaths had histologically mature kidneys, even though three of quadruplets weighed only 53, 54, and 65 g and were considered growth retarded although without congenital anomalies. They died in the first 3 days from maternal neglect and pneumonia. They were the offspring of a mother who had previously produced two malformed, growth-retarded litters. Maternal neglect and/or predation by one parent accounted for the majority of neonatal deaths and occurred on the first day of life in 18 cases. Two apparently predated animals had umbilical herniation and despite intervention died with peritonitis. Five neonates died from aspiration pneumonia while an attempt was made to rescue them from maternal neglect. Another animal with bronchopneumonia had unexplained foci of calcifications in cardiac papillary muscles (Fig. 15). Unexplained partial calcification of a pulmonary vein wall with osseous metaplasia was found in a neonatal death of triplets. Two neonates weighing 74 and 91 g with mature renal morphology died with foci of polymorphonuclear leukocytes widespread throughout the body (heart, lung, liver, adrenal, kidneys, and testes), suggesting septicemia. Special bacterial stains proved negative, but the histologic features suggested infection with encephalitozoon. Antibody titers in sibling and mother, however, were negative (courtesy Dr. J. Shadduck). Two of triplets with growth retardation (55 and 65 g) had malformations (hydrocephaly and scoliosis) and died on the third and fourth days of life.

Of 11 neonatal deaths in the *V. v. r.*, three infants had immature kidneys (73, 76, and 41 g). The twin of the first survived, while the cotriplet of the latter two was stillborn. One died from maternal neglect with bronchopneumonia. Of a set of quintuplets three survived, one was a 78-g stillborn, and another a 90-g neonatal death with scoliosis and also cataracts. The death at 3 weeks of a 237-g quintuplet was unexplained. A 3 month-old neonate died with salmonellosis following traumatic injury to the legs inflicted by cagemates. Another hand-raised quadruplet, the smallest of four, died at 5 months from intestinal candidiasis and other infections. A borderline mature 70-g neonate suffered massive hepatic, splenic, and adrenal necrosis whose cause could not be established. A male *V. v. r.* was euthanized at age 6 weeks because of progressive neuromuscular weakness and general deterioration. Despite extensive study the cause of the disease remained obscure, and the cagemates in the nursery remained normal. Finally, the smallest of a set of triplets (31 g) died neonatally; the two cotriplets weighing over 100 g survived. This neonatal death was not only severely retarded in growth, it also had immature kidneys histologically and a fibrous interstitial replacement of the testes. Superfetation or a disease leading to growth retardation are considered to be possible explanations.

Fifteen of 19 *L. c.* neonatal deaths were due to maternal neglect and/or trauma. They were all histologically mature and all but two occurred in the first 3 days. One lived as long as 6 weeks, when it finally succumbed from its wounds and pneumonia; the other lived to be 3 weeks old. The lowest weight recorded in this group was 44 g, a twin to a 45-g animal, both without milk in their intestine when they died on the third day of life. Two neonates died with omphalitis, and one additional 56-g term neonate developed aspiration pneumonia while being hand raised. The largest infant to die of undertermined causes on the first day of life weighed 71 g. Of interest is the fact that its fetal zone of the adrenal had ongoing necrosis, an event that does not usually commence until age 1 day and is therefore presumably indicative of prenatal "stress." No anomalies were found in 25 *L. c.* perinatal deaths, but 12 were members of twin pairs.

Three *L. macaco* experienced neonatal trauma inflicted by one of the parents, one living as long as 3.5 weeks when it died from aspiration pneumonia. Another large singleton (75 g) died on the first day of undetermined causes. The single *L. fulvus* neonate died from bite wounds.

This review of perinatal deaths allows several generalizations. It is evident that abortions are uncommon and that stillbirths are particularly frequent among ruffed lemurs and are associated with anomalies or growth retardation or are secondary to maternal predation. Among neonatal deaths maternal nelgect, trauma, and large litter size were the principal causes, and since an overwhelming majority occurred during the first 2 days, special vigilance by personnel during the birth season may be important. This is all the more crucial since almost all of these animals were structurally normal. Since lemurs are born at night, supervision may be difficult. Moreover, in view of the frequency of aspiration pneumonia in hand-reared infants, security and warmth (perhaps provision of nesting materials) during these critical first days should be considered in the management of lemur colonies.

V. Congenital Anomalies

Congenital anomalies are an important consideration in the evaluation of perinatal deaths, particularly when dealing with a possibly limited genetic base and faced with the dangers of inbreeding. One such anomaly, pectus excavatum, does not make its appearance until later in life. This condition has been identified in our colony of *V. v. v.* and will be discussed later. It cannot be diagnosed in perinatal deaths and its possible role in contributing to the large number of anomalous infants of *V. v. v.* is uncertain. Nevertheless, several ancestors in this pedigree (Fig. 16) have abnormal chests. No anomalies were detected in the offspring of animals in the colony of *L. fulvus, L. macaco,* and *L. catta* even though the size of the latter group is appreciable. Only two anomalous infants were present among 17 *V. v. r.* perinates and these were animals with cataracts. Histopathology of the eyes performed by Dr. G. Wickham indicated the presence of white blood cells and fibrin in the vitreous net around the lens. Moreover, there were unusual vacuoles (free of fat, mucopolysaccharides, and collagen) in the

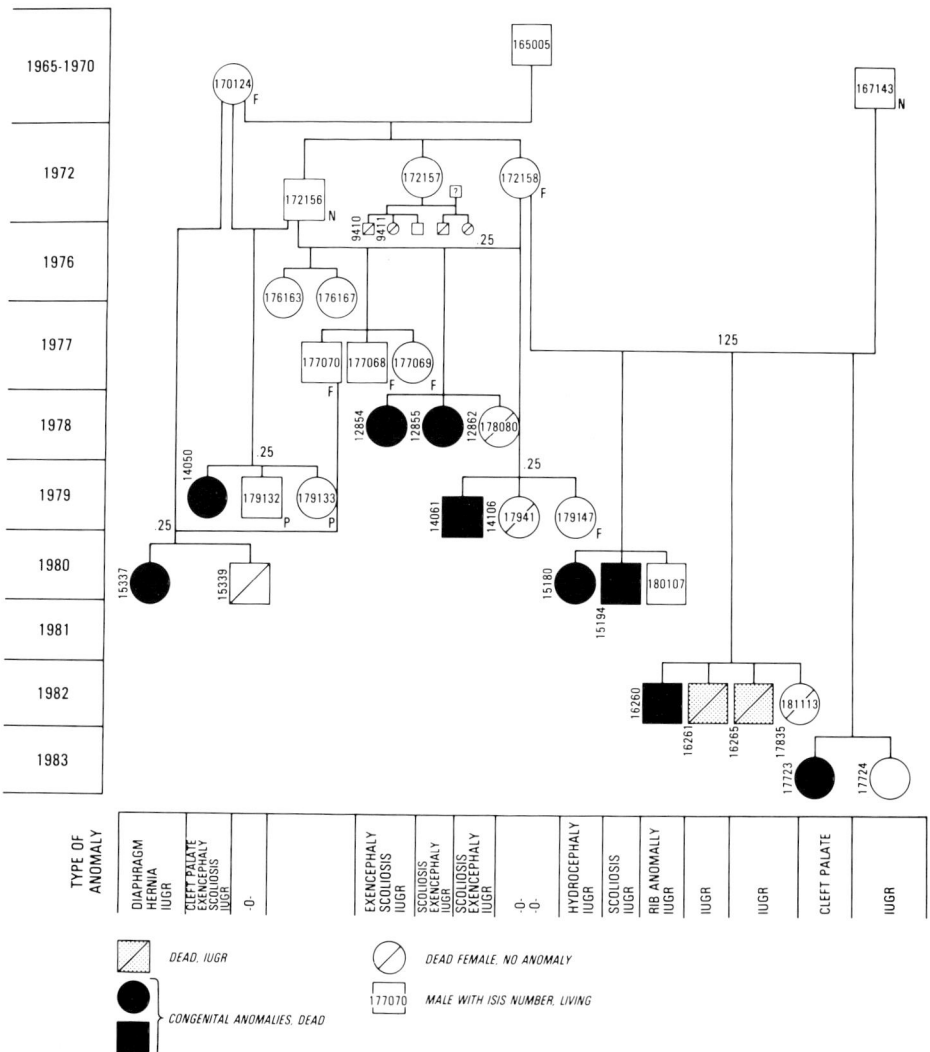

FIG. 16. Partial pedigree of *V. v. variegata* with anomalous infants. The ISIS numbers refer to the International Species Inventory System. (From Seal and Makey, 1976.) N, normal chest; P, pectus excavatum; F, flat chest; IUGR, intrauterine growth retardation; 0.25, inbreeding coefficient; the vertical numbers are autopsy numbers.

vitreous that were unexplained. The suggestion of trauma or healing infection was made. One of these quintuplets also had slight scoliosis. Although normal at birth, a red ruffed lemur died with a neuromuscular disorder for which no anatomic explanation could be given. It should not be considered an anomaly in this context.

The majority of anomalies occurred in our black and white ruffed lemur colony. The records list three newborns with umbilical hernia. On examination, however, these were undoubtedly traumatic, inflicted by the mother after birth. The isolated structural anomalies observed were right diaphragmatic hernia in a macerated, growth-retarded immature twin, cleft palate in the larger (96 g) of a set of stillborn twins (the other weighing 71 g and having growth retardation but no anomalies), a bifid left sixth rib in a set of growth-retarded quadruplets, and hydrocephaly in a growth-retarded triplet, one other of which had multiple anomalies. There were five black and white ruffed lemurs with lethal multiple congenital anomalies. Their relationship is shown in the pedigree (Fig. 16). The anomalies of four animals has been described previously (Benirschke et al., 1981). Since then one additional case has been born (Autopsy No. 15194) by the same mother who produced the previous anomalous offspring. This fetus had fusion of thoracic hemivertebrae T8-11 (Fig. 17) and was severely growth retarded (65 g). In summary, the anomalies included exencephaly, hydrocephaly, scoliosis, aplasia of the lung, cor biloculare, cleft palate, hypoplasia of the kidney, and hepatic fibrosis as well as testicular and adrenal involution associated with growth retardation.

The reason for assuming a genetic origin has been given previously and may be briefly reviewed here. The anomalies are confined to only this one species of lemurs; the different species are housed and managed similarly, and the most severely affected offspring come from brother × sister matings. Since the isolated structural anomalies are also confined to this species and occur in the same part of the pedigree, we assume that a genetic background is their basis as well. A chromosome analysis of two malformed neonates was normal. The father of one group (Autopsy No. 172156) has a kinked tail with fusion of some of its vertebrae, possibly representing part of the spectrum of anomalies. Cleft palate and scoliosis have been identified in squirrel monkeys and in that species they were also held to have a genetic background (Baker et al., 1977). A variety of skeletal anomalies and other defects can be produced experimentally, for instance, by hyperthermia *in utero* to bonnet monkeys (Hendrickx et al., 1979). Heat may act as a threshold factor in a genetically susceptible genotype; however, the complete

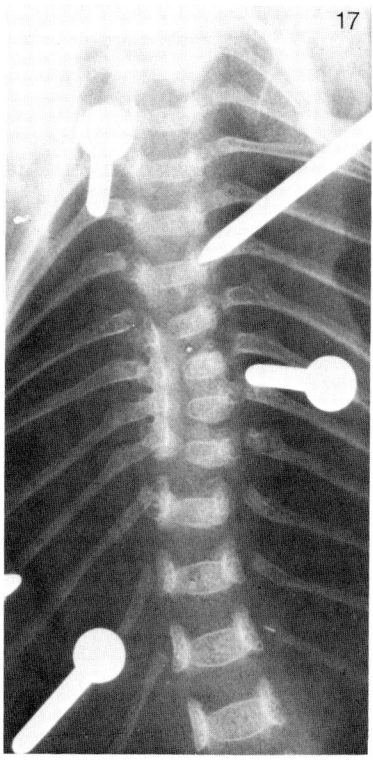

FIG. 17. Scoliosis with hemivertebrae T8-11 showing partial fusion in a 4-day-old *Varecia v. variegata* with growth retardation (Autopsy No: 15194).

pathogeneses of the frequent anomalies in this pedigree are not yet fully understood.

When the types of anomalies are compared with those in the AC/J strain of rabbits (Sawin, 1955), many similarities are noted. Thus, scoliosis, cleft palate, muscle fibrosis and contractures, hydrocephaly, and hypoplasia of the lung have all been recorded in subsequent breeding experiments by R. J. Webber (personal communication, 1984). The roentgenographic appearance of his rabbit fetuses is nearly identical to those of the severely affected lemurs. Webber considered autosomal recessive inheritance as the most likely explanation for the defects.

When the perinatal mortality of prosimians is compared with that of cercopithecids, cebids, and callithricids, several differences are noted. Price *et al.* (1973) reviewed the causes of death in 82 neonates from a primate research center. Although a majority of deaths also occurred on the first day of life, most were due to infection and perinatal distress. Trauma also occurred frequently but anomalies were found in only 1.2%, perhaps because of genetic heterogeneity.

VI. Infections

Various infectious diseases caused the death of adult prosimians. They can be roughly divided into three categories: those occurring in unacclimated animals, intercurrent infections in acclimated colonies, and unusual types (not related to intestinal disorders).

Among unacclimated animals, foremost were the rapid deaths of five sifakas. All had severe enteritis with much undigested food to which the animals had not acclimated. Microfilaria and *Anaspiralis* parasites were found in two and one had pneumonia. These animals could have been saved with earlier diagnosis and more appropriate foods. Of two *L. catta* deaths one had enteritis with pneumonia, the other myocarditis and pneumonia from septicemia. Likewise, an indri died from *Citrobacter* septicemia. Two galagos died with acanthocephalans peritonitis, one with *E. coli* meningitis, and another with *Salmonella typhimurium* septicemia. Two of three *Loris tardigradus* had massive nematodes complicated by salmonellosis, while another had unexplained interstitial pneumonia. Of four adult *Nycticebus coucang* two had nematodes, of which one died with sepsis after ulcerative lesions on the hands and feet; the other had arteriosclerosis. Two died with *Pseudomonas* infection.

Parasites were virtually absent in the established colony and were never the cause of death. In this group intercurrent infections were the cause of death, often in association with other afflictions, largely liver necrosis, a condition that will be discussed under hemosiderosis (Section VII). Salmonellosis (*S. typhimurium*) caused the death of a 3-month-old *V. v. r.* following initial parental trauma. Necrotizing enteritis with septicemia followed an obstructive trichobezoar in a 12-year-old *V. v. r.* Enteric candidiasis was found in several lemurs, usually as terminal events. In a 5-month-old *V. v. r.* it had led to ulcerations which caused mesenteric thrombi and septicemia. In a 3.5-year-old *V. v. v.* the only notable findings were gastritis associated with organisms of the *Physaloptera* sp. and pulmonary thrombi. Overwhelming peritonitis and rectal bleeding were the sequelae of intus-susception in an 8-year-old *V. v. v.* but without either intestinal tumors or bezoars as identifiable causes. Another black and white ruffed lemur died at 14 months from unexplained hepatitis with necrosis, colitis, and unidentified flagellated intestinal protozoa.

Five unusual infectious diseases were notable occurrences. A 14-month-old *L. c.* died from overwhelming toxoplasmosis, primarily in the lung, spleen, lymph nodes, and liver. The brain was not involved; accidental intestinal amoebae were found. The animal had been raised in an outdoor facility and serologic study of companion lemurs identified most to have markedly elevated toxoplasma titers. The presumptive source of infection was raw-meat-fed birds in the same enclosure. Four other lemurs had a granulomatous disease, one of which was due to disseminated cryptococcosis in a black lemur complicating hepatoma (Fig. 18). In two other animals with widespread granulomatosis only small foci of calcification were present that could not be proven to be cryptococci, although this was the suspected antigen (Fig. 19). One, an 11-year-old *V. v. v.*, had longstanding lick-ulcers on the tail. Kidneys, spleen, intestine, liver, and nodes had numerous granulomata with calcific spherules (Figs. 20 and 21). A 1-year-old *V. v. v.* surviving quadruplet (Autopsy No. 181113, Fig. 16) died with diffuse hepatic necrosis and widespread granulomata, also thought to be due to cryptococci. This animal also had granulomata with silicates and anthracotic pigment in the lung. Finally, an adult ringtailed lemur, also with areas of hepatic necrosis, had splenic granulomata, scrotal abscesses, and lymphadenitis. The etiologic agent remains obscure.

Toxoplasmosis in lemurs has been singled out as an important threat by Coulanges *et al.* (1979), who found 6 of their 126 deaths to be due to this disease. How the animals acquired the disease in Madagascar is not described. In our case the route of transmission is reasonably certain to be from raw meat. That the disease need not be fatal is attested to by the finding that 9 of 12 animals had specific high antibody titers, indicating recent infection, but it was found only in animals of the same enclosure. Meat loaf supplements in a colony of squirrel monkeys were also suspected to be the source of the organism in an explosive outbreak of fatal toxoplasmosis in a report by Dickson *et al.* (1983). Upon cooking the meat loaf, infections ceased. It should be pointed out, however, that on occasion the oocysts may be ingested with water contaminated by infected wild cats (Benenson *et al.*, 1982). A sifaka died with toxoplasmosis after 16 years of captivity at another facility (Chang *et al.*, 1980). The cagemate remained well and a source of infection could not be identified in this case. This animal also had severe cerebral involvement. Other reports on toxoplasmosis in *L. catta* and other lemurs are discussed by these authors as well.

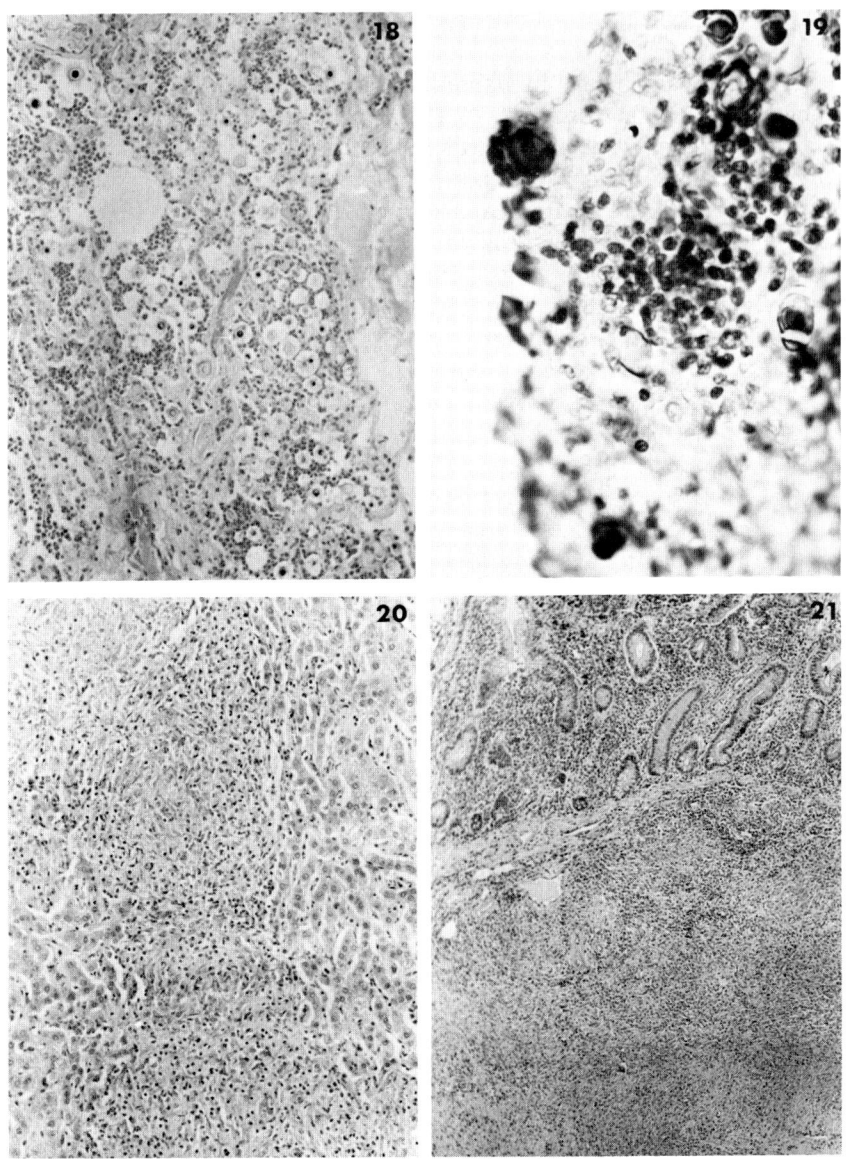

FIG. 18. Cryptococcal pneumonia in a *Lemur macaco* that also had hepatoma (H & E, ×120). Autopsy No: 8266.

FIG. 19. Lymphadenitis with calcific, PAS-positive spherules of *Varecia v. variegata* having disseminated granulomatosis. The spherules are considered to be remnants of cryptococci (H & E, ×480). Autopsy No: 18243.

FIG. 20. Liver of the same animal in Fig. 19 showing nearly confluent granulomata (H & E, ×120). Autopsy No: 18242.

FIG. 21. Intestine of the same animal as Figs. 18 and 19 with massive granulomatosis in submucosa (H & E, ×48). Autopsy No: 18243.

Cryptococcosis is rare in warm-blooded animals unless their immunologic response is impaired. At the San Diego Zoo this infection has occurred in a variety of animals, particularly in proboscis monkeys (Griner, 1983). In one of the black lemurs reviewed here, pulmonary cryptococcosis was the final cause of death even though it was complicated by hepatoma and extensive hemosiderosis. Possibly these conditions allowed the fungi to get established. In the two cases of widespread granulomatosis, cryptococcal antigens could not be detected during life and the histologic findings were only suggestive. Nevertheless, no other etiology could be identified despite exhaustive search. Sporadic reports exist on poorly defined granulomatous inflammations. Thus, in a dusky langur it was attributed to *Mycobacterium bovis* (Himes et al., 1982) and in an immune-deficient child to an unnamed Gram-negative bacterium (Seger et al., 1982). Of course, it is frustrating that in three cases of fatal granulomatosis no causative organism could be identified. Similarly, undoubtedly viral infections remain undiagnosed. A relevant suspect is the recurrent vulvar lesions of *V. v. v.* Although grossly these depigmented lesions have the appearance of papillomas, biopsies have the characteristics of herpetic blisters (Fig. 22). Despite repeated attempts at isolating viruses by a variety of culture methods and a search for typical inclusion bodies, no virus etiology was ever proven. The animals are clinically well.

Finally, it is of interest that parasitism does not usually exist in the established lemur colonies, despite an extensive list of parasites reported in the literature. G. E. Cosgrove (personal communication, 1984) finds reports on protozoa, Babesia, malaria, Prosthenorchis, hydatid cysts, Cysticercus, filaria, Ascaris, Primanebulura, Protofilaria, Linguatulid nymphs, ectoparasites, mites, cestodes, and a variety of other nematodes too numerous to list. Apparently, captive management has effectively eliminated these organisms.

VII. Hemosiderosis; Hepatoma

Iron deposits are a striking feature of the organs of all adult lemurs in captivity. Animals in several different centers and zoos other than the participating institutions have similar iron storage. Thus, the Jersey Island Trust, the St. Louis Zoo, the Duke Primate Facility in North Carolina, and the Oregon Primate Center all allowed review of some of their material, and in all adult lemurs iron depoists were found. In our experience *L. macaco* has the most and *L. catta* the least, with ruffed and brown lemurs being intermediate. The iron storage

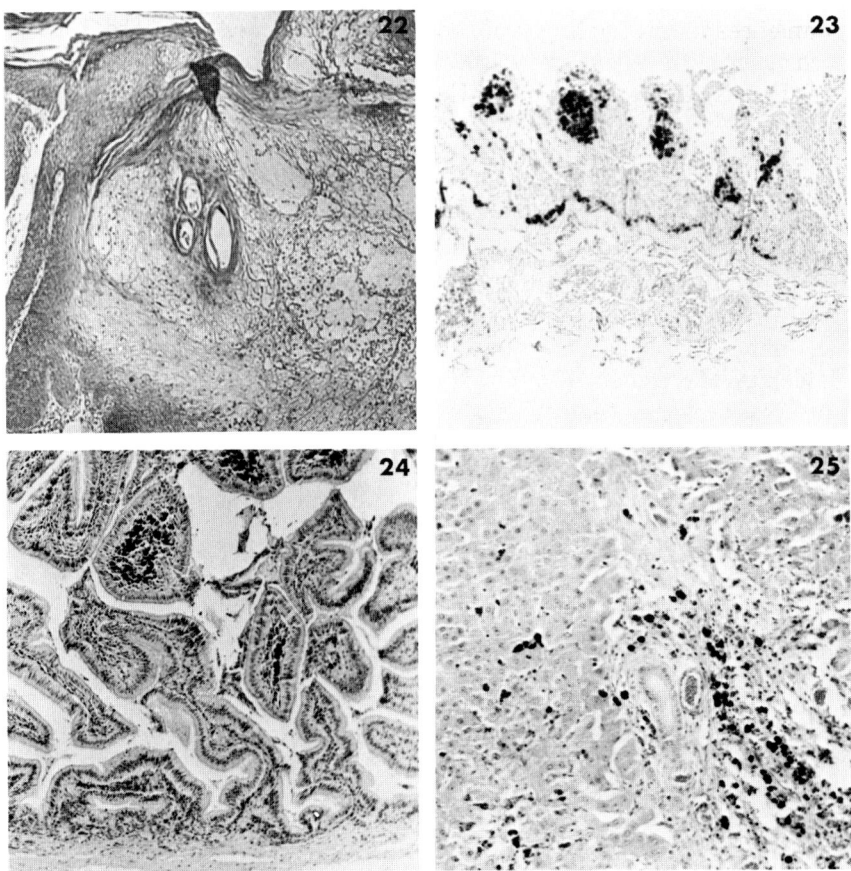

FIG. 22. Recurrent vulvar blister of a *Varecia v. variegata* (H & E, ×48). Autopsy No: S-289.

FIG. 23. Duodenum with marked iron storage in macrophages primarily in the tips of villi but also at the base of the mucosa in a 15-year-old *V. v. v.* dying with hepatoma (iron stain, ×48). Autopsy No: 14929.

FIG. 24. Iron deposits (dark) in villi of jejunum of a 11-year-old *V. v. v.* dying with granulomatosis (H & E, ×120). Autopsy No: 18243.

FIG. 25. Liver of an adult *L. macaco* with marked periportal iron deposits and fibrosis. Grossly the liver appeared cirrhotic; there were two biliary stones in dilated bile ducts (jaundice) with cholangioma. Marked hemosiderosis was evident in the nodes, spleen, liver, and duodenum. Arteriosclerosis with aortic aneurysm was found (H & E, ×120). Autopsy No: 11394.

commences in macrophages of the duodenal mucosa and here reaches such quantity that the first 10–20 cm of duodenum of old animals has a dark brown gross appearance of the mucosa. Later the iron is abundant in the spleen, the liver, and some lymph nodes. It is rarely found in other organs, except occasionally in the renal interstitium and commonly within the base of the endometrium. No iron is detected in the endocrine tissues as is common in human "bronze diabetes." The earliest accumulation noted was in a 6-week-old and a 3-month-old *V. v. r.* It is never found in neonates. While the iron is clearly predominately within macrophages, it does slowly accumulate in liver parenchymal cells and, of course, is best demonstrated with special stains. In the duodenum the demarcation is strikingly sharp at the pyloric junction. The iron accumulates first in the tips of villi but later is found in between Brunner's glands and then remains generally limited by the muscularis mucosae (Fig. 23). Rarely does it penetrate into the muscular layers in cases of excessive storage. Fibrosis or other structural changes are absent in the duodenum. Toward the jejunum the iron deposits gradually diminish but are often still present irregularly (Fig. 24). They are absent in the ileum and colon. The splenic iron deposit occurs in the perifollicular tissue and is in large macrophages. Little fibrosis takes place and there is virtually no evidence of erythrocytophagocytosis. Often, though, the spleen is enlarged in older animals with extensive hemosiderosis. This can be clinically obvious (and has led to biopsies in our colony) and is interpreted to be secondary to hepatic disease. In the liver iron accumulates predominantly in Kupffer cells and clearly can result in periportal fibrosis (Fig. 25), although it must be admitted that no direct correlation exists between the amount of iron deposited and the extent of fibrosis. In other cases extensive hemosiderin deposits are associated with focal necrosis and disorganization bordering on neoplastic transformation (Fig. 26). In several cases frank hepatocellular hepatomas were present (Fig. 27), which then lack iron pigment. Mitoses were uncommon but aneuploid nuclei and disorganization of the architecture were striking.

In this autopsy series there were three cases of hepatoma (one *L. f.*, one *L. m.*, and one *V. v. v.*) and three cases of cholangioma (one *L. m.*, one *V. v. v.*, and one *L. c.*). The hepatoma of the *L. f.* occurred in a 14-year-old male, wild-caught 11 years before death. It also had extensive atherosclerosis of the aorta. The tumor measured 4.5 cm, was multinodular, and had a large hematoma adjacent (Fig. 28). Large areas of tumor had undergone necrosis, iron was found in the nonneoplastic liver, duodenum, spleen, and nodes. The hepatoma of the 12-year-old black lemur measured 8 cm, was partially necrotic and calcified, and

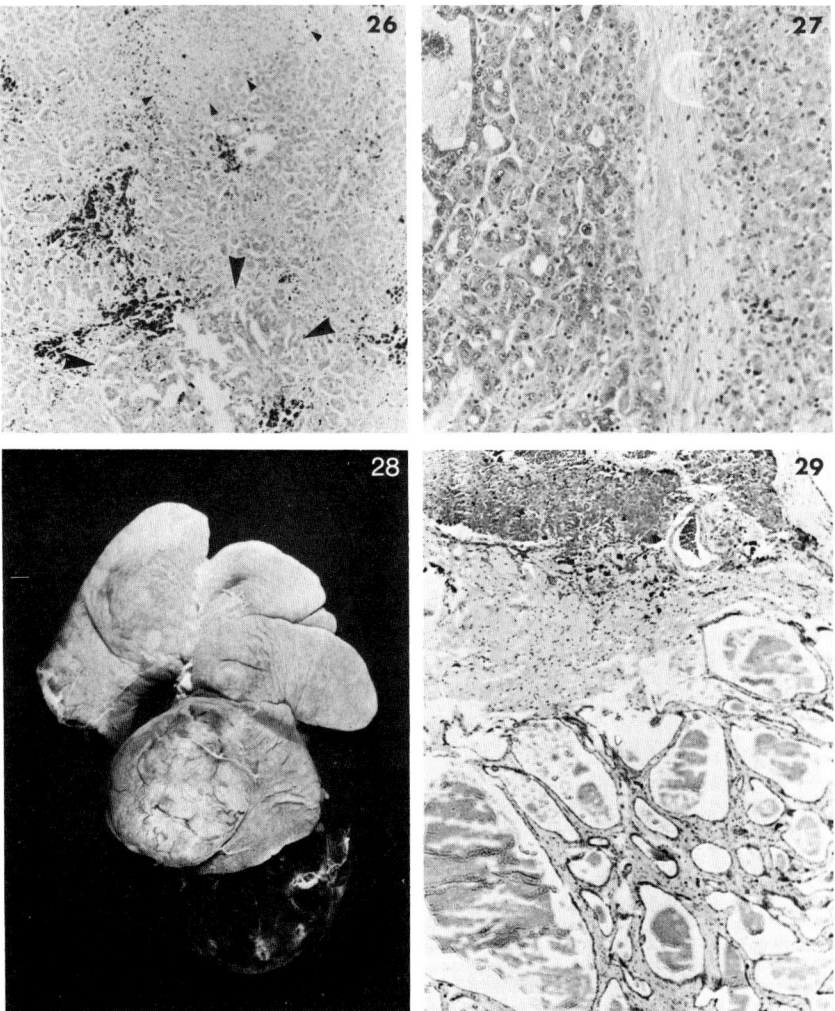

FIG. 26. Liver of an adult *Varecia v. variegata* with extensive hemosiderosis focal nodular hyperplasia (large arrowheads) and extensive areas of necrosis (small arrowheads). The animal had extensive iron deposits in the spleen, nodes, duodenum, pancreas, heart (slight), and salivary gland. Adenoma of the bile ducts and jaundice was found (H & E, ×48). Autopsy No: 12783.

FIG. 27. Liver of a 15-year-old *Varecia v. variegata* with hemosiderosis, fibrosis, multilobular hepatoma (left), bile duct proliferation, and foci of acute necrosis. The hepatoma was diagnosed by ultrasound and anesthesia. The animal died from euthanasia after pneumonia. There were no metastases (H & E, ×120). Autopsy No: 14929.

FIG. 28. Hepatoma (top of right lobe) in a 14-year-old male *Lemur fulvus* with adjacent large hematoma. The liver was cirrhotic and had much hemosiderin and the tumor was partially necrotic. Autopsy No: 15574.

FIG. 29. Cholangioma in an icteric adult female *Lemur macaco* containing two calculi (liver above). Same animal as Fig. 25, with hemosiderosis. Autopsy No: 11394.

was free of iron. The normal liver, nodes, and spleen had massive hemosiderosis and the animal died from pulmonary cryptococcosis. This tumor was the least well differentiated but had not metastasized. The black and white ruffed lemur was also adult and had a well-differentiated multinodular tumor that was iron free, even though much siderosis was present in the liver, duodenum, spleen, kidney, and endometrium. Fibrosis and bile duct proliferation were present.

The cholangioma of the old female black lemur occurred at the porta hepatis and contained two calculi. It was quite benign and consisted of a series of hugely distended ducts (Fig. 29). The animal had widespread hemosiderosis and focally severe intrahepatic bile duct proliferation. The cholangioma of the adult *V. v. v.* was a more typically proliferative lesion albeit of benign nature (Fig. 30). The animal had much cirrhosis, hepatic necrosis, bile duct proliferation, and hemosiderosis. The lesion of the 22-year-old male *L. c.* was more controversial. Marked bile duct proliferation, cholangitis with ectasia, and proliferation of pancreatic ductules were at the borderline of reactive response and neoplasia. This animal died with metastatic pheochromocytoma, cirrhosis, candidiasis, and marked hemosiderosis.

Extensive bile duct proliferation with hepatitis and hemosiderosis was also found in a 12-year-old female slow loris (*Nycticebus coucang*) that also had end-stage renal disease and collapsed vertebrae. In most of these cases there were also variably extensive foci of liver necrosis, almost invariably without attending inflammation. In addition, there were nine cases with idiopathic hepatic necrosis that in some instances was overwhelming and remains unexplained. It occurred in two *V. v. v.*, one as young as 14 months old with enteritis, hemosiderosis, bile stasis, the other an adult female with granulomata and hemosiderin. In two ringtails necrosis was found, one in an adult female with a fatty liver and hemosiderosis also with an adenomatous mucosal proliferation in the small bowel, the other associated with septicemia. The lesions were most acute and severe in black lemurs. In one case it complicated septicemia, in all others there was massive siderosis and widespread hepatic necrosis without inflammation or evidence of cardiac disease. Electron microscopy in one case of necrosis and one case of hepatoma gave no evidence of viral or bacterial etiology. A typical case is shown in Fig. 31. This 6.5-year-old female *L. m.* was slightly icteric and in an excellent nutritional state. At death the only lesions were pancreatic and midzonal lesions and central hemorrhagic liver necrosis.

Palotay (1978) also described death in eight older lemurs (*L. m., L. f.,* and *L. mongoz*) from massive liver necrosis. Like our animals, his

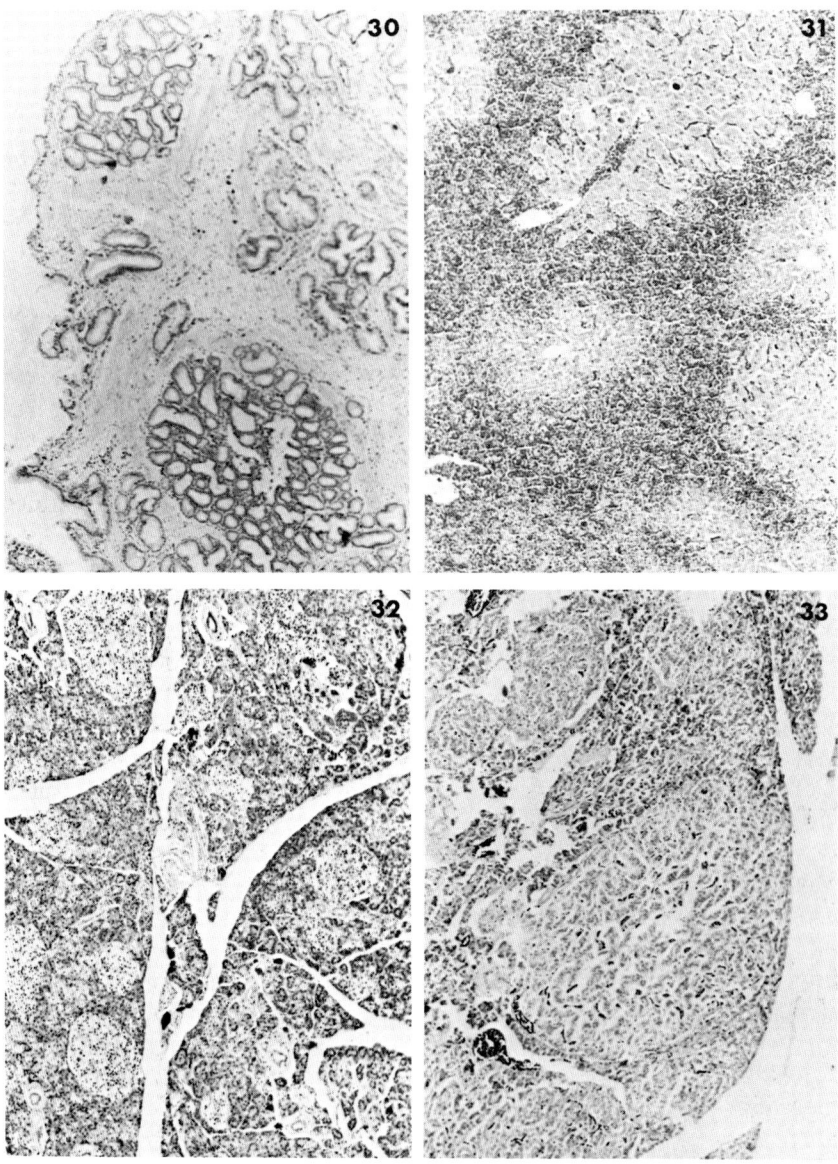

FIG. 30. Cholangioma of an adult *Varecia v. variegata* with cirrhosis and hemosiderosis (H & E, ×48). Autopsy No: 12783.

FIG. 31. Hemorrhagic liver necrosis in a female *Lemur macaco* also having pancreatic necrosis, jaundice, and marked hemosiderosis (H & E, ×48). Autopsy No: 12251.

FIG. 32. Hyperplastic islets of Langerhans (pale ovoid structures) in *L. macaco* with hepatoma and cryptococcosis (same animal as Fig. 16) (H & E, ×48). Autopsy No: 8266.

FIG. 33. Hyperplastic islets of Langerhans in an 11-year-old *L. macaco* with hemosiderosis, renal disease, and leg fractures (H & E, ×48). Autopsy No. 14596.

subjects were well one day and dead the next and a cause was not found.

The susceptibility of prosimians to iron storage and liver disease is striking. As has been pointed out previously, it is a finding made in all lemur facilities and presumably it is indicative of some biologic difference of these species when compared with simians. To be sure, occasional other primates in our autopsy series have had some iron storage, but it has never been as uniform and was not as massive or accompanied by tumors or liver necrosis. The facts that five imported adult sifakas that died in quarantine had no iron accumulation whatever, that the storage commences in the duodenal mucosa within a few months of birth and is progressively increasing, and that its quantity differs among lemur species have all suggested to us that prosimians have a peculiar way of handling ingested iron. It has led us to undertake experiments with the uptake of radioactive iron, including comparisons of *V. v. v.* juveniles with rhesus monkeys (Gonzales et al., 1984). No difference in the avidity for oral iron could be demonstrated to exist between juvenile lemurs and rhesus. The reason may be that at this stage of rapid growth both species take in all iron available to the mucosa, and similar studies in adults will be necessary. We failed to follow ferritin levels because no antibodies for lemur ferritin are currently available. Initially the sources of excess iron was conceived to be water from rusty pipes, which combined with the reductive power of citrus fruit would make iron available for absorption. Replacement of pipes, with a remarkable reduction of water iron content, did not alleviate the problem. Rehg et al. (1980) and Frye (1982) described an essentially similar iron overload in the rock hyrax (*Procavia capensis*), and the assumption was made by Frye that the primate chow diet might provide the excess iron. For the same reasons and having analyzed the iron content (high) of primate bisquits (Gonzales et al., 1984), we are now feeding an experimental group of lemurs chow with markedly lower iron content. It should be pointed out that hemosiderin macrophages accumulate in the mucosa of the small intestine of several species, e.g., horse, guinea pig, macaque, baboon, and man (review Ochoa et al., 1983), and that the view of some investigators holds that they form an obligatory stage of iron absorption (Cattan, 1983). Nevertheless, the quantities observed here were excessive as, of course, were the deposits in other organs. It was considered that the iron accumulation was the result of hemolytic processes since lemur erythrocytes show significantly greater osmotic fragility than those of man (Mason, 1981). Against this hypothesis is the absence of erythrocytophagocytosis and anemia and the lack of other evidence of chronic anemia (e.g., blood counts, absence of extramedullary hematopoiesis). Moreover, we administered by gastric tube a large bolus of distilled water to an adult *L. c.* and followed sequentially hematologic values such as RBC, Hgb, MCV, MCHL, bilirubin, and reticulocytes (with P. T. Robinson and R. Taetle) and found no evidence in favor of hemolysis. Excessive iron accumulation with extensive liver disease and occasional hepatoma has also been reported commonly in Mynah birds (*Gracula religiosa*), also for reasons that are not yet defined (Randell *et al.*, 1981). Here again a genetic difference in handling dietary iron may underlie this phenomenon since other birds fed similar diets do not suffer from hemosiderosis. Whether the disease should be labeled hemochromatosis in analogy with the human condition is conjectural. Clearly, the iron absorption is confined to only some species and it causes liver injury. On the other hand, many organs (e.g., heart, endocrine glands) that are commonly involved in human hemochromatosis are spared in these animals. Different opinions exist as to whether iron per se damages the liver. Brissot *et al.* (1983) in experimental iron overload of baboons found little hepatic damage, while acute damage to rabbit liver cells was induced by intravenous iron sulfate injection (Witzleben and Chaffey, 1966). Our view is that the frequent acute liver necrosis found in prosimians, the fibrosis and bile duct proliferation, as well as the cholangiomas and hepatomas are indicative of hepatic damage and are related to the excessive iron storage with which they were invariably associated. A locally metastatic cholangiocarcinoma has previously been described in an aged *Lemur catta* (Chang *et al.*, 1979). Unfortunately, these authors do not refer to any hemosiderin storage but point to the rarity of this neoplasm in any species. A widely metastatic cholangiocarcinoma is reported by Brown *et al.* (1980) to have occurred in an aged capuchin monkey without reference to hemosiderin storage, while that occurring in a long-time captive pallid bat (Beck *et al.*, 1982) was associated with excessive hepatic iron deposits. Attempts at identifying mycotoxin-producing fungi failed. True spontaneous hepatocellular cancers are equally uncommon in wild animals, as are cholangiomas. It is thus noteworthy that in addition to that reported by Brygoo *et al.* (1964) in a black lemur with "bronze cirrhosis," this report contains three additional cases. In all cases, as in the tumor found in siderotic mynahs (Randell *et al.*, 1981), the tumor itself was free of iron. This phenomenon is well known in human hemochromatosis with hepatomas; likewise, lipofuscin is absent in the frequent spontaneous hepatomas of captive sand rats described by Ungar and Adler (1978). Only little hemosiderin was found in their animals, and mycotoxins as etiologic agents were ruled out. The rare extrahepatic tumors reported in lemurs (renal cancer, prostatic adenoma, osteosarcoma, and uterine leiomyoma) have been referred to by Chang et al. (1979). In this series of autopsies only one other tumor, a pheochromocytoma, was observed. It occurred in a male ringtailed lemur, wild born in 1959 and coming to San Diego from the Cologne Zoo in 1962. It died in 1981 at age 22 (Reichard et al., 1981) with metastases to nodes and thymus. The animal was emaciated with terminal candidiasis and had hyperglycemia, bile duct proliferation with ectasia, and marked hemosiderosis. It is remarkable that this large (106 g) primary tumor had much iron storage, in contrast to the hepatomas. The possibility exists that this represents an example of the higher incidence of extraphepatic carcinoma associated with human hemochromatosis (Amman et al., 1980).

VIII. Hyperplasia of the Islets of Langerhans

Nine animals (one *V. v. v.*, five *L. m.*, and three *L. c.*) with hemosiderosis had unusual pancreatic findings. In the sections available the exocrine tissue was unusually prominent, apparently hyperplastic, and at times had huge islets. The *V. v. v.* was 1 year old and died with enterocolitis; all five *L. m.* were of older age and had various hepatic lesions, while the three *L. c.* were adults with sepsis in two and renal tubular necrosis in the other. One of the *L. m.*, the animal with cholangioma, cirrhosis, and biliary stones, had prominently congested, nearly hemorrhagic islets. The lesion of two black lemurs is illustrated in Figs. 32 and 33. The percentage of islets to exocrine tissue was determined by planimetry in these two black lemurs and two appropriate controls of the same species. The results in the controls were 6.1 and 7.6%, those in the affected were 14.5% (Fig. 32) and 24% (Fig. 33). Immunoperoxidase reactions for insulin, glucagon, and somatostatin were performed on one control and the two cases depicted (courtesy A. Dreilinger). Intensive reactions occurred with glucagon and insulin antibodies but not with somatostatin antibodies (lack of antigenic homology?). The enlarged islets were almost completely composed of β-cells.

It is difficult to classify the hyperplasia of islets in these lemurs. McClure and Chandler (1982) reviewed pancreatic lesions in 1000 primates, including 32 prosimians, and found 8 animals (6 macaques and 2 chimpanzees) with "islet cell adenoma," a lesion apparently similar to those described here. Four of the animals had been irradiated and one was "experiment related." The cause of the adenomas in the other is obscure. Fujita *et al.* (1976) found hyperplastic pancreatic lesions in rats in response to soybean or trypsin inhibitor continuously given per os. It may be that the unusual β-cell hyperplasia seen in these lemurs is related to hemosiderosis or diet. Clearly, lemurs in captivity obtain a different diet than in the wild. It is probably less fibrous, richer in carbohydrates, and higher in iron content. High sugar content apparently enhances iron uptake (Buck *et al.*, 1976) and clearly stimulates insulin secretion. Recent studies (Gabbe *et al.*, 1982), on the other hand, suggest that "high-fiber, high-carbohydrate diets improve glucose tolerance." Thus, different dietary supplies to captive prosimians seem to be of great importance in the future. There seems to be no evidence that the lesions represent so-called nesidioblastosis (Gould *et al.*, 1983), although they are superficially similar.

IX. Pectus Excavatum

Pectus excavatum is also known as funnel chest or cobbler's chest in humans and has been observed frequently in our colony of *Varecia v. variegata*. No other prosimians have been found to be so affected. The anomaly is manifest as a severe depression of the lower portion of the sternum with a bowing-in of the ribs (Fig. 34). It often displaces the heart laterally but on occasion the depression of the manubrium impacts directly upon the heart and leaves a deformity with focal cardiac fibrosis (Fig. 35). Funnel chest is not apparent at birth but can first be visualized radiographically at about age 1 year.

Pectus excavatum in humans occurs frequently, both sporadically and on a genetic basis. The survey by Heinonen *et al.* (1977) gives incidences of 12.6 per 1000 in some populations and 0.5 per 1000 in others. Snyder and Curtis (1934) were the first to suggest an autosomal

FIG. 34. Lateral chest X ray of an 8-year-old female *Varecia v. variegata* (ISIS No. 175109) that died from intussusception and hemosiderosis. The depth of the pectus excavatum is indicated by the arrow. Note the normal calcification of the tracheal and mainstem bronchial cartilages. Autopsy No: 19635.

FIG. 35. Depression of the anterior myocardium (indicated by arrow) in the same animal as Fig. 34. In contrast to other lemurs, this animal's heart was not laterally displaced. Autopsy No: 19635.

FIG. 36. Dissected thorax of the animal in Figs. 34 and 35. Note the pectus excavatum (arrow) and normal diaphragm (D). Autopsy No: 19635.

FIG. 37. Inside view of the anterior chest of the animal in Figs. 34, 35, and 36. Note the prominence of the pectus (P) and the normal appearance of the diaphragm. Autopsy No: 19635.

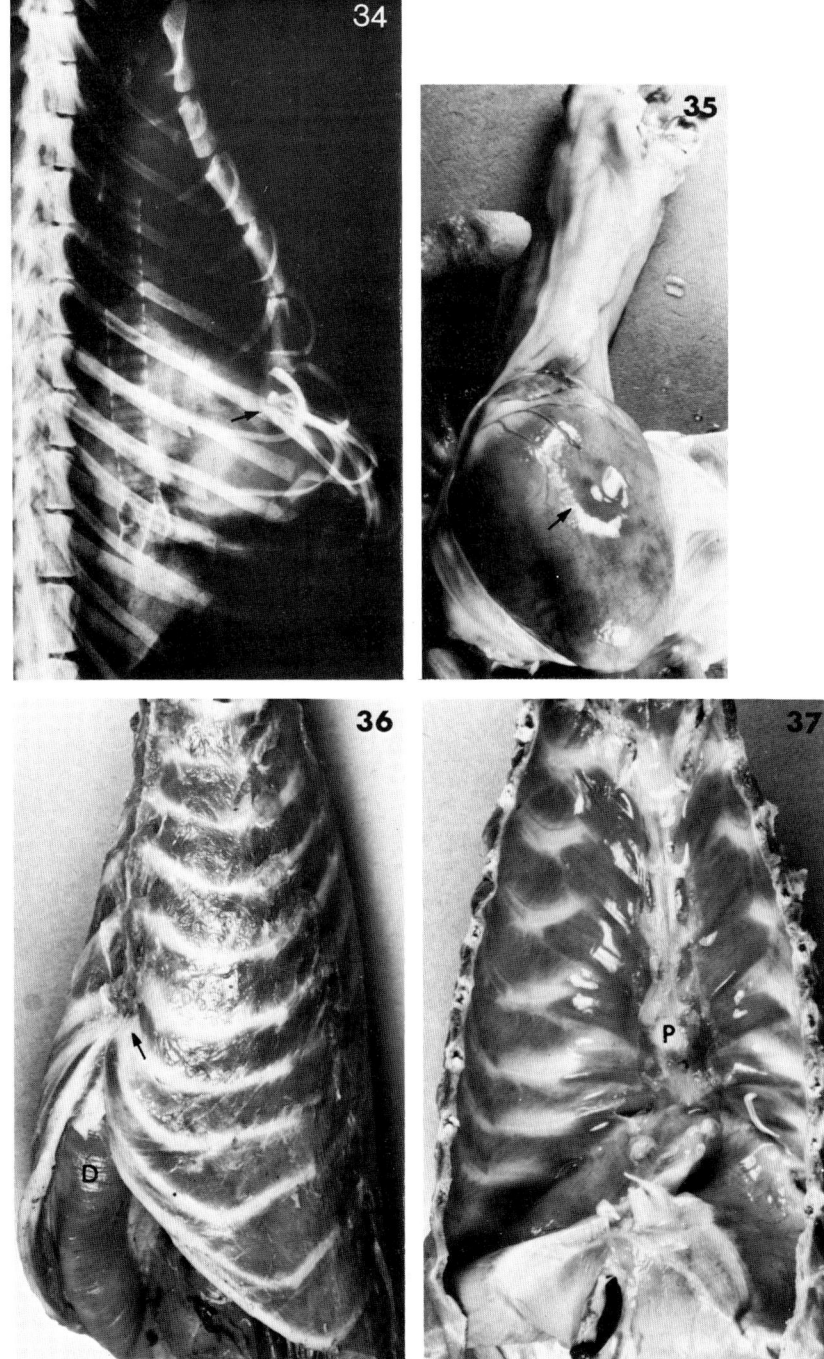

dominant inheritance in man, a suggestion that was borne out on a much larger pedigree by Stoddard (1939). In these family studies funnel chest was interchangeable with flat chest as having the same genetic basis. The same is true of *V. v. v.* (Benirschke, 1980). An apparently normal female (mother to Autopsy No. 170124 in the pedigree of Fig. 16) disseminated the trait to the San Diego lemur colony. The initial pedigree resulting from this introduction was shown in Fig. 1 of Benirschke (1980). Subsequent radiologic study has shown the condition to be inherited as an autosomal dominant condition. Other owners of *V. v. v.* have examined their animals radiographically and have kindly made the radiographs or findings available to us. No cases unrelated to our original female import (Autopsy No. 167144 (ISIS) have been identified. Thus, the introduction of the gene seems to be clearly due to this female import and suggests that it must have existed in the wild population. Inasmuch as no significant health hazard has come to light from this anomaly, we now regard it as a cosmetic defect. The same is true of humans, where the sporadic reports of respiratory or cardiac interference are not generally accepted as being secondary to pectus excavatum (Polgar and Koop, 1963; Orzalesi and Cook, 1965). Koop (1956) recommended that surgery be performed in only very severe cases; however, cosmetic repair is often undertaken in childhood.

The pathogenesis of pectus excavatum is not fully understood. Transiently it is found in neonates with severe respiratory distress. Fan and Murphy (1981) suggested that it may result from upper airway obstruction for which, however, no correlation exists in lemurs. Perhaps such an explanation can apply to the sporadic case reported in a Douc langur (Sedgwick, 1981) with emphysema, pneumonia, lung mite infestation, and a healing fracture of the sternum. In the hereditary form the precise abnormality remains obscure. The various theories have been examined in our fatalities. No abnormalities in cartilage

FIG. 38. Roentgenograph of the dissected anterior chest of a 2½-year-old female *Varecia v. variegata* (ISIS No. 178072) dying from gastric dilatation and pectus excavatum. The chest was markedly malformed, possibly contributing to respiratory dysfunction. The costochondral junctions are normal. Autopsy No: 15694.

FIG. 39. Closed sixth costochondral junction of a then 4-year-old female *Varecia v. variegata* with pectus excavatum (ISIS No. 175109). No abnormalities are noted (H & E, ×50). The biopsy was performed courtesy of T. Canti and P. T. Robinson. Autopsy No: 175109 (ISIS).

FIG. 40. Closed costochondral junction of the sixth rib in an 11-year-old normal *Varecia v. variegata* for comparison with Fig. 39 (H & E, ×64). Same animal as in Figs. 19, 20, 21, and 24. Autopsy No: 18243.

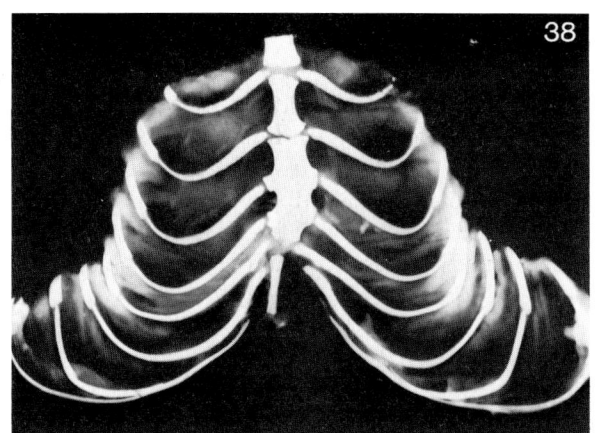
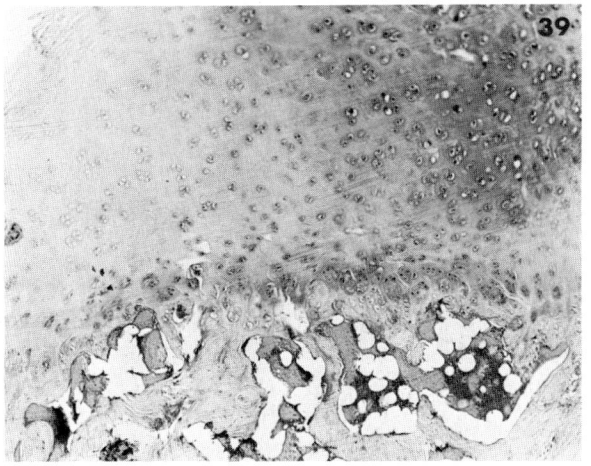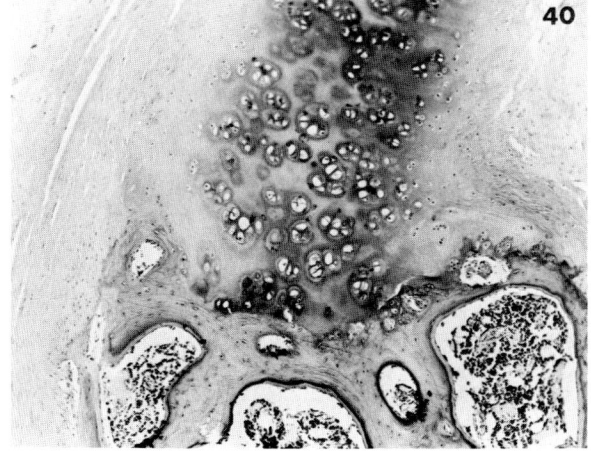

and costochondral bone formation have been seen in resected biopsies or at death. The diaphragm in all cases had normal insertion, and no fibrous replacement or muscular disease was identified (Figs. 36, 37, 38, 39, and 40). Pearson (1973), who described the anomaly in dogs, suggested that "the ventral portion of the diaphragm is deficient in musculature." This was certainly not the case in our lemurs. The condition we describe, however, may differ in other ways from that reported by Pearson in three Setter littermates. These animals were deformed at birth; three of four littermates were dead within 7 days, and the parents had no deformity. Despite detailed examination of our pedigree it is still unclear whether the gene for pectus excavatum bears a relationship to the lethal anomalies reported earlier to occur in neonates (Figs. 16 and 17). The father to many of the anomalies has a malformed tail (Fig. 41) but a normal chest. He is the littermate of the mother to several anomalous babies who also has a flat chest (Fig. 16). Another reason for a possible relationship between the anomalies and the gene for pectus excavatum is the sporadic occurrence of similar constellations in other species. For instance, Ravitch and Matzen (1968) described an 11-year-old child with funnel chest, agenesis of the left lung, scoliosis, ectromelia of the hand, and club feet. Only long-term observation and correlation with pedigrees will resolve these still outstanding questions.

X. Miscellaneous Conditions

The majority of prosimians not accounted for in the previous sections died from various infectious diseases, e.g., enteritis or pneumonia, that are not specific for this group of mammals. There were a few noteworthy findings, however, that need to be included in this review.

An adult *V. v. v.* (see Figs. 23 and 27) had empyema from an area of chronic pneumonia, in the center of which was a cavity with a piece of wood, apparently from a very old trauma. As in many other lemurs, old placental site lesions (hyalinization of vessels, hemosiderin) were

FIG. 41. Roentgenograph of the tail of an adult male *Varecia v. variegata* (ISIS No. 172156) showing fusion of three vertebrae to cause the kink. Autopsy No: 172156 (ISIS).

FIG. 42. Uterus of a 12-year-old *Varecia variegata ruber* showing an old placental site in thinned endometrium, i.e., markedly thickened, hyalinized blood vessels. Hemosiderin is present at the base between large vessels (H & E, ×60). Autopsy No: 10321.

FIG. 43. Same animal which died from intestinal obstruction, as in Fig. 42. Incidental findings are renal tubular and glomerular distension, obviously of long standing (H & E, ×60). Autopsy No: 10321.

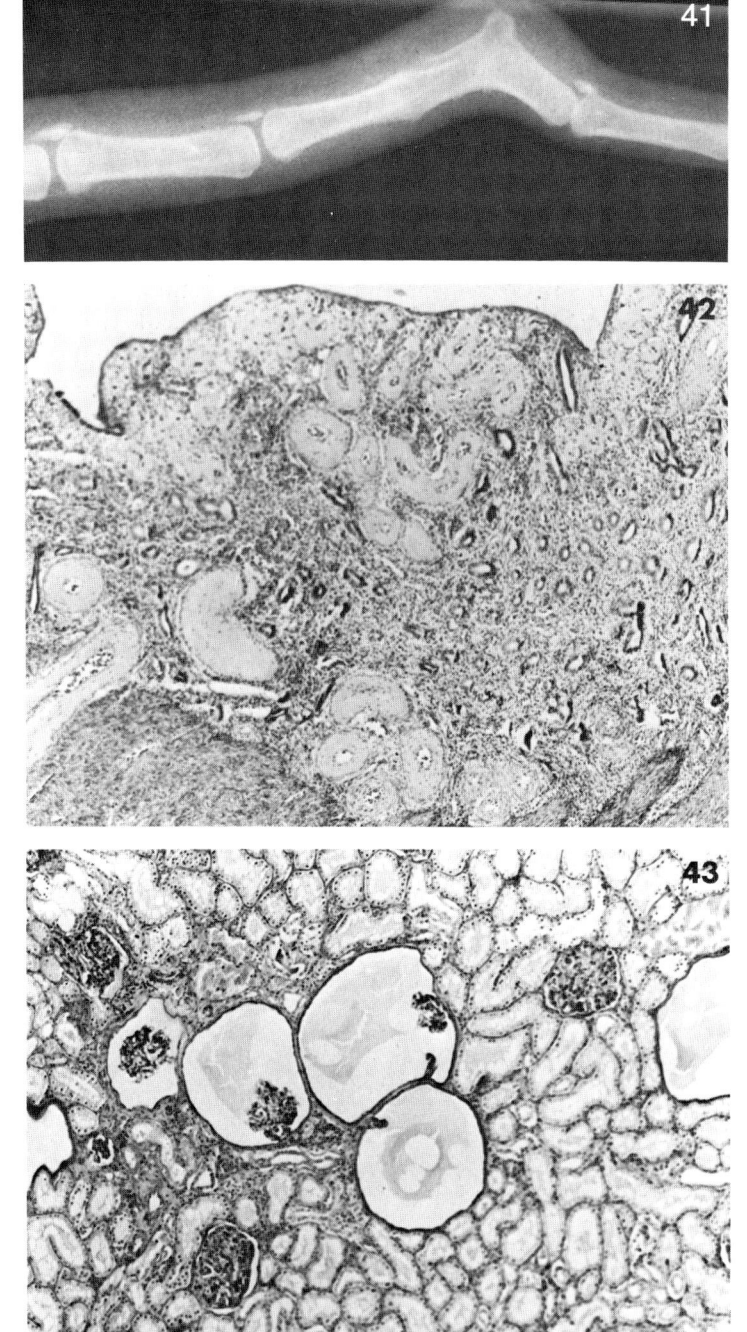

found. Intestinal obstruction killed two animals. One was the 8-year-old *V. v. v.* with hemosiderosis and funnel chest (Figs. 34, 35, 36, and 37) whose distal ileum and proximal colon had intussuscepted and become necrotic. The other was a 12-year-old red ruffed lemur with two trichobezoars in the stomach and one obstructing the ileocolic junction. This led to massive intestinal dilatation. Aside from the typical uterine placental site lesions (Fig. 42), there were numerous renal tubular cysts with casts, glomerular capsular distension, and focal glomerular fibrosis for unexplained reasons (Fig. 43). Chronic nephritis, here used for lack of a better designation, was the principal pathologic finding in seven other animals. It was very severe in an 8-year-old male *Lemur coronatus* that died from cardiac tamponade following rupture of an aortic aneurysm. Two black lemurs had renal disease, a female 11-year-old with bite injuries and the 12-year-old male that died from cryptococcosis (Fig. 18) and hepatoma. The degree of chronic nephritis in this animal was striking (Fig. 44) and was presumably related to myocardial scarring and thickening of one aortic valve leaf as well as the aortic atherosclerosis. One slow loris, one potto, and one slender loris had mild renal sclerosis. Minimal renal disease affected the 2-year-old female *V. v. v.* with pectus excavatum (Fig. 38). A different renal disease killed a 13.5-year-old female *Lemur catta*. This animal had been treated for bilateral pleural effusions (200 ml) and elevated serum creatinine and BUN. In addition to the hemosiderosis and nesidioblastosis of the pancrease mentioned earlier, both kidneys had diffuse acute tubular necrosis with mitotic repair. The cause is presumed to have been toxic but was not identified.

Several older prosimians had aortic atherosclerotic plaques but only two had aneurysms, a condition that others related to parasites. None was found in this material. One was the 8-year-old male *Lemur coronatus* with severe chronic nephritis. Two 3-cm-long thoracic aortic

FIG. 44. Chronic nephritis of a 12-year-old male *Lemur macaco* that also had hepatoma and cryptococcosis (Fig. 18). All glomeruli are severely scarred, the tubules are filled with protein and irregularly distended, and there is interstitial fibrosis (H & E, ×48). Autopsy No: 8266.

FIG. 45. Dissecting aortic aneurysm in an 8-year-old *Lemur coronatus* that had led to cardiac tamponade. Intima above left, adventitia below, dissecting dark red cells and fibrin in the center (H & E, ×48). Autopsy No: 17567.

FIG. 46. Aortic atherosclerosis of an adult *L. macaco* with aortic aneurysm, hemosiderosis, and cholangioma (see Figs. 25 and 29) (H & E, ×48). Autopsy No: 11394.

FIG. 47. Sifaka testis from an animal freshly imported in September 1965 showing meiotic activity and vacuolar degeneration of interstitial cells (H & E, ×120). Autopsy No: 895.

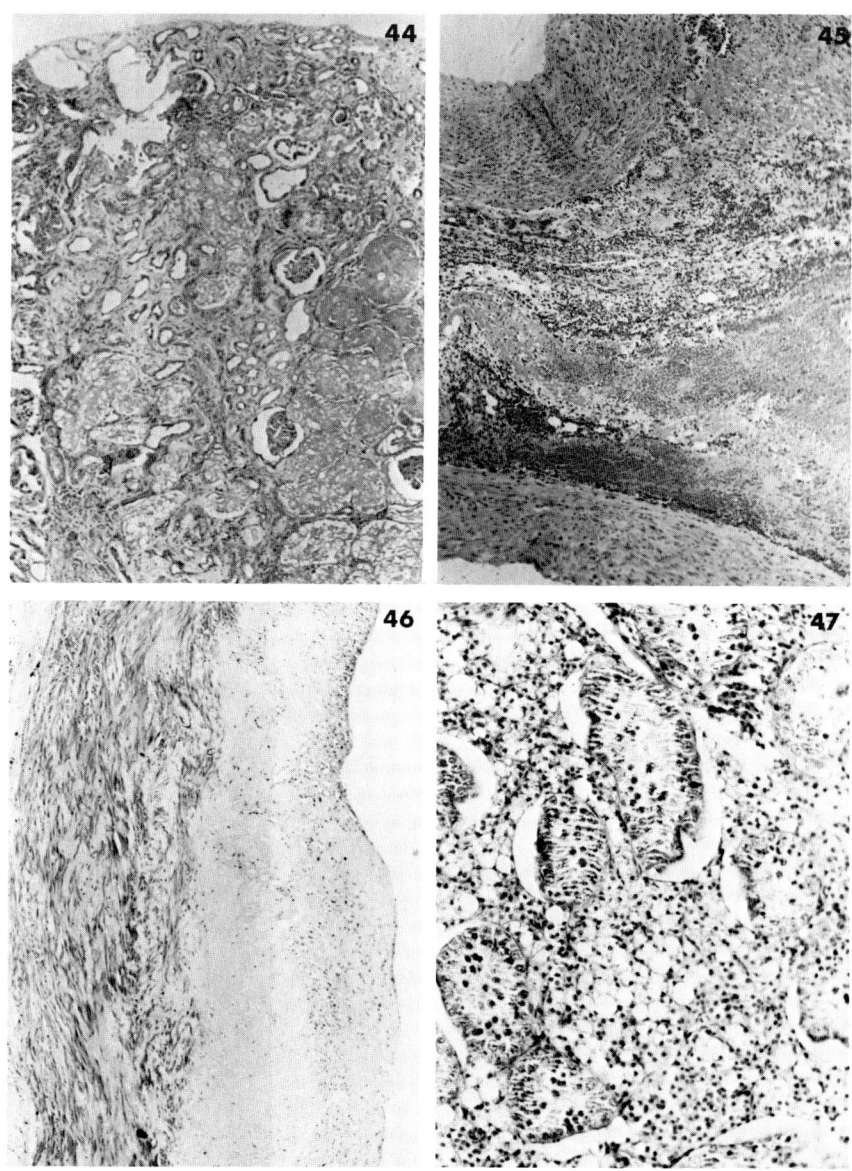

aneurysms were present, the proximal one having ruptured into the epicardium. There was typical medial necrosis with fresh hemorrhaging, as is seen in humans (Fig. 45). One must assume that this animal was hypertensive. An adult female wild-caught black lemur had a 10-cm-long thoracic aortic aneurysm with focal atheromatosis, calcification, and medial necrosis (Fig. 46) in addition to the cholangioma and hemosiderosis discussed earlier (Figs. 25 and 29). Both animals had left myocardial hypertrophy, presumably due to hpertension. A recently imported male sifaka died with enteritis and filariasis and had scattered foci of myocardial interstitial calcification, perhaps related to the parasitism. Surprising in this case was that in September when this fresh import died, there was meiotic testicular activity (Fig. 47). In lemurs that are adapted to the Northern Hemisphere, the testes are totally inactive in the summer and are easily mistaken as abnormal (Bogart et al., 1977a). The vacuolated interstitial tissues of the testis in this sifaka are distinctly abnormal and may betray the seasonal regression, although it is late. Jolly (1967) observed that the birthing season for these animals in Madagascar is July.

At the San Diego Zoo, reproductive success has been particularly good in $V. v. v.$, $V. v. r.$, and $L. c.$, as can be seen in Table I. It has been less accomplished in black lemurs, for which reason the pathologic findings in an adult female with no known history is important. She died in August 1979 with hemosiderosis, hemorrhagic enteritis, and widespread liver necrosis. The endometrium of both uterine horns was multicystic, focally fibrotic, and had numerous hemosiderin macrophages (Fig. 48). There were numerous peritubal adhesions and the tubal plicae were adherent to one another with salpingitis isthmica nodosa focally present. The ovaries had numerous Graafian follicles and two degenerating corpora lutea. Clearly, a chronic pelvic inflammatory process had led to the sterility of this animal. The most remarkable findings were made in a nearly 12-year-old slow loris. This animal had hemosiderosis, hepatic fibrosis, and pancreatic ductal and bile ductular proliferations. It died because of collapse of six distal thoracic and lumbar vertebrae. There was longstanding osteoclastic activity, fibrosis, necrosis, and some regeneration without evidence of infection. It was thought that the vertebral collapse was due to dissolution of intervertebral disks, but much more likely it relates to the end-stage chronic glomerulonephritis found and suspected hyperparathyroidism. The ovaries of this animal showed a most unusual calcification of nearly all ova and follicles (Fig. 49). There were no corpora albicantia and the uterus was infantile.

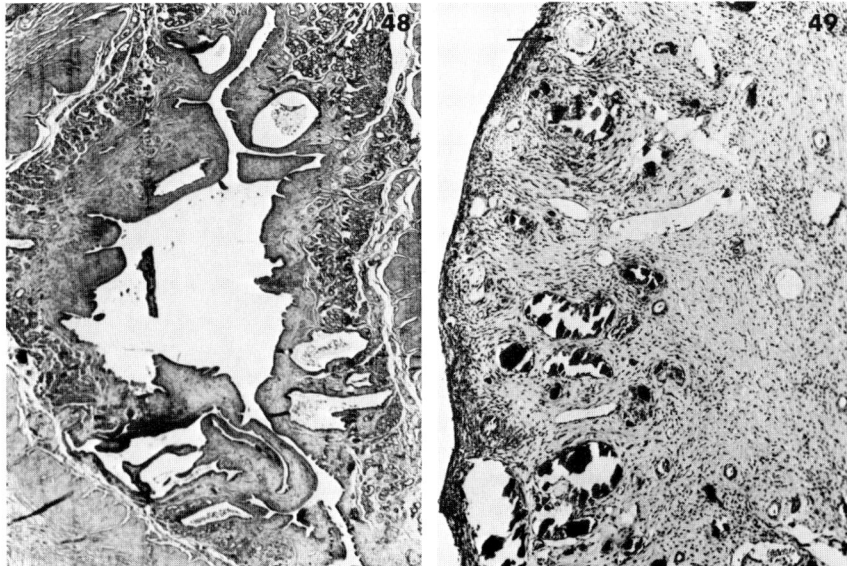

Fig. 48. Uterine horn of a *Lemur macaco* with extensive cystic changes of the endometrium (H & E, ×12). Autopsy No: 14583.

Fig. 49. Ovary of a 12-year-old *Nycticebus coucang* showing calcification of most follicles and ova. Only one normal follicle remains (arrow); there are no corpora albicantia (H & E, ×48). Autopsy No: 18790.

XI. Conclusions

The anatomic findings in our studies of prosimians provide interesting challenges for the pathologist. The reproductive tract exhibits pronounced seasonality and prenatal gonadal development differs from that of simians. In particular, the interstitial cells of the testis in normal fetuses are strongly stimulated only to atrophy upon birth, as does the fetal zone of the adrenal. Perinatal mortality is a major problem in captive colonies and is mainly the result of maternal neglect, perhaps due to their inexperience or insecurity. Congenital anomalies and spontaneous abortions are uncommon occurrences. A constellation of lethal anomalies, combined with growth retardation in black and white ruffed lemurs, may well have a genetic basis. It may be related to the autosomally determined pectus excavatum in the same species, which does not appear to have a deleterious impact on their survival.

Adult prosimians in captivity soon become free of parasites but are very susceptible to developing toxoplasmosis and diseases from the usual infectious organisms. Cryptococcosis and candidiasis were seen in animals with other lethal afflictions. Boredom apparently leads to fur chewing and the frequent development of trichobezoars with obstruction. It can be prevented by dosing with mineral oil. All proximians in our colony and those from other centers develop extensive hemosiderosis with ultimate hepatic fibrosis. Presumably on that basis hepatomas and cholangiomas form. Many of these animals also have extensive pancreatic islet hyperplasia. Chronic glomerulonephritis and aortic arteriosclerosis are common findings in older animals. This review of prosimian deaths gives firm directions for improved colony management.

Acknowledgments

Support for the pectus excavatum study came from NIH Grant RR 01261. Our gratitude is expressed to those colleagues from other centers who made their findings available to us.

References

Amman, R. W., Muller, E., Bansky, J., Schuler, G., and Hacki, W. H. (1980). *Scand. J. Gastroenterol.* **15**, 733–736.
Anonymous (1983). *Z. Köln. Zoo* **26**, 18.
Baker, C. A., Hendrickx, A. G., and Cooper, R. W. (1977). *J. Med. Primatol.* **6**, 13–22.
Beck, M., Beck, J., and Howard, E. B. (1982). *J. Wildlife Dis.* **18**, 365–367.
Benenson, M. W., Takafuji, E. T., Lemon, S. M., Greenup, R. L., and Sulzar, A. J. (1982). *N. Engl. J. Med.* **307**, 666–669.
Benirschke, K. (1980). *Int. Symp. Erkrank. Zootiere* **22**, 169–172.
Benirschke, K., and Miller, C. J. (1981). *J. Zoo Anim. Med.* **12**, 107–111.
Benirschke, K., Bloch, E., and Hertig, A. T. (1956). *Endocrinology* **58**, 598–625.
Benirschke, K., Adams, F. D., Black, K. L., and Gluck, L. (1980). *In* "The Comparative Pathology of Zoo Animals" (R. J. Montali and G. Migaki, eds.), pp. 471–489. Smithsonian Institution Press, Washington, D.C.
Benirschke, K., Kumamoto, A. T., and Bogart, M. H. (1981). *J. Med. Primatol.* **10**, 38–45.
Bogart, M. H., Cooper, R. W., and Benirschke, K. (1977a). *Int. Zoo Yearb.* **17**, 177–182.
Bogart, M. H., Kumamoto, A. T., and Lasley, B. L. (1977b). *Folia Primatol.* **28**, 134–143.
Boraski, E. A. (1981). *Vet. Pathol.* **18** (Suppl.), 1–5.
Brissot, P., Campion, J. P., Guillouzo, A., Allain, H., Messner, M., Simon, M., Ferrand, B., and Bourel, M. (1983). *Dig. Dis. Sci.* **28**, 616–624.
Brown, R. J., O'Neill, T. P., Kessler, M. J., and Andress, D. (1980). *Vet. Pathol.* **17**, 626–629.
Brygoo, E. R., Levaditi, Y., Destombes, P., and Guillon, J. C. (1964). *Bull. Soc. Pathol. Exot.* **57**, 228–235.
Buck, W. D., Osweiler, G. D., and Van Gelder, G. A. (1976). *In* "Clinical Diagnostic Veterinary Toxicology" (G. A. Van Gelder, ed.), 2nd Ed., pp. 315–317. Kendall/Hunt, Dubuque, Iowa.
Buss, D. H., Cooper, R. W., and Wallen, K. (1976). *Folia Primatol.* **26**, 301–305.

Butler, H. (1969). *Recent Adv. Primatol.* **II,** 15–21.
Cattan, D. (1983). *Lancet* **2,** 106.
Chang, J., Wagner, J. L., and Kornegay, R. W. (1979). *Lab. Anim. Sci.* **29,** 374–376.
Chang, J., Wagner, J. L., Mikat, E. M., and Hackel, D. B. (1980). *In* "The Comparative Pathology of Zoo Animals" (R. J. Montali and G. Migaki, eds.), pp. 347–352. Smithsonian Institution Press, Washington, D.C.
Coulanges, P., Zeller, H., Clark, Y., Rodhain, F., and Albignac, R. (1979). *Bull. Soc. Pathol. Exot.* **72,** 272–278, 1979.
Dickson, J., Fry, J., Fairfax, R., and Spence, T. (1983). *Vet. Rec.* **112,** 302.
Fan, L., and Murphy, S. (1981). *Am. J. Dis. Child.* **135,** 550–552.
Frye, F. L. (1982). *J. Zoo Anim. Med.* **13,** 152–156.
Fujita, T., Yanatori, Y., and Murakami, T. (1976). *In* "Endocrine Gut and Pancreas" (T. Fujita, ed.), pp. 347–356. Elsevier, Amsterdam.
Gabbe, S. G., Cohen, A. W., Herman, G. O., and Schwartz, S. (1982). *Am. J. Obstet. Gynecol.* **143,** 514–517.
Gonzales, J., Benirschke, K., Saltman, P., Roberts, J., and Robinson, P. T. (1984). *Zoo Biol.* **3,** 255–265.
Goodwin, L. G. (1980). *J. Zool.* **190,** 555.
Godwin, L. G. (1982). *J. Zool.* **197,** 17.
Gould, V. E., Memoli, V. A., Dardi, L. E., and Gould, N. S. (1983). *Pediatr. Pathol.* **1,** 7–31.
Griner, L. A. (1983). "Pathology of Zoo Animals." Zool. Soc. of San Diego, San Diego, California.
Heinonen, O. P., Slone, D., and Shapiro, S., eds. (1977). *In* "Birth Defects and Drugs in Pregnancy," pp. 256–259. Publishing Sciences Group, Littleton, MA.
Hendrickx, A. G., Stone, G. W., Henrickson, R. V., and Matayoshi, K. (1979). *Teratology* **19,** 177–182.
Hill, C. A. (1973). *Mammalia* **37,** 101–104.
Himes, E. M., Wendt, W. A., Lucksinger, D. W., and Jarnagin, J. L. (1982). *J. Am. Vet. Med. Assoc.* **181,** 1355–1357.
Jackson, C. E., Weiss, L., and Watson, J. H. L. (1974). *Pediatrics* **54,** 201–207.
Janssen, D. L., Robinson, P. T., and Meier, J. E. (1979). *Proc. Am. Assoc. Zoo Vets.,* 87–88.
Jolly, A. (1967). *In* "Social Communication Among Primates" (S. A. Altman, ed.), p. 11. Univ. of Chicago Press, Chicago.
Keller, G. L., Kramer, L., Butler, W. B., and Knapke, F. B. (1979). *J. Zool Anim. Med.* **13,** 148–151.
Koop, C. E. (1956). *Surg. Clin. N. Am.* **36,** 1627–1637.
McClure, H. M., and Chandler, F. W. (1982). *Vet. Pathol.* **19** (Suppl. 7), 193–209.
Mason, G. A. (1981). *J. Med. Primatol.* **10,** 287–289.
Moser, H. G., and Benirschke, K. (1962). *Anat. Rec.* **143,** 47–59.
Ochoa, R., Kolaja, G. J., and Klei, T. R. (1983). *Vet. Pathol.* **20,** 641–643.
Orzalesi, M. M., and Cook, C. D. (1965). *J. Pediatr.* **66,** 898–900.
Palotay, J. L. (1978). *Oregon Primate Res. Center Newslett.* **9,** 41.
Pasztor, L. M., and van Horn, R. N. (1976). *J. Hum. Evol.* **5,** 333–337.
Pearson, J. L. (1973). *Vet. Med. Small Anim. Clin.* **68,** 125–128.
Petter-Rousseaux, A. (1964). *In* "Evolutionary and Genetic Biology of Primates" (J. Buettner-Janusch, ed.), Vol. II, p. 91. Academic Press, New York.
Petter-Rousseaux, A., and Boulière, F. (1965). *Folia Primatol.* **3,** 241–244.
Poley, D. (1969). *Dtsch. Tierärztl. Wochenschr.* **76,** 695–697.

Polgar, G., and Koop, C. E. (1963). *Pediatrics* **32,** 209–215.
Price, R. A., Anver, M. R., and Hunt, R. D. (1973). *Vet. Pathol.* **10,** 37–44.
Randell, M. G., Patnaik, A. K., and Gould, W. J. (1981). *J. Am. Vet. Med. Assoc.* **179,** 1214–1217.
Ratomponirina, C., Andrianiva, J., and Rumpler, Y. (1982). *J. Reprod. Fertil.* **66,** 707–721.
Ravitch, M. M., and Matzen, R. N. (1968). *Dis. Chest* **54,** 58–62.
Rehg, J. E., Burek, J. D., Strandberg, J. D., and Montali, R. J. (1980). *In* "The Comparative Pathology of Zoo Animals" (R. J. Montali and G. Migaki, eds.), pp. 113–120. Smithsonian Institution Press, Washington, D.C.
Reichard, T. A., Ensley, P. K., and Henrick, M. J. (1981). *Proc. Am. Assoc. Zoo Vets.,* 44–45.
Ruch, T. C. (1959). "Diseases of Laboratory Primates." Saunders, Philadelphia.
Sawin, P. B. (1955). *Adv. Genet.* **7,** 183–226.
Schneider, H. E., Blaschke-Hellmessen, R., Klemm, G. M., Thess, G., and Pohle, V. (1983). *Int. Symp. Erkrauk. Zootiere* **25,** 299–308.
Seal, U. S., and Makey, D. G. (1976). *Int. Zoo Yearb.* **16,** 180–184.
Sedgwick, C. J. (1981). *J. Zoo Anim. Med.* **12,** 124–127.
Seger, R. A., Hollis, D. G., Weaver, R. E., and Hitzig, W. H. (1982). *J. Clin. Microbiol.* **16,** 821–825.
Shideler, S. E., and Lindburg, D. G. (1982). *Zoo Biol.* **1,** 127–134.
Shideler, S. E., Czekala, N. M., Benirschke, K., and Lasley, B. L. (1983). *Biol. Reprod.* **28,** 963–969.
Snyder, L. H., and Curtis, M. (1934). *J. Hered.* **25,** 445–447.
Stoddard, S. E. (1939). *J. Hered.* **30,** 139–141.
Swanson, H. H. (1980). *Lab. Anim.* **14,** 143–147.
Tomson, F. N., and Lotshaw, R. R. (1978). *J. Am. Vet. Med. Assoc.* **173,** 1103–1106.
Ungar, H., and Adler, J. H. (1978). *Am. J. Pathol.* **90,** 399–410.
Wadsworth, P. F., Gobinath, C., and Jones, D. M. (1980). *Vet. Pathol.* **17,** 386–388.
Witzleben, D. L., and Chaffey, N. J. (1966). *Arch. Pathol.* **82,** 454–461.

Methods for Evaluating Reproductive Function in Exotic Species

BILL L. LASLEY

Research Department, San Diego Zoo, San Diego, California

I. Introduction 209
II. The Estrogen/Testosterone Ratio 212
III. Evaluation of Estrogenic Components 214
IV. Bioactive Luteinizing Hormone Measurements 220
V. Direct Assays for Steroid Conjugates 222
VI. Pregnanediol-3-Glucuronide 223
VII. Estrone Conjugates 226
References 228

I. Introduction

Most of the information that is available relating to comparative mammalian reproductive physiology is derived from a relatively small number of species. The number of well-characterized species probably represents less than 1% of the total number of mammalian species and includes the common domesticated and laboratory animals. If the definition and characterization of the female reproductive cycle includes the complete hormone profile which reflects ovarian cyclicity, the total number of well-characterized species is probably less than 20. Since each species that is well characterized in terms of hormone profile exhibits a species-specific or unique pattern of hormonal events, it seems clear that many more species need to be defined for there to be a good representation of the spectrum of differences that naturally occur.

Two serious limitations have prevented investigators from making progress in this area. First, the lack of access to many animals outside of zoos or wild animal sanctuaries prevents the development of well-defined research protocols that can be acted upon. In some cases opportunistic access to certain individuals will provide enough information to accumulate data for a cross-sectional analysis of reproductive function. These kinds of data seldom provide sequential hormone profiles which demonstrate the animal-to-animal differences. The second limitation is the result of a tradition that has developed concerning sample collection. Many investigators believe that measurements of circulating hormones provide the best evaluation of endocrine function since, by definition, a hormone is a chemical messenger that exerts its effects as a result of the circulatory system. The desire to measure the active hormone at functional concentrations, along with the development of radioimmunoassays which are practical in this regard, has led to the general practice and wide acceptance of using circulating levels of hormones to define reproductive events. Since sequential blood samples are seldom available from nontractable species, there has been little opportunity to characterize the circulating hormone profiles in exotic or nondomesticated species for comparison to profiles of the well-characterized domestic or laboratory species.

The measurement of hormone metabolites in the urine, which was widely accepted prior to the development of evaluative methods for measuring circulating hormones, is becoming popular again. Although this approach will never completely replace the direct measurement of circulating hormones, urine monitoring has several advantages when compared to serum measurements. Practicability for longitudinal sampling and economy in terms of the cost of actually processing the samples are the most important attributes of urinary monitoring. The ease of collecting daily urine samples compared to collecting blood samples on a daily basis makes urine collection more attractive in tractable species and a necessary choice for nontractable, pugnacious species. The higher concentration of hormone metabolites in urine, compared to the levels of active hormone in circulation, is the basis for the development of simple, direct, and economical urine assays. Finally, urine evaluations provide integrated measurements of the hormone production over an extended period of time. In some cases this integration of minute-to-minute changes in hormone excretion may dampen the influence of rapid dynamics in hormone production. In general, this is not a disadvantage but instead provides a clearer indication of glandular function since the episodic nature of hormone secretion does not influence individual measurements.

Caution must be exercised when urinary measurements are used in place of circulating hormone concentrations. Since total excretion or

24-hr urine collections are usually so impractical that this strategy is seldom useful, smaller, short-time collections of individual voidings are, therefore, the necessary limitation, and concentrations of hormones in less than the total volume of urine is not necessarily informative. In serum homeostatic mechanisms keep component substances within a relatively narrow range of variation, but in urine concentrations of solutes largely reflect the clearance of water and inorganic salts through the kidney. Measurements of urinary concentrations of hormone metabolites are therefore relative to water balance dynamics and only indirectly reflect changes in hormone production. Adjustments of urinary hormone metabolite concentrations are usually required in order to normalize the concentration of hormone metabolites so that they are less dependent on general urine concentration and more reflective of hormone production rate changes. Two approaches can be used, and examples of both are presented in this review. The first combines independent measures of diametrically opposed hormonal components to generate a dimensionless ratio independent of concentration. This approach has been used for estrogen and testosterone measurements to generate an estrogen/testosterone ratio in determining the functional sex of exotic birds. The second and more common approach uses creatinine measurements of the urine to index the hormone concentration of the sample. This latter method assumes that creatinine clearance is constant for the individual, and this assumption should be verified for all species but, unfortunately, this is seldom the case (Fig. 1).

The objective of this report is to bring together recent reports of progress in one area of comparative reproductive endocrinology with an emphasis on exotic species. The information contained in this report, for the sake of convenience, is taken from a single laboratory and has been generated over the last 6 years. There is no implication that the data contained here totally represent the field. Rather, the data presented represent applications of the same or similar techniques in order to demonstrate the versatility of the approach and the advantage of similar strategies for making species-to-species comparisons. The techniques presented are exclusively evaluations of hormone metabolites in the excreta since this approach lends itself to the study of exotic species. In general, the chronological progression of this review represents the development of different aspects of the methodologic approach. This progression suggests that most, if not all, mammalian species can now be characterized in terms of reproductive endocrinology with techniques which are both practical and revealing.

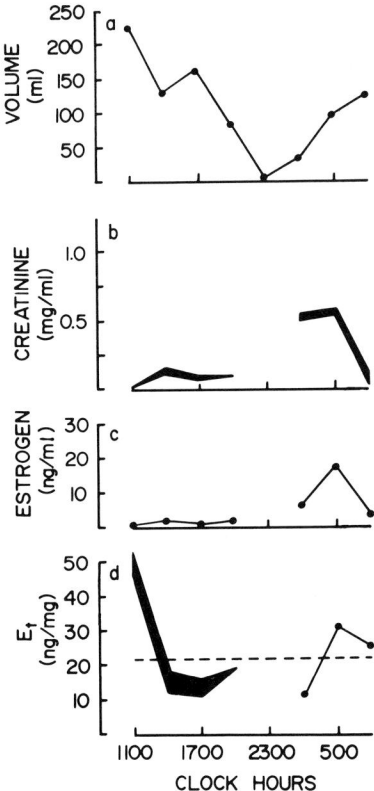

FIG. 1. The diurnal shift in urine production of a nonhuman primate (a) and the resulting effects on creatinine concentration (b) as well as estrogen concentration (c) are presented. Part (d) shows the results of dividing the estrogen concentration by the creatinine concentration at each data point. The dashed line on the bottom panel denotes the value obtained when the total urine for 24 hr was mixed together and an aliquot was taken to obtain a single measurement of estrogen indexed by creatinine. These data demonstrate that when urine volume is high (late morning) creatinine and estrogen measurement are near the limit of sensitivity, resulting in exaggerated levels of estrogen per milligram of creatinine. At night, urine production decreases and few measurements can be made. In the early morning hours, when creatinine and estrogen levels are highest, the estrogen level indexed by creatinine at each time interval closely approximates the value obtained by evaluating the combined 24-hr pool.

II. The Estrogen/Testosterone Ratio

The two major problems associated with measurements of excreted hormone metabolites are differential metabolism of the active hormones and changes in excretion rate. Even when changes in hormone excretion reflect the known physiologic event, it is difficult to be sure that the excretion profile is an accurate reflection of hormone production. Simultaneous measurements of circulating active hormones and excreted metabolites, together with clearance studies of the radiolabeled precursor, are generally required to validate the excretion profile. In nontractable animal species, such validations are often difficult and the monitoring strategy itself must be such that metabolism and excretion rates are not major contributors to the final result. The combined measurements of metabolites of diametrically opposed precursor hormones for the evaluation of gonadal function is a strategy that has been used to evaluate the functional sex of "monomorphic" avian species which avoids excretion rate in the final result (Bercovitz et al., 1978).

A surprisingly high percentage of bird species are not sexually dimorphic with respect to size, coloration, or other visible clues. These monomorphic species present a problem to the bird breeder because when pairing is necessary for breeding, pairs are often chosen by guess, with the results of the guess revealed by the breeding success or failure. Direct observation of the gonad is an efficient method for resolving the question of sex, and laparoscopic techniques are used in most cases. Since laparoscopy requires capture and restraint as well as some amount of trauma, a less stressful approach is preferable for the extremely delicate or rare species. This need is effectively met by fecal steroid evaluations. Fecal samples can be collected from the floor of an enclosure without imposing any stress on the bird or any change in management procedure. Such samples can be collected opportunistically and as often as needed. Storage in a normal freezer compartment without preservatives allows for the retrospective evaluation of samples collected from distant sites and sent in a frozen state to the laboratory for evaluation.

The assay procedure is simple, requiring enzyme hydrolysis, extraction, and simultaneous assay of estrogen and testosterone metabolites. The results of each assay are first expressed as concentrations of the original sample and then combined to generate a ratio of estrogen and testosterone which has no units or dimension. Since the original fecal sample has no direct relation to gonadal function, its size is independent of questions relating to hormone content. However, concentrations of steroid measured are directly related to the original sample size and in this case can influence the final result. The process of dividing the estrogen metabolite concentration by the testosterone metabolite concentration removes concentration from the quotient and therefore removes the influence of sample size from the result. At the same time, the ratio generated magnifies smaller quantitative differences that resulted from separate, independent comparisons of estrogen and testosterone (Fig. 2 and Table I).

The example shown here was for birds, not mammals, and in this way deviates from the specific topic of this review, which is comparative mammalian reproductive physiology. The concept, however, is independent of this example and could have similar applications in exotic mammalian species. Certainly, circulating estrogen/progesterone ratios have been used to assess ovarian and placental function in primates. In a similar way, estrogen and progesterone metabolite ratios could be used for similar evaluations of urine or feces to monitor the stage of the ovarian cycle in carnivores, where much of the steroid clearance is through the gut rather than the kidney.

III. Evaluation of Estrogenic Components

The measurement of total immunoreactive estrogens, as described above for fecal sex steroid evaluations, requires the ability to simultaneously measure all contributing estrogen components. This can be achieved by using an antiserum that exhibits cross-reactivity to all

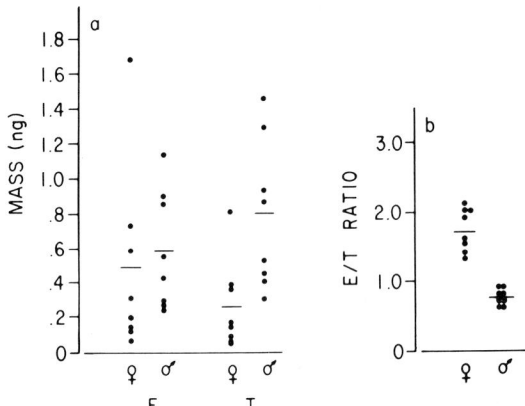

FIG. 2. Comparison of measurements of immunoreactive estrogen (E) and testosterone (T) in the droppings of male and female cockatiels. Part (a) shows the mass in nanograms of each steroid in the total dropping and demonstrates that the range of values for estrogen and testosterone overlap between the sexes. Part (b) displays the same data after dividing the estrogen value by the testosterone value for each dropping. The resulting E/T ratio ranges of values do not overlap when the sexes are compared, and female ratios are approximately twice that of male ratios.

TABLE I

Estrogen/Testosterone (E/T) Ratios for a Wide Range of Species in which Sex Was Determined at the Time of Autopsy[a]

Species	Sex	E/T ratio
Sparrow Hawk (*Falco sparverius phalaena*)	F	3.0
Bob White Quail (*Colinus virgianus texanus*)	M	0.5
	F	3.2
Bare-throated Francolin (*Pternistes leucosecpus infuscatus*)	F	9.8
Pigeon (*Columba livia domestica*)	F	9.0
	F	6.7
	M	1.0
Blue-naped Mouse Bird (*Colius macrourus pulcher*)	F	3.7
Razor-billed Curasow (*Mitu mitu*)	M	0.8
White-headed Piping Guan (*Aburria pipile cumanensis*)	M	0.3
E. African Crowned Crane (*Balaerica pavonina gibbericeps*)	F	2.5
Red-winged Tinamou (*Rhynchotus rufescens*)	M	0.8
Crested Seriema (*Cariama cristata*)	M	1.1
Burmeister's Seriema (*Chunga burmeisteri*)	F	3.9
Van Oort's Cassowary (*Casuarius casuarius*)	F	4.1
	F	2.8
	M	0.3
Blue Grey Tanager (*Thraupis v. virens*)	M	1.4
Maleo (*Macrocephalon maleo*)	F	3.9
	M	0.2
Maguari Stork (*Euxenura galeata*)	M	0.6

[a] For females, with $n = 11$, mean $\pm$ SE $= 4.8 \pm 0.8$; for males, with $n = 10$, mean $\pm$ SE $= 0.7 \pm 0.1$; the level of statistical significance $p < 0.001$.

steroidal estrogens but which is specific for estrogens compared to C-19 androgens and C-21 progestins and corticoids. The Abraham S-310 #5 antiserum is extremely useful for this purpose, as demonstrated by Hodges et al. (1979). Using a single radioimmunoassay, the algebraic sum of estrone, estradiol, and estriol in a wide range of species can be quantified accurately independent of the ratio of the contributing components. This methodologic approach not only simplifies the laboratory procedures involved in monitoring quantitative changes in estrogen production but also provides the basis for characterizing the qualitative differences in estrogen components contained in a given sample, as described below.

The utility of a simple method to evaluate the total immunoreactive estrogen level is that it provides a reliable and informative method for appraising changes in total estrogen production. This method has been applied to a number of exotic species and has been found to reflect general estrogen excretion (Hodges et al., 1979; Czekala et al., 1981). It does not, however, reflect the differences in estrogenic components between samples and, more importantly, between species. Since individual estrogen components may provide more specific information than all components measured together, a separation system was developed and combined with the total estrogen assay to provide the ability to evaluate all estrogenic components as separate entities. Since the polarities of estrogens from estrone to estriol are extremely wide in comparison to most families of molecules, high-performance liquid chromatography (HPLC) provides the only practical system which allows all steroidal estrogens to be separated by a continuous elution of a single solvent system.

A cochromatogram of radiolabeled steroidal estrogens together with the concomitant measurement of the immunoreactive components provides an immediate evaluation of the relative contribution of steroidal estrogen components in any biological sample (Fig. 3). This approach has been extremely useful in comparing the nature of estrogen metabolism and excretion in a wide range of primate species as well as in providing an early impression of major estrogen metabolites in other exotic species which were not previously defined. An example of the utility of this technique is the comparison of the human and gorilla pregnancies reported by Czekala et al. (1983). A lower total estrogen profile in hydrolyzed urine samples in the gorilla compared to the human pregnancy was puzzling at first and indicated that either estrogen production rates or estrogen excretion patterns were different in the two species. To examine these possibilities, the separated urinary estrogen components were compared at various times of gestation as just described. The results of these evaluations indicated that the major difference between human and gorilla estrogen excretion was in estriol excretion in the second and third trimester. Since estriol excretion is largely a result of fetal adrenal weak androgen production, a difference at this level was investigated by comparing fetal adrenal weights and percentage fetal zone in both the human and gorilla. Consistent with the urinary estrogen profiles, the gorilla fetal adrenal was found to be smaller than that of the human in both absolute and relative weight relationships. More to the point, the relative width of the fetal zone of the gorilla and chimpanzee fetal adrenal had the same relationship to the fetal zones of the human and orangutan, as did the estrogen excretion during pregnancy of the two pairs of hominoids.

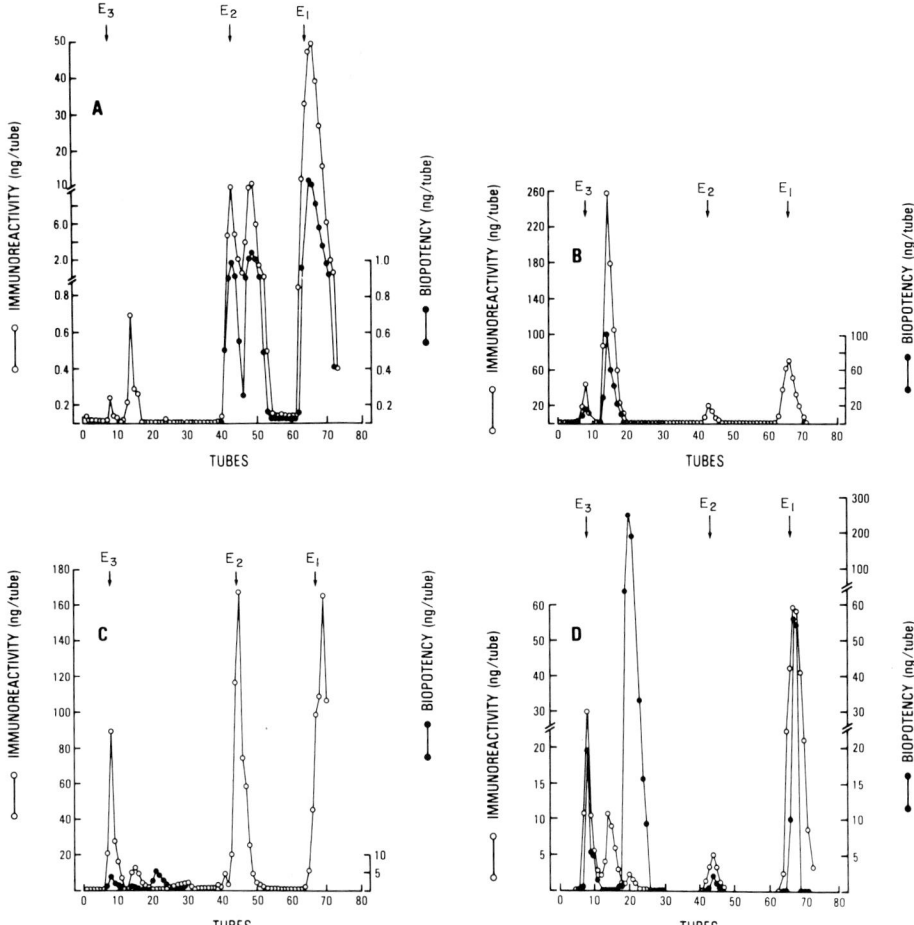

FIG. 3. The separation of estrogen components using high-performance liquid chromatography with immuno (○) and receptor activity used (●) as end points. The panels show the components found in pregnancy urine of (A) lemur (*L. varecia*), (B) capuchin (*C. albifrons*), (C) spider monkey (*A. fuciceps*), and (D) macaque (*M. silenus*). The election of the tracer estriol (E_3), estradiol (E_2), and estrone (E_1) is shown by the arrows and corresponds to major immuno- and receptor-binding activities. The peak following estradiol-17β in panel (A) was shown to be estradiol-17α by mass spectrometry. Similarly, the large receptor peak in panel (D) was shown to be equol, a phytoestrogen.

These data suggest that the orangutan pregnancy may be more similar to the human pregnancy in terms of fetal steroid production than either the chimpanzee or the gorilla pregnancy.

A more practical use of evaluating total urinary estrogen components is identifying specific estrogen compounds which will best reveal specific physiologic events. Kassam and Lasley (1981) demonstrated that the Indian rhinoceros excreted larger amounts of estrogen prior to ovulation than most other mammalian species. By differential hydrolysis and subsequent high-performance liquid chromatography, it was further demonstrated that the major estrogen component in Indian rhinoceros urine was estrone sulfate. Using this information the same workers have subsequently shown that a direct radioimmunoassay for urinary estrone conjugates can be used as a rapid and economical method to monitor ovulation and pregnancy in the rhinoceros and related species, i.e., the horse and tapir. The same logic and a similar procedure has been applied to primate species, resulting in a very versatile direct assay for estrone conjugates in the urine of several primate species. This aspect will be addressed later in this article.

Beyond the rapid identification of known estrogenic components in a given sample, the chromatographic procedure described above offers an approach for investigating the possibility of the presence of molecules which are not classical steroidal estrogens but which contribute estrogenic potential. Erb et al. (1982) combined, as an endpoint, the evaluation of estrogen receptor binding to the previous method of simply evaluating immunoreactive components. This process provides clear resolution of all expected estrogenic components with three independent evaluations. First, the retention time (Rf) with respect to known radiolabeled tracers provides an internal marker in terms of elution time from the column. Second, the immunoreactivity of anticipated peaks provides a quantitative evaluation of mass observed with respect to the amount of radiolabeled tracer added. Third, the receptor binding profile not only confirms the purity of the anticipated estrogenic peaks but confirms or denies the presence of other substances that may be putative estrogens on the basis of binding to the estrogen receptor (Table II).

In at least three instances the comprehensive evaluation of estrogen components has led to new information that has potential physiologic significance. In exotic carnivores urinary immunoreactive estrogen profiles provide little information in terms of female reproductive physiology. In contrast, urinary components which are detected by the receptor but not by the immunoassay accurately reflect ovarian stimulation by gonadotropin therapy (Ensley et al., 1982). Additionally, a previously unidentified estrogen-like component in the urine of pregnant macaques was isolated, characterized, and later identified to be the phyto-estrogen equol by this method (Monfort et al., 1984). Since this compound is well described as a cause of infertility in sheep, its

TABLE II

THE STEROIDAL ESTROGENS THAT HAVE BEEN CHARACTERIZED BY HIGH-PERFORMANCE LIQUID CHROMATOGRAPHY RETENTION (Rf), IMMUNOREACTIVITY (IMMUN), AND ESTROGEN RECEPTOR ACTIVITY (RECEPT)[a,b]

Estrogen	Chemical name	Immun	Recept	R/I	Rf
Estrone	3-Hydroxy-1,3,5(10)-estratrien-17-one	0.9	0.4	0.44	8.0
Estradiol-17β	1,3,5(10)-Estratriene-3,17β-diol	1.4	1.0	0.70	5.4
Estradiol-17α	1,3,5(10)-Estratriene-3,17α-diol	0.30	0.10	0.33	6.7
Estriol	1,3,5(10)-Estratriene-3,16α,17β-triol	1.0	0.2	0.20	1.0
2-Methoxyestriol	1,3,5(10)-Estratriene-2,3,17β-triol 2-methylether	0.00016			1.3
2-Hydroxyestriol	1,3,5(10)-Estratriene-2,3,17β-triol	0.0008	0.0167	20.8	4.6
2-Methoxyestrone	2,3-Dihydroxy-1,3,5(10)-estratrien-17-one 2-methylether	0.00009	0.0005	5.23	
2-Hydroxyestrone	2,3-Dihydroxy-1,3,5(10)-estratrien-17-one	0.005	0.02	4.00	1.75
15α-Hydroxyestrone	3,15α-Dihydroxy-1,3,5(10)-estratrien-17-one	0.0035	0.002	1.75	1.53
16-Ketoestradiol	3,17β-Dihydroxy-1,3,5(10)-estratrien-16-one	0.83	0.02	0.024	1.2
16α-Hydroxyestrone	3,16α-Dihydroxy-1,3,5(10)-estratrien-17-one	0.64	0.013	0.02	2.13
16,17-Epiestriol	1,3,5(10)-Estratriene-3,16β,17α-triol	0.27	0.167	0.62	2.7
16-Epiestriol	1,3,5(10)-Estratriene-3,16β,17α-triol	1.2	3.33	2.78	3.33
17-Epiestriol	1,3,5(10)-Estratriene-3,16α,17α-triol	0.6			3.7
d-Equilenin	d-3-Hydroxy-1,3,5(10),6,8-estrapentaen-17-one	0.06			6.0
Equilin	3-Hydroxy-1,3,5(10),7-estratetraen-17-one	0.28			6.0

[a] From Erb et al. (1982).
[b] The relative receptor activity was divided by the immunoreactivity to derive the R/I ratio. Each steroidal estrogen can be identified by its retention time and R/I ratio, and all estrogen components in a single sample can be partially identified and characterized simultaneously.

presence at high levels in captive macaques warrants further investigation of its dietary source and potential physiologic impact (Fig. 3). Other putative estrogenic compounds which have been revealed by this method include a compound found in testicular profusates of young dogs which later develop benign prostatic hyperplasia (Ewing *et al.*, 1984). Not detectable in testicular profusates from normal dogs or older dogs with the disease, this putative estrogen appears at the time that prostatic programming or induction for hyperplasia is taking place. The possibility that this substance is related to the induction of hyperplasia is currently being investigated.

IV. Bioactive Luteinizing Hormone Measurements

There are several situations where measurements of pituitary and/or chorionic gonadotropin are important in general comparative reproductive physiology. However, unlike steroid hormones that retain their basic structure through phylogeny, the protein and glycoprotein hormones demonstrate species-specific structural differences. As a consequence of this, immunoassays which are extremely useful for steroid hormones in divergent species are not always useful for measuring gonadotropin levels except in closely related species and, even then, require the development of heterologous immunoassay systems.

In vitro bioassays which are reliable and economical have been developed and can be used to quantify small amounts of luteinizing hormone. Since the active portion of luteinizing hormone is highly conserved throughout mammalian physiology, species differences in the primary structure of the complete molecule are a minor consideration when bioactivity is assessed. Using either dispersed rat Leydig cells or minced mouse testes, pituitary extracts from a wide range of species accelerate testosterone production, which is parallel to the dose–response production of testosterone by WHO human pituitary luteinizing hormone. This approach, therefore, allows for the quantitative appraisal of luteinizing hormone bioactivity in samples from the total range of mammalian species (Fig. 4).

Some confusion may be generated by the application of a bioassay since most investigations are comfortable with immunoassay results and immunoreactivity is considered to reflect the active hormone. Studies comparing immuno- versus bioassay results show that, although the two assay systems detect different populations of luteinizing hormone components, the qualitative aspects of the hormonal pro-

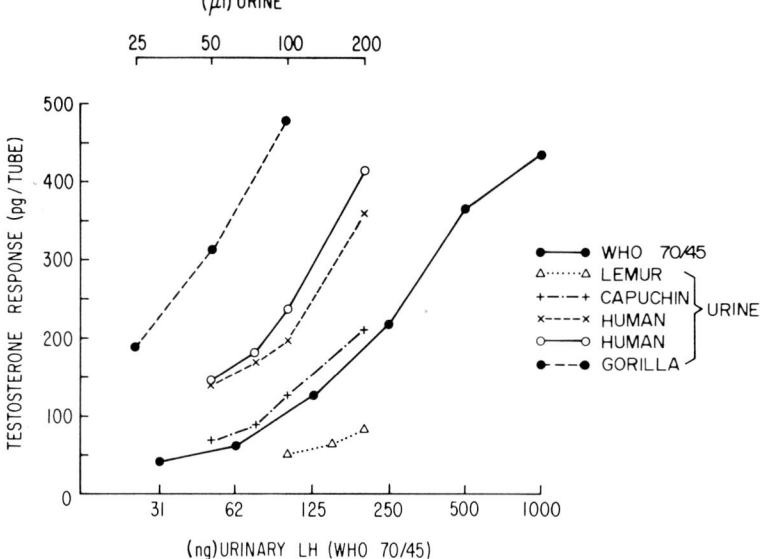

FIG. 4. The dose–response dynamics of serially diluted urine from a wide range of species is compared to the WHO 70/45 standard of human gonadotropin. Urine samples from a wide range of primate species were selected as those representing the preovulatory luteinizing hormone surge by evaluating complete ovarian cycles. These data support the concept that a single assay can be employed to monitor changes of luteinizing hormone production by the direct measurement of luteinizing hormone bioactivity using a dispersed Leydig cell preparation. Testosterone production was evaluated after a 3-hr incubation of dispersed rat Leydig cell wells of each serial dilution of urine or standard.

files generated are comparable (Sawyer-Steffan et al., 1982). The advantage of a single strategy for evaluating luteinizing hormone in all mammalian species far overshadows the minor differences in quantification because relative differences are considered more important. Furthermore, it might be argued that bioactivity rather than immunoreactivity should be the measurement of choice since it has a greater likelihood of revealing the secretion rather than the degradation of the protein moiety.

The application of these bioassays for measuring pituitary luteinizing concentrations in serum is well documented in the literature and is beyond the scope of this review. Instead, the focus here is on the specific application of the bioassay for luteinizing hormone in urine to complement the steroid assays for monitoring reproductive events in exotic species. As a complement to urinary estrogen measurements, Hodges et al. (1979) demonstrated that luteinizing hormone bioactivity measured in small samples of unprocessed urine and indexed by creatinine accurately reflected circulating luteinizing hormone levels in most primate species. Since chorionic gonadotropin is largely composed of luteinizing hormone in biological activity, this approach provides a single simple strategy for measuring both the preovulatory pituitary release of luteinizing hormone as well as the production and excretion of trophoblastic gonadotropin at the time of implanatation.

The combination of urinary estrogen and luteinizing hormone measurements has enabled the characterization of the ovarian cycle and pregnancy of about 15 different primate species. This approach has not only extended our knowledge of primate reproductive physiology, it provides comparable data, using the same technique, for species across the entire order. Furthermore, the ability to use urine samples instead of blood has allowed many more species to be evaluated, including the very small or fragile species which are difficult to bleed on a daily basis. The direct evaluation of ovulation and implantation has been useful in narrowing the lengths of gestations reported for a number of poorly defined primate species since previous numbers were based largely on the last observed mating. Ultimately, the accumulation of these kinds of hormone profiles will be helpful to colony managers by enabling quick and efficient evaluation of both reproductive status and perhaps reproductive potential of the brood stock.

V. Direct Assays for Steroid Conjugates

The measurements of free or unconjugated steroids in urine have two major weaknesses in terms of efficiency as a laboratory strategy. The first weakness is the time element. Since most steroids in urine are present as a conjugate, these conjugates must be hydrolyzed to free the steroid moieties so that they can be extracted and measured by immunoassays. These processes require a minimum of 12 to 24 hr and remove any possibility of the development of a rapid evaluation test with this approach. The second weakness concerns the efficiency of the hydrolysis procedure. Many reports have suggested and even indicated that neither acid nor enzyme hydrolysis of urinary steroids is efficient or reliable; nonetheless, the process is widely accepted and the results are informative.

The development of antisera directed to steroid conjugates made the direct measurements of urinary steroids possible without first hydrolyzing and extracting the sample. These direct assays not only save time, they obviate the worry of inefficient or differential hydrolysis.

Unprocessed urine diluted by assay buffer can be added directly to the assay tube to give results within a few hours. Resulting hormone profiles from direct conjugate assays show that conjugate concentrations are, in general, much higher than would have been predicted by the measurement of free steroids after hydrolysis. This supports the contention that hydrolytic procedures in urine are less than efficient and are prone to underestimations and uncontrolled variations. More importantly, the direct evaluations of steroid conjugates produce hormone profiles which have greater resolution than profiles generated by methods requiring hydrolysis. Some urinary hormone profiles using direct assays are comparable and perhaps more informative than serum profiles. This result was not expected and may not be readily accepted, since it indicates that some urinary evaluations will become measurements of choice rather than alternatives to circulating hormone determinations.

As the following sections demonstrate, the evaluation of urinary steroid conjugates provides a simple and broadly applicable strategy for monitoring ovarian and trophoblastic events in a wide range of species. The simplicity of a direct radioimmunoassay for substances that exist in relatively high concentration in urine enhances the possibility for the development of other, more adaptable tests which could be used outside of the endocrine laboratory. For example, enzyme assays have already been developed for free steroids, and this technique lends itself well to the measurement of steroid conjugates. Direct enzyme-linked assays for steroid conjugates should be available in the very near future, providing portable and objective evaluations of urine from most exotic species.

VI. Pregnanediol-3-Glucuronide

Approximately 30% of the circulating progesterone is cleared into the urine as pregnanediol-3-glucuronide in the human female. The evaluation of pregnanediol-3-glucuronide has been well established as a simple urinary test for luteal function in women. Similarly, the same test can be used to monitor luteal function in the gorilla and orangutan since, like the human, this steroid conjugate accurately reflects circulating progesterone levels (Mitchell *et al.*, 1982). When total estrogen excretion, as described earlier, is monitored in conjunction with pregnanediol-3-glucuronide levels in daily urine samples, a complete hormonal profile of the hominoid ovarian cycle can be obtained. This approach has allowed direct comparison of the human and gorilla menstrual cycles and demonstrates a major difference in the time course of preovulatory estrogen and progesterone metabolites (Mitchell et al., 1982). Whether or not these differences in the periovulatory period represent important differences in physiology, the approach provides the basis for longitudinal studies to be performed and compared in two species which otherwise could not be compared.

Abnormal ovarian cycles in the gorilla have also been characterized using the same approach (Mitchell et al., 1982). These data underscore the importance of sequential sampling which, with animals like gorillas, is not practically approached with a blood-collecting strategy. The ability to precisely and objectively indicate the time of ovulation and the quality of luteal function in the female gorilla offers useful information relating to fertility as well as provides new comparative data relating to ovarian defects in the hominoids.

Pregnanediol-3-glucuronide is not the major urinary metabolite of progesterone in Old World monkeys and therefore is generally considered not to offer promise as an endocrine tool in species not closely related to the hominoids. Thus, it was somewhat surprising to find that pregnanediol-3-glucuronide levels in the urine of some exotic hoofed species are useful and informative in revealing ovarian and, more specifically, luteal function. Since the follicular or preluteal phase of the ovarian cycle of hoofed species is compressed compared to that of primates, the monitoring of luteal function is of primary concern because the regression of the corpus luteum immediately precedes ovulation in a polyestrous hoofed species. Loskutoff et al. (1982) demonstrated the utility of this approach by monitoring repetitive cycles and pregnancy in the okapi (Fig. 5). These studies provide the insight on how to assess and characterize the ovarian cycles of the giraffe, oryx, and rhinoceros (Loskutoff et al., 1983). This strategy probably has more immediate clinical and conservation merits than scientific impact since the relative proportion of progesterone metabolites reflected by pregnanediol-3-glucuronide in various species is still not known. Nevertheless, the ability to longitudinally evaluate and assess reproductive status and function as an adjunct to intensive breeding programs will lead to an accumulation of normative profiles, which will gradually add to our understanding of comparative reproductive endocrinology.

Antisera to pregnanediol-3-glucuronide frequently show cross-reactivity to a wide range of urinary progesterone metabolites, and these can be used to detect urinary metabolites of progesterones other than pregnanediol-3-glucuronide. One example of this strategy is the report of Shideler et al. (1985), in which the luteal phase was monitored in the

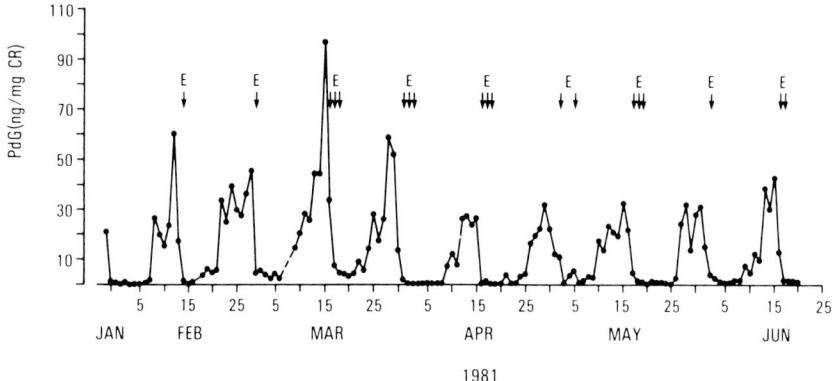

FIG. 5. Levels of immunoreactive pregnanediol-3-glucuronide indexed by creatinine in daily urine samples from a female okapi (*O. johnstonii*). The arrows represent the time periods that the animal was judged to be in estrus, although mating was not allowed. Peaks of pregnanediol-3-glucuronide precede each estrus and allow the evaluation of ovarian activity as well as the anticipation of ovulation. (Loskutoff et al., 1982; by permission of *Zoo Biology*.)

lion-tailed macaque. Antisera to pregnanediol-3-glucuronide were used with 20α-hydroxyprogesterone label to devise a semiquantitative assay for progesterone metabolites in the urine. This system, which does not meet the requirements of a valid, quantitative assay, provides an approach for evaluating progesterone excretion in macaque monkeys through a direct assay using unprocessed urine for the first time. Procedures are currently underway to characterize and identify the cross-reactive substance in order to develop a specific, and therefore quantitative, assay for progesterone metabolite excretion in all macaques.

Cochromatography of macaque urine with radiolabeled pregnanediol-3-glucuronide and pregnanediol-3-glucuronide immunoreactivity using the assay described above demonstrate clearly that the material measured does not elute with pregnanediol-3-glucuronide. This simple test clearly demonstrates that pregnanediol-3-glucuronide is not present in the sample and at the same time isolates the cross-reacting substance. Dose–response dynamics of the peak eluate tube from the HPLC separation show a nonparallel curve compared to the 20α-OH progesterone metabolites, thus necessitating the classification of the assay system as semiquantitative. More importantly, the ability to isolate such cross-reacting peaks allows for a direct strategy to purify and identify progesterone metabolites in a wide range of exotic species. This process will be helpful in developing specific and quantitative assays for urinary progesterone metabolites without the use of a radiolabel in *in vivo* metabolic studies. Since most exotic species are not available for such investigations, this strategy seems ideal for broad comparative studies.

VII. Estrone Conjugates

In most situations estrone conjugates represent the largest pool of urinary estrogens because estradiol has a tendency to be converted to estrone prior to excretion. There are some exceptions where estradiol or estriol predominates in the urine, but these generally reflect a pregnancy in which all estrogens are highly elevated. Since estrone is excreted predominantly as one of two conjugates, an antiserum that cross-reacts with both the estrone-3-glucuronide and estrone-3-sulfate should measure the predominant urinary estrogen in a wide range of species. This, in fact, is true and provides the basis for the development of a simple assay which has broad utility.

Shideler *et al.* (1983) compared the urinary estrogen profile of the lion-tailed macaque using the original total estrogen assay as described by Hodges *et al.* (1979) and Czekala *et al.* (1981) to a direct assay of estrone conjugates (Fig. 6). The resulting profiles were qualitatively similar but quantitatively disparate. The direct mea-

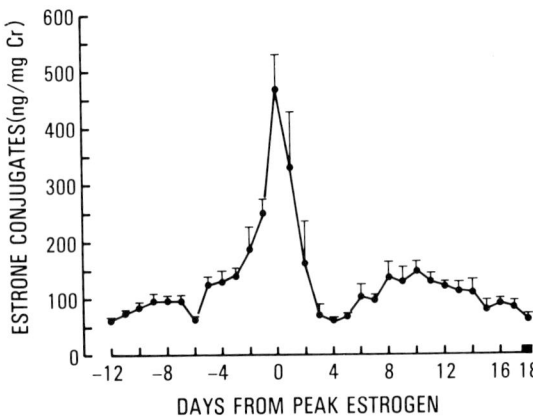

FIG. 6. Urinary estrone conjugates measured by direct radioimmunoassay of daily random urine samples from 10 mature female macaques. The individual animal profiles were aligned to the day of the highest preovulatory level of estrone conjugates (day 0). (From Shideler *et al.*, 1983, *Biology of Reproduction* **29,** 905 with permission.)

surement of estrone conjugates produced individual values several-fold higher than the measurement of all estrogen components combined. As previously noted, other workers have suggested that enzyme hydrolysis or acid solvolysis of urinary estrogen components is a relatively inefficient process, and this could account for the differences observed. Regardless of the differences in the mass of steroid measured, the direct measure of estrone conjugates provided a more resolute profile since peak values were higher than baseline values for the conjugates in comparison to the peak and baseline values for total estrogens following hydrolysis. More importantly, the direct assay for estrone conjugates required only 3 laboratory steps compared to 18 steps for hydrolysis, extraction, monitoring recovery, and assay for total urinary estrogens.

As would be predicted from Kassam and Lasley (1981), the estrone conjugate assay can be used to monitor follicular growth and ovulation in the Indian rhinoceros, as mentioned earlier. It would therefore follow that this method would be useful in other odd-toed species like the horse and tapir. When horse urine is evaluated for estrone conjugates, the trophoblast is revealed by a rapid rise in estrone sulfate 37 days postovulation. Estrone conjugate levels fall within hours of fetectomy by either surgery or prostaglandin injection, while circulating free estrogens and pregnant mare serum gonadotropin show little or no change. These results are consistent with the concept that the horse conceptus is directly responsible for the early rise in estrogen production between days 16 and 35 postconception. A more general implication is that a simple measure of urinary estrone conjugates reflects the presence or absence of a viable fetus when pregnant mare serum gonadotropin, circulating estrogen, and/or progesterone may not provide a clear indication. This approach may not replace rectal palpation for detecion of pregnancy in domestic horses, but it is rapidly gaining appreciation in zoos for the evaluation of zebras, tapirs, and rhinoceroses (Evans *et al.*, 1984; Kasman *et al.*, 1985).

The development of more efficient methods for hydrolyzing steroid conjugates provides the basis for the development of techniques that are even more revealing. Preliminary data indicate that as much as 50% of the conjugated estrogens are not cleaved by enzyme or acid hydrolysis. Bain *et al.* (1984) demonstrated that increasing the effciency of the hydrolytic reaction leads to the ability to extract and measure more estradiol than previously reported on well-defined urine samples. The results are consistent with the concept that estradiol is frequently disulfated, and this conjugate is poorly hydrolyzed by acid and enzyme hydrolysis. Since the more efficient ammonolysis reaction is highly efficient in cleaving both the 3 and 17 position sulfates, the estradiol disulfate is converted to free estradiol. This additional estradiol pool that can now be accurately evaluated in urines will hopefully allow urine monitoring to better reflect estrogen production.

ACKNOWLEDGMENTS

This work was supported by NIH Grants HD-01337, HD-16263, RR-09002, and HD-10190, NSF Grant PCM 78-16833, grants from The Charles Ulrick and Josephine Bay Foundation and The Ellen Browning Scripps Foundation, and the Rolex Award for Enterprise. The veterinary, curatorial, and keeper staffs that collected the samples are listed in the individual publications cited. The author is grateful to Sharon Dinwiddlie for preparation of the manuscript as well as for the editorial advice from Dr. K. Benirschke, L. Kasman, N. M., Czekala, and Drs. M. Thompson and S. E. Shideler.

REFERENCES

Bain, J., Kasman, L., Bercovitz, A. B., and Lasley, B. L. (1984). *Steroids* 43, 603–619.
Bercovitz, A. B., Czekala, N. M., and Lasley, B. L. (1978). *J. Zoo Anim. Med.* 9, 114–124.
Czekala, N. M., Hodges, J. K., and Lasley, B. L. (1981). *J. Med. Primatol.* 10, 1–15.
Czekala, N. M., Benirschke, K., McClure, H., and Lasley, B. L. (1983). *Biol. Reprod.* 28, 289–299.
Ensley, P. K., Wing, A. E., Gosink, B. B., Lasley, B. L., and Durrant, B. (1982). *Zoo Biol.* 1, 333–343.
Erb, L., Lasley, B. L., Czekala, N. M., and Monfort, S. L. (1982). *Steroids* 39, 33.
Evans, K. L., Hughes, J. P., Couto, M., Kasman, L. H., and Lasley, B. L. (1984). *Theriogenology* 22, 615–620.
Ewing, L. L., Thompson, D. L., Cochran, R. C., Lasley, B. L., Thompson, M. A., and Zirkin, B. R. (1984). *Endocrinology* 114, 1308–1314.
Hodges, J. K., Czekala, N. M., and Lasley, B. L. (1979). *J. Med. Primatol.* 8, 349.
Kasman, L. H., McCowan, B., and Lasley, B. L. (1985). *Zoo Biol.* 3.
Kassam, A. A. H., and Lasley, B. L. (1981). *Am. J. Vet. Med.* 42, 251–255.
Loskutoff, N. M., Ott, J. E., and Lasley, B. L. (1982). *Zoo Biol.* 1, 45–53.
Loskutoff, N. M., Ott, J. E., and Lasley, B. L. (1983). *J. Zoo Anim. Med.* 14, 3–12.
Mitchell, W. R., Loskutoff, N. M., Czekala, N. M., and Lasley, B. L. (1982). *J. Zoo Anim. Med.* 13, 143.
Mitchell, W. R., Presley, S., Czekala, N. M., and Lasley, B. L. (1982). *Am. J. Primatol.* 2, 167.
Monfort, S. L., Thompson, M. A., Czekala, N. M., Kasman, L. H., Shackleton, C. H. L., and Lasley, B. L. (1984). *Steroid Biochem.* 20, 869.
Sawyer-Steffan, J. E., Lasley, B. L., Hoff, J. D., and Yen, S. S. C. (1982). *J. Reprod. Fertil.* 65, 45.
Shideler, S. E., Czekala, N. M., Benirschke, K., and Lasley, B. L. (1983). *Biol. Reprod.* 28, 963.
Shideler, S. E., Czekala, N. M., Kasman, L. H., Lindburg, D. G., and Lasley, B. L. (1983). *Biol. Reprod.* 29, 905–911.
Shideler, S. E., Mitchell, W. R., Lindburg, D. G., and Lasley, B. L. (1985). *Zoo. Biol.* 4, 65.

Index

A

Acetylcholine, platelets and, 150
Acid hydrolases, in neutrophils, 93, 94, 108
Activation, of neutrophils, 111
Adenine nucleotides, in platelets, 140–143
Adenosine diphosphate, platelets and, 141–143
Adenovirus, 12, 13
Adrenal, estrogen excretion and, 216–217
Adrenal cortex, fetal zone, neonatal maturity of prosimians and, 174, 176
Aggregation, of platelets, 137–138
Anesthetics, platelet acquisition and, 132–134
Aneurysms, in prosimians, 202, 204
Angiotensin, neutrophils and, 121
Antibodies
 absence in bursectomized birds, 75
 neutrophil phagocytosis and, 114, 119–120
Antigens, MDV-specific, in arteries, 48, 56
Antiheparin, in platelets, 136
Antiidiotype antibody, vaccines and, 31–32
Antimicrobial systems, of neutrophils
 oxygen-dependent, 104–106
 oxygen-independent, 106–110
Antiserum
 for estrogen components, 215
 to pregnanediol-3-glucuronide, other progesterone metabolites and, 224–226
Arachidonic acid pathway, in platelets, 144–148, 154
Arenaviruses, 12
 protein vaccines and, 18
Arginase, neutrophils and, 108
Arterial lesions
 MDV-induced
  evidence for, 55–56
  grossly visible, 45
  microscopic, 45–48
Arteries, alteration of SMC lipid metabolism by MDV
 cholesterol and cholesteryl esters, 56–57
 mechanisms of, 57–58
Arylsulfatase, in neutrophils, 101
Atherosclerosis
 in humans, preliminary evidence for herpesvirus role in, 62
 initial experiments on herpesvirus infection
  arterial lesions, 45–48
  conclusions, 51–52
  experimental design, 42
  Marek's disease: index of MDV infection, 43–45
  MDV-specific antigens in arteries, 48
  serum cholesterol levels, 42–43
 MDV-induced
  immunization as protection against, 60–62
  pathogenic mechanisms
   alterations of arterial SMC metabolism, 56–58
   conclusions, 58–59
   pathogenesis experiments, 52–56
Azurophil granules, neutrophils of domestic animals and, 93

B

Bacillus subtilis, as host for chimeric DNA vectors, 5
Bacterial diseases, recombinant DNA protein vaccines for, 21–23
Birds
 estrogen/testosterone ratio in, 215

monomorphic, determination of sex of, 213–214
B-L antigens, analogy to Ia$^+$ antigens, 71
Blood
  circulating, neutrophils of, 117–118
  hormone levels, reproductive function in exotic mammals and, 210
B lymphocytes
  identifying nonbursal site and associated cells, 76–82
  precommitted, 83
  precursor, secretory cells and, 78–79
  progenitor cells, 68, 69
Bone marrow, granulocytopoiesis and, 116–117
Bothrops jararaca venom, platelet agglutination and, 155
Bovine papilloma virus, 12
  vaccine for, 13
Brucella abortus, protein vaccine and, 22–23
Bunyaviruses, 12
  protein vaccines and, 18–19
Bursa of Fabricius, ontogeny and microenvironment, 68–73
Bursectomy, *in ovo,* specific antibody production and, 74

C

Caecal tonsil, secretory cells and, 77
Calcium
  neutrophil migration and activation, 110, 111, 112
  platelets and, 150, 154
Caliciviruses, 12
  protein vaccines and, 17
Carbonic anhydrase, in neutrophils, 107
Cathepsins, neutrophils and, 109
Cattle
  neutrophils of, 97, 99, 100
  protection by FMD protein vaccine, 10, 11
Cell cycle, thymic cells and, 86
Centrosome, of neutrophils, 112
Chalone, neutrophil maturation and, 116

Chemical synthesis, of vaccines, 24–27
Chemotactic factors, neutrophil migration and, 110, 111, 112–113, 118
Chickens
  infected, normocholesteremic, microscopic arterial lesions in, 53
  for study of MDV infection, 42
Cholesterol
  dietary, arterial lesions and, 45–46, 51–52
  metabolism in arterial SMC, MDV-induced atherosclerosis and, 56–57
Cholesterol acyltransferase, in MDV infected cells, 58
Chronic nephritis, in prosimians, 202
Citrate, platelet acquisition and, 132
Coccidiosis, protein vaccine and, 23
Collagen, platelets and, 152–153, 155
Colony-stimulating factors, neutrophil maturation and, 116
Complement, cleavage products, chemotactic factors and, 108
Complement receptors, neutrophils and, 120
Congenital anomalies, in prosimians, 180–184, 200
Connective tissue, destruction, neutrophils and, 108
Coronavirus, 12
  protein vaccines and, 17–18
Coxsackie virus B3, 12
  protein vaccine for, 17
Creatinine, as index to hormone concentration in urine, 211, 222
Cryptococcosis, in lemurs, 185, 187
Cyclic adenosine monophosphate, platelet sensitivity and, 151–152, 154
Cyclic nucleotides, neutrophil migration and, 110, 112
Cyclooxygenase
  arachidonate metabolism in platelets and, 145
  neutrophil activation and, 111
Cyclophosphamide
  agammaglobulinemia and, 76
  bursal development and, 69, 71
Cytokine
  absence of bursa and, 81
  bursal development and, 68, 71

Cytomegalovirus
  arterial endothelium and, 41
  crystalline accumulations in arterial SMC cultures and, 62
Cytotoxicity, neutrophils and, 120–121

D

Deaths, neonatal, in prosimians, 178–180
Degranulation, of neutrophils, 114–115
Dendritic cells, in spleen of birds, 77
Dense granules, of platelets, 135
  constituents of, 140
Deoxyribonucleic acid ligases, in thymic cells, 86
Deoxyribonucleic acid viruses
  double-stranded, protein vaccines for, 11–14
  single-stranded, protein vaccines for, 15
Deoxyribonucleoprotein viruses, double-stranded, protein vaccines for, 14
Dexamethasone, thymic cells and, 86
Dextran sulfate, immunoglobulin production in bursectomized birds, 74–75
Diet, of prosimians, 196
Diphtheria toxin, synthetic vaccine and, 27
Disease
  neutrophil chemotaxis and, 113, 118
  platelet membrane glycoproteins and, 156–157
  of prosimians, 168–171

E

Ellipsoid-associated cell
  secretory cell and, 77–78
  transmission of antigenic messages and, 81–82
Endotoxin, platelet agglutination and, 155–156
Enzymes
  in azurophil granules of neutrophils, 93–94
  in neutrophil membranes, 103
  secretion by neutrophils, 115–116
  in tertiary granules of neutrophils, 100
Epinephrine
  as gain controller, platelets and, 154–155
  platelet response to, 152–154
Epstein-Barr virus, 12
  protein vaccine for, 13
Equol, identification of, 218, 220
Escherichia coli
  cloning of FMD protein VP_1, gene in, 8–10
  enterotoxogenic, protein vaccine for, 4, 21–22
  as host for chimeric DNA vectors, 5
Estrogenic components
  evaluation of, 214–220
  identified by HPLC, 219
Estrogen/testosterone ratios, in urine of exotic mammals, 212–214
Estrone conjugates, measurements of, 226–227
  pregnancy and, 227
Exotic animals
  estrogen/testosterone ratio in urine of, 212–214
  pregnanediol-3-glucuronide in, 223–224

F

Feces, steroid evaluation in, 213
Feline herpesvirus, urinary obstruction and, 40
Flavoprotein oxidase, in neutrophils, 105
Foot-and-mouth disease virus
  infectious vaccines and, 2–3
  recombinant DNA protein vaccine for, 6–10, 16–17
  synthetic vaccine for, 26
N-Formylated methionyl-leucyl-phenylalanine, neutrophil chemotaxis and, 113

G

Genes, immunogenic, preparation for cloning, 5–6

Genetic origin
  of congenital anomalies in prosimians, 182–183
  of pectus excavatum, 197–198
β-Glucuronidase, in neutrophils, 101
Glutathione peroxidase, in neutrophils, 105
Glycogen granules, in neutrophils, 102
Glycolysis, in neutrophils, 107
Glycoproteins, of platelet membranes, 156–157
Glycosidases, neutrophils and, 108
Goats, FMD protein vaccine and, 16
Golgi apparatus, of neutrophils, 102, 112
Gonads, of neonatal prosimians, 176
Granules
  of neutrophils, 92–102
  of platelets, 135–136
Granulocytopoiesis, in neutrophils, 116–117

H

Hemodialysis, neutrophil function and, 118
Hemosiderosis, in prosimians, 187, 189, 191, 193
Heparin, platelet acquisition and, 132
Hepatitis B, 32
  protein vaccine for, 3, 4, 20–21
  simian virus 40 and, 29
  synthetic vaccine for, 25
  vaccinia virus recombinant and, 28
Hepatoma, in prosimians, 189
Herpes simplex viruses, 12
  protein vaccine for, 14
  synthetic vaccine for, 26
  vaccinia virus recombinant and, 28
Herpesvirus
  initial experiments
    arterial lesions, 45–48
    conclusions, 51–52
    experimental design, 42
    Marek's disease: index of MDV infection, 43–45
    MDV-specific antigens in arteries, 48
    serum cholesterol levels, 42–43
  preliminary evidence for role in human atherosclerosis, 62

Herpesvirus of turkeys, 12
  immunization by
    prevention of MDV-induced atherosclerosis and, 60–62
  protein vaccine for, 13
Herpes zoster virus, 12
Hexose monophosphate shunt, in neutrophils, 105
High-performance liquid chromatography, for separation of estrogen components, 216–217
Horses, neutrophils of, 95, 97, 100, 113
Human, atherosclerosis in, 39–40
  preliminary evidence for herpesvirus role in, 62
Hydrogen peroxide
  oxygen-independent metabolism in neutrophils and, 107
  production by neutrophils, 105–106
Hydrolysis, of estrogen conjugates, 227–228
Hydroxyeicosatetraenoic acids
  formation in platelets, 145, 146
  neutrophil activation and, 111, 112
Hydroxyl radical, neutrophil metabolism and, 105, 109
5-Hydroxytryptamine, thymus cells and, 85
Hypochlorous acid, neutrophil metabolism and, 105, 106

I

Immune system, control, neutrophils and, 109
Immunization, protection against MDV-induced atherosclerosis
  conclusions, 61–62
  experimental plan, 60
  results, 60–61
Immunoglobulin(s), synthesis, nonbursal site of, 73–75
Immunologic processes, neutrophil function and, 119–121
Infections, in prosimians, 184–187, 200
Infectious bovine rhinotracheitis virus, 12
  protein vaccine for, 13
Inflammatory processes, neutrophil function and, 118–119

Influenza virus, 2
  protein vaccine for, 3, 4, 18
  reassortants and, 30
  synthetic vaccines for, 25–26
  vaccinia virus recombinant and, 28
Interleukin 2, T cell growth and, 86–87
Intestinal obstruction, in prosimians, 202
Iron, metabolism by prosimians, 193–194
Islets of Langerhans, hyperplasia in prosimians, 195–196

L

Lactate, production in neutrophils, 107
Lactoferrin, in neutrophils, 93, 94, 97, 109, 110
Lemurs
  causes of mortality in, 168–169
  reproductive cycle in, 171–172
Lesions
  arterial
    evidence of MDV infection in cells of, 59–60
    MDV-induced atherosclerosis and
      gross, 52–53
      microscopic, 53–55
  microscopic, arterial
    comparisons in various groups of chickens, 53–55
Leukocidin, phosphatase and, 103
Leukokinins, production of, 108
Leukotrienes, neutrophil function and, 119
Lipid metabolism, of arterial SMC by MDV
  cholesterol and cholesteryl esters, 56–57
  mechanisms, 57–58
Lipid peroxidation, in neutrophils, 106
Lipoxygenase
  arachidonate metabolism in platelets and, 145
  products, neutrophil activation and, 111–112
Luteinizing hormone, bioactive, measurements of, 220–222
Lymphocytes, thymic, enzymatic changes in, 85–86
Lymphokines, neutrophil function and, 119
Lysosomes, azurophil granules and, 93–94

Lysozyme, in neutrophils, 93, 97, 101, 107, 108, 109, 110

M

Maloney leukemia virus, synthetic vaccine and, 25
Marek's disease, 12
  evidence of infection in cells comprising arterial lesions, 59–60
  index of infection, 43–45
  pathogenic mechanism of atherosclerosis induced by
    alteration of arterial SMC metabolism and, 56–58
    conclusions, 58–59
    pathogenesis experiments, 52–56
  protein vaccine for, 13
  viral antigens in arteries, 48
Maternal neglect, neonatal death in prosimians and, 178, 179, 180
Membranes
  of neutrophils, 102–103
  smooth, of platelets, 136–137
Microbicides, in neutrophils, 93, 97
Microtubules
  in activated neutrophils, 112
  neutrophil phagocytosis and, 114
Migration, of neutrophils, 110
Mortalities, distribution in prosimians, 175
Mutants, deletion, vaccines and, 30–31
Myeloperoxidase, in neutrophils, 93, 97, 101, 106, 108, 109

N

Neisseria gonorrhoeae, protein vaccine for, 22
Neoplasias, in prosimians, 169, 170–171
Neurolymphomatosis, atherosclerosis in chickens and, 41
Neutrophils
  of circulating blood, 117–118
  function in inflammatory and immunologic processes, 118–121
  granulocytopoiesis and, 116–117
  metabolism and antimicrobial systems, 103–104

oxygen-dependent, 104–106
oxygen-independent, 106–110
migration and activation of, 110–113
morphology
  cytoplasmic organelles other than granules, 102
  granules, 92–102
  membranes, 102–103
  nucleus, 92
phagocytosis and degranulation, 114–116
Newcastle disease virus, 2
  protein vaccine for, 19
Nicotinamide adenine dinucleotide phosphate, neutrophil metabolism and, 105
5'-Nucleotidase, in neutrophils, 103
Nucleus, of neutrophils, 92

O

Orbiviruses, 12
  protein vaccines and, 15–16
Organelles, of neutrophils, 102
Orthomyxoviruses, 12
  protein vaccines and, 18

P

Paramyxoviruses, 12
  protein vaccines and, 19
Parasitic diseases, recombinant DNA protein vaccines for, 21–23
Parvoviruses, 12
  protein vaccines for, 15
Pathogenesis experiments, MDV-induced atherosclerosis and
  evidence of arterial injury, 55–56
  gross lesions, 52–53
  microscopic arterial lesions, 53–55
Pectus excavatum, in prosimians, 196–200
Perinatal mortality, in prosimians, 173–180
Peroxidase, in neutrophils, 93

pH, in phagocytic vacuoles of neutrophils, 107
Phagocytosis, by neutrophils, 114
Phosphatases, in neutrophils, 94, 100, 101, 103
Phospholipids
  cleavage, neutrophil activation and, 111
  release of aracidonate from, 144–145
Picornaviruses, 12
  protein vaccines for, 16–17
Pili, vaccines and, 21–22
Plasmodium knowlesi
  protein vaccine and, 23
  vaccinia virus recombinant and, 28–29
Platelets
  acquisition of blood samples for study of, 132–134
  agglutinating agents
    endotoxin, 155–156
    von Willebrand factor, 155
  basic response, 138–140
    additional agonists, 150
    arachidonic acid pathway, 144–148
    dense granule pathway, 140–144
    platelet-activating factor, 148–150
    summary, 150–151
  function of, 131–132
  inflammation and, 119
  membrane glycoproteins of, 156–157
  modulators and
    epinephrine, 152–154
    epinephrine as gain controller, 154–155
    PGI_2 and cAMP, 151–152
  thrombocytopenia and, 158, 159
  tumor cells and, 157–159
  ultrastructure, 134–138
Platelet-activating factor
  nature and formation of, 148–149
  role in platelet aggregation, 149–150
  systemic effects of, 149
Poliovirus
  protein vaccine for, 17
  synthetic vaccines for, 26–27
Pregnancy, in primates, estrogen excretion and, 216–217
Pregnanediol-3-glucuronide, as test for luteal function, 225–226

Primates, pregnancy in, estrogen excretion in, 216–217
Prosimians
  causes of death in, 169
  congenital anomalies in, 180–184, 200
  general considerations, 172–173
  hemosiderosis and hepatoma in, 187–195
  hyperplasia of islets of Langerhans in, 195–196
  infections in, 184–187, 200
  miscellaneous conditions in, 200–205
  pectus excavatum in, 196–200
  perinatal mortality in, 173–180
  review of literature, 168–172
  taxonomic considerations, 167–168
Prostacyclin, platelet sensitivity and, 151
Prostaglandins
  formation in platelets, 145, 146
  granulocytopoiesis and, 116
  as modifiers, 151
Proteases, in neutrophils, 100, 108–109, 115
Protein(s)
  cationic, in neutrophils, 107–108, 110
  of FMD, 7–8
Pseudoplatelets, neutrophils and, 92
Pseudorabies virus, 12
  protein vaccine for, 13

R

Rabbitpox virus, 12
  vaccines and, 14
Rabies virus, 32
Radioimmunoassay, for estrogen components, 214–216
Reassortants, vaccines and, 29–30
Receptor binding, estrogen components and, 218
α Receptors, of platelets, 153
β Receptors, of platelets, 153
Recombinant deoxyribonucleic acid subunit vaccines, 4–5
  for bacterial and parasitic diseases, 21–23
  for foot-and-mouth disease, 6–10
  for other viral diseases, 10–21
  preparation of immunogenic genes for cloning, 5–6
Recombinant virus vaccines, vaccinia virus and, 27–28
Renal cortex, as guide to neonatal maturity in lemurs, 174
Reoviruses, 12
  protein vaccines for, 15
Reproductive cycle, in lemurs, 171–172
Reproductive success, of captive prosimians, 204
Respiratory burst, in neutrophils, 104–105
Reticuloendothelial cells, soluble factor from, thymus cell differentiation and, 84–85
Retroviruses, 12
  protein vaccines and, 20
Rhabdoviruses, protein vaccines and, 19–20
Rheumatoid arthritis, parvovirus and, 15
Rhinoceros, estrogen excretion in, 218
Ribonucleic acid viruses, single-stranded, protein vaccines for, 16–18
Ribonucleoprotein viruses
  double-stranded, protein vaccines for, 15–16
  nonsegmented, single-stranded, protein vaccines and, 19–20
  retroviral protein, vaccines for, 20
  segmented, single-stranded protein vaccines and, 18–19
Risk factors, for atherosclerosis, 40–41
Ristocetin, platelet agglutination and, 155
Rosettes, formation by neutrophils, 117–118
Rotaviruses, 12
  protein vaccines and, 16

S

Sabin poliovirus vaccines, reversions of, 2
Salmonella, deletion mutants of, 30–31
Secretory cells
  B cell ontogeny and, 68, 73
  structure of, 76

Serotonin, in platelets, 135, 140, 141, 143–144
Serum cholesterol levels, MDV infection and, 42–43
Simian virus 40, 12, 13
  recombinant virus vaccines and, 29
  synthetic vaccine for, 24–25
Singlet oxygen
  neutrophil metabolism and, 105, 106
Species, neutrophils
  enzymes of, 101, 103
  granules of, 93, 100
  nucleus of, 92, 100
  organelles, 100
Spleen, secretory cells and, 77
Stem cell, multipotential, 82–83
Steroid conjugates, direct assays for, 222–223
Stillbirths, in prosimians, 176, 178
Storage-pool deficiency, of platelets, occurrence of, 140
Strategies, for new vaccines, 1–2
Superoxide-anion-producing enzymes, in neutrophils, 103, 105
Superoxide dismutase, in neutrophils, 105
Swine, protection by FMD protein vaccine, 10, 11

T

Terminal deoxyribonucleotidyltransferase, in thymic cells, 85–86
Testosterone propionate, elimination of bursa and, 73
Thrombin, platelet activation and, 142
Thrombocytopenia, platelets and, 158, 159
Thromboxanes, formation in platelets, 145, 146, 147, 150
Thymus
  avian, role of, 82
  microenvironment of, 84–87
  ontogeny of, 83–84
T lymphocytes, precommitted, 83
Tobacco mosaic virus, synthetic vaccine and, 24
Togaviruses, 12
  protein vaccines and, 17

Toxic granules, in neutrophils, 100, 102
Toxoplasmosis, in lemurs, 185
Treponema pallidum, protein vaccine and, 22
Trypanosoma rhodesiense, vaccine for, 23
Trypanosomiasis, 32
  immunotolerance to, 23
Tumor(s), in prosimians, 195
Tumor cells, platelets and, 157–159

U

Ultrastructure
  of neutrophil nucleus, 92
  of platelets, 134–138
Urine, hormone metabolites in, reproductive function in exotic mammals and, 210–211

V

Vaccines
  conventional, disadvantages of, 2–3
  new, impetus for, 2–3
  prospects for, 3–4
  other approaches to, 23
    antiidiotype antibody vaccines, 31–32
    chemically synthesized, 24–27
    genetically engineered reassortants and deletion mutants, 29–31
    recombinant virus vaccines, 27–29
Vaccinia virus, 12
  vaccines and, 14, 27–29
Vascular permeability, neutrophils and, 119
Vasopressin, platelets and, 150
Vibrio cholerae
  deletion mutants of, 31
  synthetic vaccine and, 27
Viral diseases, recombinant DNA protein vaccines for, 10–11
  DNA and DNP viruses, 11–15
  RNA and RNP viruses, 15–20
  unclassified viruses, 20–21
Viruses
  isolation of specific genes from, 5–6

unclassified, 12
  protein vaccines and, 20–21
von Willebrand factor
  function of, 157
  platelet aggregation and, 155

Y

Yeasts, as hosts for chimeric DNA vectors, 5

RAYMOND H. FOGLER LIBRARY
DATE DUE